50 YEARS AFTER DEINSTITUTIONALIZATION: MENTAL ILLNESS IN CONTEMPORARY COMMUNITIES

ADVANCES IN MEDICAL SOCIOLOGY

Series Editor: Brea L. Perry

Series Editor for Volumes 5–6: Gary L. Albrecht

Series Editor for Volumes 7–8: Judith A. Levy

Series Editor for Volumes 9–15: Barbara Katz Rothman

Recent Volumes:

Volume 5: Quality of Life in Health Care – Edited by Ray Fitzpatrick

Volume 6: Case and Care Management – Edited by Gary L. Albrecht

Volume 7: Emergent Issues in the Field of Drug Abuse – Edited by Judith A. Levy, Richard C. Stephens and Duane C. McBride

Volume 8: Social Networks and Health – Edited by Bernice A. Pescosolido and Judith A. Levy

Volume 9: Bioethical Issues, Sociological Perspectives – Edited by Barbara K. Rothman, Elizabeth M. Armstrong and Rebecca Tiger

Volume 10: Patients, Consumers and Civil Society – Edited by Susan M. Chambré and Melinda Goldner

Volume 11: Understanding Emerging Epidemics: Social and Political Approaches – Edited by Ananya Mukherjea

Volume 12: Sociology of Diagnosis – Edited by P. J. McGann and David J. Hutson

Volume 13: Sociological Reflections on the Neurosciences – Edited by Martyn Pickersgill and Ira van Keulen

Volume 14: Critical Perspectives on Addiction – Edited by Julie Netherland

Volume 15: Ecological Health: Society, Ecology and Health – Edited by Maya K. Gislason

Volume 16: Genetics, Health and Society – Edited by Brea L. Perry

ADVANCES IN MEDICAL SOCIOLOGY VOLUME 17

50 YEARS AFTER DEINSTITUTIONALIZATION: MENTAL ILLNESS IN CONTEMPORARY COMMUNITIES

EDITED BY

BREA L. PERRY
Department of Sociology, Indiana University, Bloomington, IN, USA

Emerald

United Kingdom – North America – Japan
India – Malaysia – China

Emerald Group Publishing Limited
Howard House, Wagon Lane, Bingley BD16 1WA, UK

First edition 2016

British Library Cataloguing in Publication Data
A catalogue record for this book is available from the British Library

ISBN: 978-1-78560-403-4
ISSN: 1057-6290 (Series)

Printed and bound by CPI Group (UK) Ltd, Croydon, CR0 4YY

ISOQAR certified Management System, awarded to Emerald for adherence to Environmental standard ISO 14001:2004.

ISOQAR
REGISTERED
Certificate Number 1985
ISO 14001

INVESTOR IN PEOPLE

CONTENTS

PART II
COMMUNITY REINTEGRATION AND THE SOCIAL ENVIRONMENT

PART III
CONFRONTING STIGMA AND ITS CONSEQUENCES

PART IV
BIOMEDICALIZATION IN THE ERA OF COMMUNITY MENTAL HEALTH

EDITORIAL ADVISORY BOARD

LIST OF CONTRIBUTORS

Wallis E. Adams	Department of Sociology, Northeastern University, Boston, MA, USA
Brandon Attell	Department of Sociology, Georgia State University, Atlanta, GA, USA
Adrianna Bagnall	Department of Sociology, Columbia University, New York, NY, USA
Gil Eyal	Department of Sociology, Columbia University, New York, NY, USA
William H. Fisher	School of Criminology and Justice Studies, University of Massachusetts-Lowell, Lowell, MA, USA
Jeffrey L. Geller	Department of Psychiatry, University of Massachusetts Medical School, Worcester, MA, USA
Sarah K. Harkness	Department of Sociology, University of Iowa, Iowa City, IA, USA
Anthony R. Hatch	Science in Society, Wesleyan University, Middletown, CT, USA
Gracie Jackson	School of Leadership and Education Sciences, University of San Diego, San Diego, CA, USA
Amy Kroska	Department of Sociology, University of Oklahoma, Norman, OK, USA
Alisa K. Lincoln	Department of Health Sciences and Sociology, Northeastern University, Boston, MA, USA
Kristen Marcussen	Department of Sociology, Kent State University, Kent, OH, USA

Will R. McConnell Department of Sociology, Indiana University, Bloomington, IN, USA

Dana L. McMannus Worcester Recovery Center and Hospital, Worcester, MA, USA

Brea L. Perry Department of Sociology, Indiana University, Bloomington, IN, USA

Bernice A. Pescosolido Department of Sociology, Indiana University, Bloomington, IN, USA

Christian Ritter Department of Psychiatry, Northeast Ohio Medical University, Rootstown, OH, USA

Teresa L. Scheid Department of Sociology, University of North Carolina-Charlotte, Charlotte, NC, USA

Russell K. Schutt Department of Sociology, University of Massachusetts-Boston, Boston, MA, USA; Harvard Medical School, Boston, MA, USA

Sandra H. Sulzer Department of Sociology, Xavier University of Louisiana, New Orleans, LA, USA

Nana Tuntiya Department of Sociology, University of South Florida, Tampa, FL, USA

Eryn Viscarra Department of Sociology, Georgia State University, Atlanta, GA, USA

Marik Xavier-Brier Department of Sociology, Georgia State University, Atlanta, GA, USA

Ashelee Yang Department of Sociology, University of California Los Angeles, Los Angeles, CA, USA

INTRODUCTION: LEGACIES OF DEINSTITUTIONALIZATION THROUGH THE LENS OF MEDICAL SOCIOLOGY

Throughout the 1960s and 1970s, a revolution in mental health policy and practice known as deinstitutionalization occurred in Europe and the United States. This movement was catalyzed in large part by criticisms of psychiatric institutions leveled by sociologist Irving Goffman and others, and resulted in the release of hundreds of thousands of people with severe mental illness from long-term care facilities into the community. It is widely acknowledged that these reforms held great promise, but have had numerous unintended negative consequences for people with mental illness and their families. Having been chronically underfunded, deinstitutionalization has strained the resources and reach of community-based mental health treatment systems, spilling into other institutions such as criminal justice and social welfare. This has led to renewed debates in the United States, the United Kingdom, and elsewhere about problems in public mental health systems, and to calls for rebuilding some functional aspects of the inpatient system that were successfully dismantled by deinstitutionalization reforms.

CONTEMPORARY ISSUES AND CALLS FOR MENTAL HEALTH SYSTEM REFORM

Much of the contemporary attention to mental health issues is positive – the culmination of efforts by high-profile political figures and celebrities. For example, in early 2016, First Lady Michelle Obama announced her collaboration with a multi-sector coalition on mental health that launched the Campaign to Change Direction. The goals of this initiative are to raise awareness of mental illness, improve recognition of symptoms for early intervention, and to "change the conversation about mental health in this country (Obama, 2016, p. 1)." Similarly, the Duchess of

Cambridge, Kate Middleton, has passionately spoken out about mental health issues, including stigma, focusing in particular on children's mental health and advocacy (Middleton, 2016). In addition to supporting numerous mental health charities, she launched M-PACT Plus in 2013 – a campaign to support children affected by parental drug and alcohol addiction. In addition, celebrities like actress Glenn Close, comedian Ruby Wax, and actor Joe Pantoliano have founded or collaborated with organizations seeking to reduce the stigma around mental illness.

At the same time, mental health issues have received substantial negative media coverage in the past decade in relation to connections (real or imagined) between mass shootings and mental illness. For example, after the 2012 shooting at Sandy Hook Elementary, there was widespread speculation that shooter Adam Lanza had undiagnosed schizophrenia, prompting media commentator Anne Coulter to declare that "Guns don't kill people, the mentally ill do (Coulter, 2013)." Similar public conversations took place following mass shootings at a Norwegian summer camp, a Columbine, Colorado school, and an Aurora, Colorado movie theater, among others.

Under the flawed assumptions that mental illness causes such crimes and that diagnosis and treatment can prevent them (Metzl & MacLeish, 2015), these tragedies spark national dialogues about deficiencies in public mental health systems. Among the chief complaints are underfunding, shortages of mental health beds, lack of coordinated care across agencies, and undue investment in behavioral wellness (i.e., mild mental illness) to the detriment of those with severe psychiatric disorders. However, while a substantial amount of mental health legislation has, in fact, resulted directly from these violent events, it is largely misplaced. Specifically, policy efforts at the state and federal level have centered on restricting access to firearms among people with a history of mental illness rather than laws that would improve the efficiency or effectiveness of the public mental health system (Rosenberg, 2014).

The "Helping Families in Mental Health Crisis Act" (Murphy, 2013), introduced to congress in 2015 and awaiting a vote in the U.S. House of Representatives, is one such example. The bill proposes some important and positive changes, such as increased funding for screening and early intervention, suicide prevention, and increased coordination of care. However, many argue that the bill represents a return to pre-deinstitutionalization era clinical and legal approaches to mental illness that are authoritarian, coercive, and not evidence-based, focusing on public safety to the detriment of public health (Harris, 2015). Moreover, this legislation would strip a large minority group of its civil and privacy rights (e.g., the right to bear arms), has little potential to improve public safety, and likely represents an attempt by conservative lawmakers to shift the focus of the debate away from gun control. For better or worse, the so-called Murphy bill is unlikely to be passed into law in its current form, given overwhelming opposition by democratic members of congress. However, it is unclear in the current political climate whether and when there will be comprehensive mental health system reform in the United States, despite some promising developments associated with the Affordable Care Act (ACA).

CONTRIBUTIONS OF MEDICAL SOCIOLOGY TO INNOVATIONS IN POLICY AND PRACTICE

Many public, professional, and scientific voices have spoken out against and in support of reform efforts like the Murphy bill. Yet, medical sociologists are in a unique position to make meaningful contributions to debates around mental health policy and practice. The shift to community-based care means that, by definition, the social conditions, interactions, and institutions that comprise the community context have become critical determinants of recovery outcomes and life chances for people with mental illness. By virtue of the breadth of this subfield and the tendency to approach social problems through multiple theoretical lenses and levels of analysis, medical sociology has made substantial progress toward understanding the failures of deinstitutionalization and identifying ways forward.

Macro-Level Perspectives on Systems of Care

Medical sociologists often study *macro-level problems* in the social structure of mental health care post-deinstitutionalization, documenting how the political economy, institutionalism, and prevailing cultural conceptions of mental illness have shaped societal response to individuals with psychiatric disorders. For example, sociologists have identified a pressing need to create integrated service delivery systems for people with severe mental illness. The work of Mechanic (2008) and others has demonstrated that for those with severe mental illness, service delivery is often characterized by an uncoordinated combination of visits to emergency departments, short-term stays in inpatient facilities, short-term treatment through jails, prisons, or forensic psychiatric units, inadequate and intermittent outpatient treatment, and resources through a mix of entitlement programs, many of which were not designed to serve the needs of people with mental illness. Thus, critical elements of a social safety net – including housing, financial aid, vocational training, medical treatment, and psychiatric services – are typically provided by multiple different agencies with distinct and sometimes conflicting institutional goals and norms (Perry & Horwitz, 2014; Scheid, 2003).

Evidence suggests that system integration and coordination of care are critical factors in the quality and cost of services, as well as patient outcomes and experiences (Morrissey et al., 1994; Peek, 2009). Fragmentation in the mental health system has created barriers to providing comprehensive and continuous long-term care for the most severely impaired and socioeconomically disadvantaged individuals (Lamb & Bachrach, 2001). Consequently, there has been an increase in untreated or poorly managed severe mental illness. Sociologists identify poverty, unemployment, and other unmet needs in this population as major contributors to visible social problems like homelessness and crime, which exacerbate stigmatization and discrimination against people with psychiatric disorders and prohibit successful community reintegration (Hartwell, 2004; Hiday, 1995; Markowitz, 2006; Schutt & Goldfinger, 2011).

Thus, a key contribution of macro-level medical sociology is the assertion that solutions for severe mental illness must go beyond the development of effective drug treatments or psychotherapies to encompass a variety of systemic and organizational factors. This ideology is now widely accepted, and coordination of care across agencies constitutes a major component of Obama's Affordable Care Act. Mechanic (2012) notes that the ACA promotes reforms and provides funding to develop and test a number of innovative programs that are consistent with the recommendations of sociologists regarding fragmentation and uncoordinated care. For example, payment reforms that bundle or package services for particular illness episodes rather than billing for each service provided encourage continuity and efficiency, incentivizing health providers to take responsibility for long-term care. Likewise, the ACA encourages and partially funds Medicaid coverage of health home providers, who manage care, provide necessary referrals, offer individual and family support, and monitor health information technology in order to integrate services across multiple providers and agencies.

Micro-Level Perspectives on the Role of Family and Community Ties

Medical sociological research also reveals *micro-level processes*, demonstrating that social interaction, social psychology, and individual agency shape and are shaped by the experience of mental illness, treatment, and recovery. For instance, sociologists have studied the social interactional consequences of a fragmented system of formal care and a prevailing philosophy of community reintegration. Specifically, although many lack the resources to provide adequate care and support, family members and other informal supporters often accept responsibility for caregiving (Carpentier, Lesage, & White, 1999). In the absence of a formal social safety net, informal caregivers must often provide housing, financial support, emotional support, medication management, and custodial care to their loved ones (Wright, Avirappattu, & Lafuze, 1999). They also act as patient advocates, navigating the mental health system to identify and obtain health and disability services for the ill person. Pescosolido and others have documented the instrumental role of family members in promoting entry into formal treatment, using persuasion, coercion, or force to compel their loved ones to seek mental health services (Pescosolido, Gardner, & Lubell, 1998). Conversely, classic and contemporary sociological research suggests that treatment delays and other barriers to recovery can occur among individuals embedded in unsupportive social networks, or those with negative orientations toward medical or mental health treatment (Corrigan & Phelan, 2004; Horwitz, 1977; Kadushin, 1966; Perry & Pescosolido, 2015).

Medical sociologists have also examined the consequences of increased responsibility for family members and other informal supporters, demonstrating that the effects of deinstitutionalization reforms extend well past individuals with severe mental illness. Gallagher and Mechanic (1996) found that simply living with someone with mental illness is associated with a range of adverse health outcomes and increased utilization of health services. Likewise, research by Karp (2002) and Cook and colleagues (1994) suggests that the level of caregiving required by family members in the post-deinstitutionalization era is associated with substantial social, emotional, and economic burden. In other words, sociologists take a broader view of the problems caused by gaps in the public mental health system, documenting the ripple effect of gaps in social and health services through families and communities.

Sociological research on micro-level social consequences in the post-deinstitutionalization era has unique and important implications for clinical and policy reforms. Namely, because recovery from severe mental illness is not merely a discrete outcome of using services, but rather an ongoing process that involves improvement in day to day functioning, return to social roles, and reengagement in meaningful social life in the community, the broader lay social context in which patients are embedded is critical (Aneshensel, 2013; Pescosolido, 1996). However, some health policies originally designed to protect patients are at odds with sociological research on the integral role of informal caregivers. For example, existing confidentiality requirements allow widespread information flow between professionals, but often preclude the sharing of information with family caregivers (Petrila & Sadoff, 1992).

Although mental health professionals are now less likely than in the past to view families as pathogenic, they often neglect family members rather than cultivating community resources and creating allies among informal supporters. Recently, evidence-based models – including community support systems approaches, consumer-centered family models, and related interventions for families (e.g., psychoeducational therapy) – have made important advances in this area, focusing on the development of more holistic and inclusive treatment models that embrace the role of lay supporters and community integration (Lucksted, McFarlane, Downing, & Dixon, 2012). These evidence-based interventions are designed to facilitate collaborative management of people with serious mental illness by professionals and family members, including coordinating treatment, ensuring medication compliance, and involving family members in treatment planning (Dixon et al., 2001). In short, sociological research has pushed the boundaries of care into families and communities, demonstrating that achieving buy-in and participation from members of lay community networks is critical for the efficacy of therapeutic interventions.

50 YEARS AFTER DEINSTITUTIONALIZATION: NEW SOCIOLOGICAL INSIGHTS AND INNOVATIONS

This volume of *Advances in Medical Sociology* confronts deinstitutionalization's legacies approximately 50 years after reintegration began in earnest. The chapters in this volume turn a critical lens toward contemporary problems and solutions related to mental illness in countries where reform occurred. Its goal is to highlight the diversity of theoretical, methodological, and substantive work related to deinstitutionalization in the subfields of medical sociology, the sociology of mental health, and health services research. Each of the authors highlights pressing issues around mental health treatment, stigma and social relationships, or the lived experiences of people with mental illness – all of which continue to be significantly influenced by deinstitutionalization reforms.

50 Years after Deinstitutionalization is divided into four parts. In Part I, *Taking Stock of the Past and Looking Toward the Future* – comparative and historical and institutional approaches are used to identify defining features and turning points in the deinstitutionalization movement that have had lasting impacts on the contemporary mental health system. In "Same Problem, Different Century: Issues in Recreating the Functions of Public Psychiatric Hospitals in Community-Based Settings," William H. Fisher, Jeffrey L. Geller, and Dana L. McMannus adopt a functionalist approach to assessing the success of the deinstitutionalization movement. These authors provide a historical account of the functions of the pre-deinstitutionalization state hospital system with respect to patients (e.g., social welfare, treatment) and communities (e.g., social control, eldercare). They argue that the failure to replicate some of these functions in the community mental health system created gaps that led to contemporary problems like homelessness and the criminalization of mental illness. Adrianna Bagnall and Gil Eyal have contributed a chapter entitled, "'Forever Children' and Autonomous Citizens: Comparing the Deinstitutionalizations of Psychiatric Patients and Developmentally Disabled Individuals in the United States." In it, they present a comparative historical analysis of key factors in the deinstitutionalization processes in these two cases, including differences in motivations, patient populations, levels of funding, and results. They conclude that the positive outcomes of the reform movement for developmentally disabled people are attributable to successful framing of the moral worth of this population. This part concludes with a forward-looking chapter by Teresa L. Scheid. In "An Institutional Analysis of Public Sector Mental Health in the Post-Deinstitutionalization Era," she analyzes the current state of the community mental health system. She describes competition between three incompatible institutional logics which have shaped the political and economic climate of mental health care in the United States, arguing that a meaningful reform solution lies in the development of a logic of social justice.

Part II, titled *Community Reintegration and the Social Environment*, highlights the critical and enduring role of social connectedness and informal community support in recovery from mental illness. Russell K. Schutt's chapter, "Social Environment and Mental Illness: The Progress and Paradox of Deinstitutionalization," traces the history of institutionalization and deinstitutionalization reform, identifying periods of concern throughout history with the role of the social environment in recovery from mental illness. He demonstrates that the most effective programs for people with mental illness have been those that create safe and humane residential environments and facilitate social integration, though these are also the most difficult to implement. In our chapter entitled, "The Revolving Door: Patient Needs and Network Turnover during Mental Health Treatment," Will R. McConnell and I examine how people with mental illness fill support gaps left by deinstitutionalization. Using data on first-time mental health clients, we find that individuals activate support from members of their personal community networks who offer resources that match their needs. However, this strategy has unintended consequences – people with elevated unmet needs tend to cycle through supporters, creating high membership turnover in their social networks. Alisa K. Lincoln and Wallis E. Adams, in their chapter entitled, "Understandings of Community among People Using Publicly Funded Community Mental Health Services," ask an important, but seldom-addressed question. Namely, how do people using community mental health services define community and conceptualize their place in it? Drawing on nearly 300 interviews, these authors identify points of intervention in mental health clients' perceptions of barriers to and facilitators of community integration.

Part III – *Confronting Stigma and its Consequences* – illuminates the profound adverse social and psychological effects and barriers to recovery associated with perceived and internalized stigma, and highlights strategies used by mental health clients to resist stigmatization. In "Revisiting the Relationships among Community Mental Health Services, Stigma and Well-Being," Kristen Marcussen and Christian Ritter investigate the consequences of labeling for people with severe and persistent mental illness in contemporary communities. Using longitudinal data and more detailed and comprehensive measures of services, stigma and recovery outcomes than previous studies, they find only moderate support for a positive relationship between nine types of mental health services and well-being and self-concept. However, while stigma has negative consequences for recovery outcomes, the authors found no evidence that labeling leads to stigmatization. Sarah K. Harkness, Amy Kroska, and Bernice A. Pescosolido, in their chapter entitled, "The Self-Stigma of Psychiatric Patients: Implications for Identities, Emotions, and the Life Course," identify consequences of self-stigmatization for people with mental illness living in the community using principles from affect control theory. A particularly important insight from this study is the finding that higher levels of self-stigma are associated with avoidance of social and community integration into role-identities, including employment, dating, marriage, and parenthood. Finally, Nana Tuntiya also addresses stigma and its relationship to the sick role in her article, "The 'Dignity of the Sick': Managing Social Stigma by Mental Patients in the Community." She presents results from an interpretive analysis of secondary qualitative data collected in the town of Geel, Belgium – a unique community where people with mental illness are taken into the homes of residents as boarders in a system known as "family care." Tuntiya suggests that Geel boarders actively manage stigma by resisting exemption from social roles typically associated with the sick role, remaining functional members of households and the community.

In Part IV of this volume, entitled *Biomedicalization in the Era of Community Mental Health*, authors provide a window into the social, clinical, and ethical problems that have emerged as a result of failures of deinstitutionalization reform, focusing in particular on biomedicalization and the overuse of pharmaceuticals. Drawing on data from 39 in-depth interviews with mental health providers, the authors of "Borderline Personality Disorder and the Biomedical Mismatch" examine how the combination of biomedicalization and deinstitutionalization has failed individuals with borderline personality disorder (BPD). Sandra H. Sulzer, Gracie Jackson, and Ashelee Yang document provider discourse around the pharmaceutical imperative and short courses of care, describing the incompatibility of these central features of the community mental health system with successful recovery of patients with BPD. In "Soldier, Elder, Prisoner, Ward: Psychotropics in the Era of Transinstitutionalization," Anthony R. Hatch, Marik Xavier-Brier, Brandon Attell, and Eryn Viscarra examine the practice and ethics of psychotropic medication prescription in total institutions following the biomedical turn in mental health practice. They argue that rather than being deinstitutionalized, many people with severe forms of mental illness have been shifted to other institutions like prisons, nursing homes, and the foster care system – a development which has led to unprecedented use of psychotropic medication for social control.

Together these chapters showcase the innovative, theoretically grounded, and critically important scholarship being conducted in medical sociology around issues of deinstitutionalization and the state of the contemporary community mental health system. This volume demonstrates that sociologists are uniquely positioned to identify and improve our understanding of the social, cultural, and institutional forces that explain both the failures and successes of mental health reform movements. Finally, the contributors illuminate social policy issues and economic and ethical dilemmas which must be confronted to create a more comprehensive and recovery-oriented system of care for people with mental illness and their families.

Brea L. Perry
Editor

REFERENCES

Aneshensel, C. S. (2013). Mental illness as a career: Sociological perspectives. In *Handbook of the sociology of mental health* (pp. 603–620). Netherlands: Springer.

Carpentier, N., Lesage, A., & White, D. (1999). Family influence on the first stages of the trajectory of patients diagnosed with severe psychiatric disorders. *Family Relations, 48*, 397–403.

Cook, J. A., Heller, T., & Pickett-Schenk, S. A. (1999). The effect of support group participation on caregiver burden among parents of adult offspring with severe mental illness. *Family Relations, 48*, 405–410.

Corrigan, P. W., & Phelan, S. M. (2004). Social support and recovery in people with serious mental illnesses. *Community Mental Health Journal, 40*(6), 513–523.

Coulter, A. (2013). Guns don't kill people, the mentally ill do. *Ann Coulter Blog*. Retrieved from http://www.anncoulter.com/columns/2013-01-16.html. Accessed on February 18, 2016.

Dixon, L., McFarlane, W. R., Lefley, H., Lucksted, A., Cohen, M., Falloon, I., & Sondheimer, D. (2001). Evidence-based practices for services to families of people with psychiatric disabilities. *Psychiatric Services, 52*(7), 903–910.

Gallagher, S. K., & Mechanic, D. (1996). Living with the mentally ill: Effects on the health and functioning of other household members. *Social Science & Medicine, 42*(12), 1691–1701.

Harris, L. (2015). Washington's horrible mental health legislation. *Huffington Post*. Retrieved from http://www.huffingtonpost.com/leah-harris/washingtons-horrible-mental-health-legislation_b_8623226.html. Accessed on February 18, 2016.

Hartwell, S. (2004). Triple stigma: Persons with mental illness and substance abuse problems in the criminal justice system. *Criminal Justice Policy Review, 15*(1), 84–99.

Hiday, V. A. (1995). The social context of mental illness and violence. *Journal of Health and Social Behavior, 36*, 122–137.

Horwitz, A. (1977). Social networks and pathways to psychiatric treatment. *Social Forces, 56*(1), 86–105.

Kadushin, C. (1966). The friends and supporters of psychotherapy: On social circles in urban life. *American Sociological Review, 31*, 786–802.

Karp, D. A. (2002). *The burden of sympathy: How families cope with mental illness*. Oxford: Oxford University Press.

Lamb, H. R., & Bachrach, L. L. (2001). Some perspectives on deinstitutionalization. *Psychiatric Services*, *52*(8), 1039–1045.

Lucksted, A., McFarlane, W., Downing, D., & Dixon, L. (2012). Recent developments in family psychoeducation as an evidence-based practice. *Journal of Marital and Family Therapy*, *38*(1), 101–121.

Markowitz, F. E. (2006). Psychiatric hospital capacity, homelessness, and crime and arrest rates. *Criminology*, *44*(1), 45–72.

Mechanic, D. (2008). *Mental health and social policy: Beyond managed care*. Boston, MA: Pearson Higher Ed.

Mechanic, D. (2012). Seizing opportunities under the affordable care act for transforming the mental and behavioral health system. *Health Affairs*, *31*(2), 376–382.

Metzl, J. M., & MacLeish, K. T. (2015). Mental illness, mass shootings, and the politics of American firearms. *American Journal of Public Health*, *105*(2), 240–249.

Middleton, C. (2016). Let's make a real difference for an entire generation of young children. *Huffington Post*. Retrieved from http://www.huffingtonpost.co.uk/her-royal-highness-the-duchess-of-cambridge/lets-make-a-real-difference-for-young-children_b_9246336.html. Accessed on February 18, 2016.

Morrissey, J. P., Calloway, M., Bartko, W. T., Ridgely, M. S., Goldman, H. H., & Paulson, R. I. (1994). Local mental health authorities and service system change: Evidence from the Robert Wood Johnson foundation program on chronic mental illness. *The Milbank Quarterly*, *72*, 49–80.

Murphy, T. (2013). Helping Families in Mental Health Crisis Act. H.R. 3717, 113th Congress, 1st Session.

Obama, M. (2016). Let's change the conversation around mental health. *Huffington Post*. Retrieved from http://www.huffingtonpost.co.uk/michelle-obama/lets-change-the-conversation-around-mental-health_b_9245816.html. Accessed on February 18, 2016.

Peek, C. J. (2009). Integrating care for persons, not only diseases. *Journal of Clinical Psychology in Medical Settings*, *16*(1), 13–20.

Perry, B. L., & Horwitz, A. (2014). Mental health services: I. Settings and programs. In B. Jennings (Ed.), *Encyclopedia of bioethics* (4th ed.). Farmington Hills, MI: Macmillan Reference.

Perry, B. L., & Pescosolido, B. A. (2015). Social network activation: The role of health discussion partners in recovery from mental illness. *Social Science & Medicine*, *125*, 116–128.

Pescosolido, B. A. (1996). Bringing the "community" into utilization models: how social networks link individuals to changing systems of care. In J. Kronenfeld (Ed.). *Research in the Sociology of Health Care*. (Vol. 13A, pp. 171–197). Greenwich, CT: JA1 Press.

Pescosolido, B. A., Gardner, C. B., & Lubell, K. M. (1998). How people get into mental health services: Stories of choice, coercion and "muddling through" from "first-timers". *Social Science & Medicine*, *46*(2), 275–286.

Petrila, J. P., & Sadoff, R. L. (1992). Confidentiality and the family as caregiver. *Psychiatric Services*, *43*(2), 136–139.

Rosenberg, J. (2014). Mass shootings and mental health policy. *Journal of Sociology and Social Welfare*, *41*, 107.

Scheid, T. L. (2003). Managed care and the rationalization of mental health services. *Journal of Health and Social Behavior*, *44*, 142–161.

Schutt, R. K., & Goldfinger, S. M. (2011). *Homelessness, housing, and mental illness.* Cambridge, MA: Harvard University Press.

Wright, E. R., Avirappattu, G., & Lafuze, J. E. (1999). The family experience of deinstitutionalization: Insights from the closing of central state hospital. *The Journal of Behavioral Health Services & Research*, *26*(3), 289–304.

PART I
TAKING STOCK OF THE PAST AND LOOKING TOWARD THE FUTURE

SAME PROBLEM, DIFFERENT CENTURY: ISSUES IN RECREATING THE FUNCTIONS OF PUBLIC PSYCHIATRIC HOSPITALS IN COMMUNITY-BASED SETTINGS

William H. Fisher, Jeffrey L. Geller and Dana L. McMannus

ABSTRACT

Purpose – *The purpose of this chapter is to apply structural functional theory and the concept of "unbundling" to an analysis of the deinstitutionalization and community mental health efforts that have shaped the current mental health services environment.*

Approach – *We examine the original goals of the institutional movement, the arguments supporting it, and the functions of the institutions that were created. We then examine the criticisms of that approach and the success of the subsequent deinstitutionalization process, which attempted to undo this process by recreating the hospitals' functions in community settings. Finally, we address the question of whether the*

50 Years after Deinstitutionalization: Mental Illness in Contemporary Communities
Advances in Medical Sociology, Volume 17, 3–25

ISSN: 1057-6290/doi:10.1108/S1057-629020160000017001

critical functions of psychiatric institutions have indeed been adequately recreated.

Findings – *Our overview of outcomes from this process suggests that the unbundling of state hospital functions did not yield an adequate system of care and support, and that the functions of state hospitals, including social control and incapacitation with respect to public displays of deviance were not sufficiently recreated in the community-based settings.*

Social implications – *The arguments for the construction of state hospitals, the critiques of those settings, and the current criticism of efforts to replace their functions are eerily similar. Actors involved in the design of mental health services should take into account the functions of existing services and the gaps between them. Consideration of the history of efforts at functional change might also serve this process well.*

Keywords: Deinstitutionalization; mental illness; mental health services; psychiatric hospitals

INTRODUCTION

Deinstitutionalization of persons with serious mental illness,[1] a process beginning in the middle of the 20th century, led to the massive downsizing of public mental hospitals,[2] both by transferring patients confined in them to "community-based settings" – that is, those operating outside the walls of institutions – and by deflecting new admissions to alternative settings. The result of this process can be seen in the declining number of persons confined in these public mental hospitals (Geller, 2000a). On an average day in 1955, some 590,000 persons resided in public mental hospitals; by 1995 that number had declined by nearly 95%. It currently hovers at just under that point (Lutterman, 2015).

The factors that led to this decline and its aftermath have been the subjects of numerous works that collectively point to a myriad of causal factors, as we shall discuss. They include a turning against institutional solutions for social problems of all kinds and toward "community-based" remedies, changes in the legal rights of confined persons, advances in the pharmacologic treatment of some of the most serious psychiatric illnesses, and financial incentives to house persons with disabilities in non-institutional settings.

Like the institutional project that was its predecessor, the deinstitutionalization process was intended to provide more humane and effective care and treatment for persons with serious mental illness at lower cost to the taxpayer. And like the institutions it sought to abolish, deinstitutionalization has been viewed with considerable negativity by many (cf. Chu & Trotter, 1974; Jacobs, 1974), with one observer characterizing it as a "psychiatric Titanic" (Torrey, 1997) and at least the partial cause of the numerous social problems involving persons with mental illness, including high rates of homelessness and incarceration. In this chapter, we briefly explore this process, using as a basis for our exploration the sociological framework provided by structural functional theory.

The Institutional Era and Its Discontents

It is difficult to enter into a discussion or analysis of deinstitutionalization without considering first the state of mental institutions preceding the start of that process. The institutional approach to managing persons with serious mental illnesses has a number of policy antecedents (cf. Grob, 1966; Morrissey, Goldman, & Klerman, 1980; Rothman, 1971), but a driving force for the creation of these institutions was the work of Dorothea Dix, who, in an 1841 visit to the East Cambridge Jail in Massachusetts, observed what she believed were persons suffering from mental illnesses who were inappropriately incarcerated and inhumanely treated. This observation set her on a multistate course of reform that would culminate in the creation of numerous institutions for housing persons with mental illness across much of the eastern half of the United States. These institutions, it was believed, would provide more humane treatment to persons with mental disabilities than had been provided in jails, almshouses, and poor farms. They would also save money by treating people and returning them to productive lives rather than housing them for life at public expense. Dix received substantial support from the psychiatric hospital superintendents of her era.

State mental hospitals quickly came to function as what economists term a "free good." Extremely liberal regulations surrounding involuntary admission and retention allowed police, family members, and others to use the state hospital as a repository for persons who were mentally ill, developmentally disabled, chemically addicted, demented, otherwise mentally impaired, or inclined to perform acts thought to be socially unacceptable. In fact, descriptions by Grob (1966) of hospitals operating in the latter part of the 19th and early 20th centuries describe a hodgepodge of patients confined in state hospitals because there were few alternative settings and because the hospital was easily accessed.

These facilities proliferated rapidly during the roughly 75 years that state and county governments actively invested in them. In Massachusetts, for example, 14 hospitals, including one used exclusively for children, were constructed between 1877 and the early- to mid-1900s. The lax legal statutes that allowed individuals to be easily admitted and retained, coupled with the attractiveness of these settings as places to send not only those with mental illness, but also the generally undesirable, led to uncontrolled growth in the hospitals' populations.

Paradoxically, as these facilities' censuses grew, they received less and less public attention. This is due in part to the stigma associated with being detained in a state hospital having a family member confined there, and also to the fact that these facilities were often sited in areas removed from large population centers. In many areas, the growing facilities became important sources of employment for local communities (Morrissey et al., 1980). Even employment in such facilities contributed to the disconnect between the public and the hospital. Doctors, nurses, and other hospital employees often were housed on the grounds of the hospital, and to accommodate employees and patients, a variety of services were provided, including movie theaters, stores, and other conveniences.

There is evidence that the optimistic view of tying the functions of state hospitals to the provision of what was the prevailing notion of humane treatment could not survive the onslaught of patient population growth. The evidence, however, is meager. The "invisibility of patients" (Grob, 1966) residing in these facilities led to little public interest in or attention to what transpired in them, and continued underfunding led to perennial short staffing. It very much appears that as long as individuals detained in public psychiatric hospitals were not in the community, few were concerned about what happened to them. The lack of effective treatments for the illnesses from which many patients suffered led to growth in the populations of what were termed the "backwards" of the hospital, which housed chronic patients whose conditions had deteriorated or failed to improve.[3]

Among the important missing functions of these facilities were both effective treatment and the resources necessary to provide those treatments that were available. A number of treatment approaches were tried in the early- to mid-20th century, including insulin coma, hydrotherapy, metrazol shock, lobotomy, and others. Some of these, of course, yielded successes, owing more perhaps to the remissions that are characteristic of the cyclical nature of some mental illnesses. An expanding population of persons with largely untreatable psychiatric illnesses and static human and capital resources led to abuses that would come to light toward the mid-20th century. Accounts of maltreatment in psychiatric facilities written by conscientious objectors who worked in state hospitals during World War II, journalists and others, such as Deutch's *The Shame of the States* (1948), revealed overcrowding, understaffing, serious abuse of patients, dietary budgets of pennies per day per patient, nakedness, and filth. Were Dorothea Dix to return to inspect the facilities her crusade had inspired she would likely have been horrified.

Overcrowding had led to continual hospital construction well into the early 1950s, but many hospitals were filled soon after opening. New York's Pilgrim State Hospital, for example, which began construction in the 1930s, would ultimately house some 15,000 patients, making it one of the largest psychiatric facilities ever built. As we noted in the introduction, by 1955, on any given day the nation's public psychiatric hospitals housed an average of more than 590,000 individuals (Lutterman, 2015), and this represented a staggering 50% of *all* hospital beds operating in the United States at the time (Gorman, 1956)

The Decline of the Public Mental Hospital

By the post-World War II era, state hospitals were plunging into disfavor. As noted, their censuses ballooned, as many more patients were admitted than were discharged (Fisher & Phillips, 1990). And, despite the fact that mere pennies per day were expended on patients, operational costs were perceived as out of control and much too great a percentage of states' budgets. Accounts of patient abuse and neglect became more widespread and more targeted to the general public, as exemplified in an exposé in *Life* Magazine in 1946 (Maisel, 1946). It had become clear that the mission of providing humane care and treatment for persons with mental illnesses had essentially failed.

Several factors brought about the impetus for change. Most commonly cited, perhaps, is the serendipitous discovery of the antipsychotic effects associated with the drug chlorpromazine or Thorazine as it came to be commercially labeled in the United States. This came about as the drug, originally formulated as a sedative, was tested on psychiatric patients, many of whom experienced reductions in their psychotic symptoms to the extent that some could be discharged. Graphic trends in the census of state hospitals typically show a significant downward deflection in that trend following the introduction of Thorazine in 1955 (Frank & Gleid, 2006).[4] The advent of Medicaid and Medicare, as well as increased availability of nursing homes that could assume some of the state hospital's long-term care function also contributed significantly to this decline (Frank & Gleid, 2006).[5]

The Community Mental Health Movement: Moving Hospitals' Functions and Services beyond Institutional Walls

In the 1950s, recognition that the institutional approach to managing persons with mental illness was no longer viable led to action at multiple levels of government, including, for the first time, the federal government. In the late 1950s, the federal government convened a panel of experts, The Joint Commission on Mental Health and Illness, who were charged with developing the blueprint for a system of localized mental health services that would not include a large psychiatric inpatient facility. The findings of this group became the substance of the landmark report *Action for Mental Health* (1961). This report recommended the creation of more focused, defined services that would support persons with mental illnesses living outside of institutions, that is, "in the community." There were to be designs for systems of care and treatment intended to allow the downsizing or closure of state hospitals. The findings of this group enabled President John F. Kennedy to address a joint session of congress in October 1963, where he argued for a "bold new approach" to the treatment of mental illness, including new psychiatric medications available for the treatment of serious mental illnesses, that promised to make it possible for "all but a small portion" of persons in large institutions to be placed in the community. To support that process, Kennedy called for the creation of what would become the federally funded community mental health program. Although he would not live to see its implementation, it nevertheless came to fruition as the Community Mental Health Centers Act of 1964.

The intent of the community mental health movement was threefold. First, by moving the locus of service delivery from the hospital to the community, many patients could be discharged and the censuses of state hospital thereby reduced. Second, many persons, it was believed, could essentially bypass the hospital altogether and receive treatment and support services in community settings. Finally, this relocation of patients and services would decrease costs of care, a cost borne almost exclusively by states (and in some states, counties) at the time.

The linchpin of the new community-based care was to be the community mental health center, which would provide medication, therapy, and support services for persons discharged from their local state hospital. As envisioned, individuals would exit the hospital with an appointment at the community mental health center, where they would be seen by psychiatrists and social workers who would provide the treatment and supports necessary to sustain them in the community.

The attractiveness of this new approach to state governments cannot be overstated. Shifting the financial burden of care and treatment, which had been born by state and county governments for nearly a century, to the federal government, which funded services provided in community mental health centers, was particularly attractive to state officials. Moreover, the advent of Medicaid and Medicare, which would allow those persons deemed eligible by low income and disability, to receive care in local general hospitals, also allowed inpatient treatment to be financed by the federal government (in the case of Medicare) or through a state-federal split (Medicaid), with the state's share depending on its per capita income (although the state never pays more than 50%). Using local general hospitals, instead of state hospitals, as the locus of inpatient treatment for persons with serious mental illness had been recommended by policy makers in the report *Action for Mental Health* and, as a practice, was incentivized fiscally by the availability of Medicaid as a form or reimbursement (Dorwart & Epstein, 1993; Fisher, Dorwart, Schlesinger, Epstein, & Davidson, 1992; Frank & Gleid, 2006; Geller, 2000b; Gronfein, 1985a). These initiatives collectively constituted the largest shifting of costs of care for those with mental illness from one level of government to another since the state took responsibility for this function in the late 19th century (Frank & Gleid, 2006; Geller, 2000a).

A STRUCTURAL FUNCTIONAL THEORETICAL APPROACH FOR EXAMINING DEINSTITUTIONALIZATION

Much of the research done in the area of deinstitutionalization and community mental health has been descriptive and empirical but not grounded in sociological or other theoretical perspective. There are important exceptions, however. Rothbard, Hadley, and Richman (1997) drew on a perspective from business and economics termed "unbundling" to describe the process of disaggregating the functions in place at the Philadelphia State Hospital and recreating them as individual service entities in community-based settings.

Here, we adopt (but liberally adapt) a longstanding sociological perspective, "structural functionalism" or, simply, "functionalism" to examine the state hospital's functions and the process of recreating them in non-institutional, community-based settings. Once a major force in sociological theory, functionalism's roots are in the work of 19th century social theorists August Comte and Herbert Spencer. This perspective flourished in the mid-20th century, most notably in the works of Parsons (1950) and Merton (1968), but has declined in influence since that time. At the risk of oversimplification, it could be argued that their work focused on large social systems, the roles and functions of key institutions and societal components, and the effects of failures of key functions to fulfill their roles. Our application of functionalism is based on an adaptation of that theoretical perspective. It focuses on the state hospital and its key functions with respect to (a) the patients housed within them, and (b) the communities to which patients would be discharged in the process of depopulating state hospitals and recreating their functions in community settings. We postulate that failure to (a) understand the key functions played by state hospitals and how they might be recreated in a "system of care" and (b) to anticipate the potential effects of legal, economic, and other factors that could affect the utilization of the state hospital would create significant social problems for patients, their families, and agents of government beyond the mental health system. Our perspective, which has been described in earlier work (Fisher et al., 2001), sees the relationship between the functions of hospitals and community-based services as dynamic and fluid, rather than static, such that the functions of the hospitals and community services co-evolve, with the hospital's function constantly shaped or reshaped by the changes in the role definitions of the community services, the resources made available to them, and their efficacy in meeting the needs of their clientele.

The Functions of State Hospitals vis-à-vis the Larger Society

Social Control of Deviance

The major function of the state hospital vis-a-vis the communities they served was and is social control. Most obviously, they provided a setting in which to place persons who were disruptive but for whom arrest and detention would not be a long-term solution. Vagrants, public alcoholics, and others who were simply bothersome could not be jailed for any length of time, but if a case could be made that a "mental condition" was at the root of their problem, they were likely to be committable to a state hospital. Criminologists use the term "incapacitation" to describe the effects of incarceration, whereby individuals are prevented from offending, at least among the general public, by virtue of their confinement in a correctional setting. Public mental hospitals, where lengthy stays could be quite common, arguably played a similar role with respect to nonoffenders by removing their socially unacceptable behaviors from the public square. Viewed in the context of the functional aspects of the state hospital, these settings provided a place where persons whose behaviors were troublesome – that is, who displayed behaviors related to mental illness, alcoholism, dementia – or who needed long-term care, the provision of which would be disruptive to family units – could be considered for admission. Public psychiatric hospitals therefore contributed to the stability not only of communities but also of families and other social groupings.

Long-Term/Elder Care

In the pre-reform era of the 1960s, state hospitals filled an important function for two classes of elders: individuals who had been admitted at a younger age and simply "aged in" and those who had developed the behavioral symptoms of dementia and who could not be cared for in other settings or by family (Morrissey et al., 1980). This was in evidence in "point in time" data collected on patient resident on one day in the 1980s at two Massachusetts state hospitals. In these populations were persons who had been hospitalized for 60 years or more (Geller, Fisher, Simon, & Wirth-Cauchon, 1990). Providing care for the elderly was an important function, given the small number of nursing homes operating in the early part of the 20th century – a number that would subsequently grow and absorb some of the long-term care functions of the state hospital.

Repositories for Persons Exhibiting Psychiatric "Symptoms"

Obviously, public psychiatric hospitals became an important setting for persons who appeared to be affected by psychiatric illnesses, but the admission process was, if couched in epidemiological terms, "sensitive but not selective." That is, individuals presenting symptoms that appeared to be related to psychosis or depression were admitted, but it appears that persons with organic brain disorders, long-term sequelae of alcohol abuse, dementias, and even tertiary syphilis were also present (*Report of the Superintendent of Worcester State Lunatic Asylum*, 1921) given the absence of other social structures that could manage the behaviors of many with these conditions.

State Hospital Functions vis-à-vis Recipients of Care

In their heyday, public mental hospitals maintained a range of functions with respect to patient populations. First and foremost, they provided the basic necessities of life – albeit sometimes of questionable quantity and quality – including food, clothing, and shelter. As such they could be considered as providers of an important "social welfare" function. State hospitals also provided all manner of work. Dowdall's (1996) account of the closure of Buffalo State Hospital shows residents of these hospitals working in the kitchen, doing housekeeping chores, farming, and other activities essential to the operation of the hospital. This necessity arose from the fact that state hospital budgets were very small and operated well because, based on hospitals' annual reports, first person accounts and pictures provided in accounts of these hospitals, many inpatients were reasonably functional and able to fill essential roles within the hospital (Dowdall, 1996; Grob, 1966, 1991; Morrissey et al., 1980).

State hospitals also provided a treatment function. Until the advent of chlorpromazine, psychiatric treatment in state hospitals was largely based on sedation, interpersonal interactions, rest, escape from environmental stressors, and meaningful work, albeit with mixed results. The centrality of treatment to the individual patient varied from high to virtually nil, depending upon each person's clinical circumstances.

Designing a Community Mental Health System

As we noted, the term "deinstitutionalization" is frequently applied to the process by which the number of patients and beds in state hospitals declined and the number of hospital themselves was reduced. But a structural functional analysis of the planning and implementation of the process – how the functions of the hospital were to be replaced by services provided elsewhere that would cohere into a system of care – arguably lends itself better to an examination of the process.

A blueprint for this process, as we have noted, was presented in *Action for Mental Health* (Joint Commission on Mental Health and Illness, 1961). This work was not intended to be a structural functional analysis, but its approach was very much consistent with that perspective. *Action for Mental Health* mandated that a range of community-based programs be designed that would provide important services for persons discharged from state hospitals. In this design, various clinical supports would be provided by community mental health services: residential programs would provide persons places to live; day treatment programs would offer habilitation and rehabilitation services; and finally, recognizing that inpatient treatment would be occasionally necessary, local general hospitals were encouraged to open acute psychiatric units. This would appear, at least, to be a reasonable blueprint for transferring the functions of the hospital vis-a-vis the population to be served. However, this blueprint was flawed in numerous ways that would lead to problems for the population of persons with mental illness as well as the communities to which they would be released.

A FUNCTIONAL ANALYSIS OF OUTCOMES

The Social Control Function

We postulated that failure to fully recreate the hospital's functions would become problematic. While community mental health approaches evolved and attempted, albeit not always successfully, to provide many of the functions once provide by the hospitals in the form of community-based services, one critical function, the incapacitation of deviance, was never fully addressed in any of the plans. As we noted, a key function of state hospitals had entailed the prevention of deviant behavior in community settings via incapacitation. Persons confined in state hospitals for lengthy periods may have engaged in deviant or troublesome behaviors, but the public was not exposed to them. Blame for the failure to create anything resembling a social control function can be attributed to two factors. First, planning for community mental health focused almost entirely on the creation of services that would fill the support and treatment functions of the hospital. In *Action for Mental Health*, for example, little attention is given to the fact that, improved treatments notwithstanding, many individuals released to the community would exhibit behaviors ranging from annoying to dangerous. And, the fact that many persons who had traditionally been admitted to state hospitals with problems that were more social than clinical was not recognized in the plans put forward for the new mental health system.

The second factor undermining the mental health system's capacity for social control came from the legal reforms surrounding the way in which individuals could be involuntarily confined in state hospitals. As mentioned earlier, prior to the early 1970s the process of involuntary civil commitment had been a relatively easy one. Many states' statutes allowed for quick commitment, largely without due process, upon the testimony of family members, physicians or police (Warren, 1982). But while involuntary hospitalization was easy, the process by which individuals could be released was difficult. This allowed hospitals to play a significant incapacitation function. But beginning in the early 1970s, increased concern for the civil rights of ethnic minorities, women, and populations generally disenfranchised led to numerous court cases challenging existing state commitment statutes, which resulted in revisions of substantive and procedural changes in commitment laws (Appelbaum, 1994). In general, these reforms required that persons have a diagnosed mental illness and that, because of that illness, they were a danger to themselves or others or unable to meet basic human needs for food, clothing, and shelter. The procedural reforms typically limited initial confinement for assessment to a few days and required court hearings for commitments exceeding these periods through a formal judicial process. The effects of civil commitment reforms have typically been evaluated within the context of changes within states (cf. Durham, Fisher, & Pierce, 1986) and all tend to show dramatic reductions in both admissions to and length of stay in state hospitals, with a concomitant reduction in the incapacitation potential of state hospitals for public deviance and illegal behavior.[6]

The "Criminalization" of Mental Illness; Consequences of Failing to Recreate the Social Control Function

One consequence of the mental health systems' failure to provide the necessary degree of social control in the post-deinstitutionalization era has been the ceding of that function to the criminal justice system. Shortly after the passage of civil commitment reforms in California, there was an apparent increase in the number of individuals with serious psychiatric illnesses appearing in the criminal justice system (Abramson, 1972; Geller & Lister,

1978). Since that time, numerous studies, using a range of techniques, have found levels of justice system involvement in this population that are well in excess of what would be observed in the community (Fisher et al., 2011; Steadman, Osher, Robbins, Case, & Samuels, 2010; Teplin, 1994). The social control function with respect to persons with mental illness has thus been shifted at least in part from the mental health system to the criminal justice system via a process that has been termed "transcarceration" (Johnson, 1992). Beginning in the 1990s, large county jails, such as Rikers Island in New York City, Cook County Jail in Chicago, and the Los Angeles County Jail surpassed psychiatric hospitals as the chief provider of institutionally based psychiatric treatment (Torrey, 1995). Currently, a person with serious mental illness has a far greater chance of spending a night in jail than in a psychiatric hospital (Morrissey, Cuddeback, & Meyer, 2007).

Structural Functional Assessment of the Deinstitutionalization Process

Earlier, we argued that a structural functional analysis of the deinstitutionalization process would find that if key functions were not recreated in the community, the deinstitutionalization process envisioned by policy makers would fail. And as we have observed, many problems have in fact emerged. A functional analysis of these problems suggests a number of things. First, the unbundled functions often did not fully reconstitute the "whole" of which they were once apart. This was due in part to the fact that the totality of a mental health system and how its component services could or should be linked was not well understood. As a result, the disaggregated, unbundled functions of the state hospital often failed to comprise a coherent structural system. Thus, while reference may have been made to a "community-based system of care," in reality what developed in many locales was not a "system" at all, at least in the sense in which this term is typically applied. Efforts to enhance system integration, which would create an entity whose function was to tie these pieces together more effectively, would become a focus of research in the mid-1980s (Goldman, Morrissey, & Ridgely, 1994) but remain unsuccessful at the time of this chapter's publication (Geller, in press).

A number of particularly negative outcomes would come to public attention as a consequence of this structural failure. The housing function was not well funded or implemented, or was in some instances designed on the basis of faulty assumptions regarding the duration of need for residential services (Geller & Fisher, 1993). In many of the urban areas where some persons with mental illness had once been able to settle a gentrification process exacerbated homelessness among many individuals with mental illness. Homelessness would, in fact, become one of the principal problems confronting mental health service providers, as exemplified in a study conducted in the 1980s which found that 84% of a sample of homeless individuals in one city met criteria for mental illness (Fischer & Breakey, 1991). Moreover, placement of persons in the community and efforts to develop residential programming was complicated by powerful stigma associated with mental illness, and only neighborhoods with little "collective efficacy" (Sampson, Raudenbush, & Earls, 1997) would be able to prevent the placement of residences for persons with mental illness (Mechanic, 2008). As a result, many individuals were placed in poor neighborhoods with high crime rates and large numbers of individuals who used and sold drugs (Alverson, Alverson, & Drake, 2001; Drake & Wallach, 1989; Drake, Wallach, & McGovern, 2005; Silver, Mulvey, & Swanson, 2002). With unemployment rates approaching 90% for persons with the most severe mental illnesses (National Governor's Association, 2002), many individuals had little money and substantial idle time, leading some to associate with persons who engaged in drug and alcohol use and in some cases petty crime. These activities contributed to the excessive criminal justice involvement of observed this population (Teplin, 1994).

Overall, two distinct efforts aimed at reforming mental health care in a way that would create a more humane systemic approach – the creation of asylums and their subsequent elimination – ultimately failed to achieve that goal.

The Status of the State Hospital in 2015

So what is the situation of the current public psychiatric hospital? Just over 41,000 persons remain in the 195 state-operated psychiatric hospitals still in operation (Lutterman, 2015). Because of the dwindling number of patients, many states have closed most of their hospitals and consolidated their inpatient populations and resources in just one or two facilities (Fisher, Geller, & Pandiani, 2009). But trends in hospital census have begun to stabilize. According to a report by the National Association of State Mental Health Program Directors Research Institute, Inc. (NRI, 2013), as of 2015, the number of persons residing in state hospitals has declined little since 2005. But the number of beds in state hospitals has declined precipitously, however, to the point where several states are reporting that their existing facilities have become significantly overcrowded and are concerned that bed closure has been overly aggressive, leading to a backlog of patients waiting for state hospital beds (NRI-INC, 2013) http://www.nri-incdata.org/ProfilesReport.cfm.

But even as many states continue to close their old, decaying facilities, the problems cited here have led some states to undertake construction of new hospitals. These facilities, as characterized by their names, are intended to fill a new function focused on recovery, rather than asylum or confinement. For example, the iconic Worcester State Hospital (Massachusetts), subject of many historical accounts (Grob, 1966; Morrissey et al., 1980), has closed and been replaced by the Worcester Recovery Center and Hospital, which was constructed on the same grounds. Other states electing to build new public psychiatric hospitals include Arizona, California, Nevada, New Hampshire, New Jersey, North Carolina, Ohio, Vermont, Virginia, and West Virginia. This trend forces us to recognize the continued role for state hospitals, and points to the existence of a patient population that is not well served elsewhere. It also suggests that the co-evolution of the hospital and other systemic components have defined the function of the hospital as similar to what it has always been, but with a much smaller served population.

As we consider this trend, we are led to ask, "In mental health systems that have seen investments in an array of community services and supports, and which likely include general hospitals with psychiatric units, what functions do state hospitals now fill? What is their case mix? What is the system's plan for these facilities and the patients they serve?" As is the case in Massachusetts, many of the hospitals that remain open are not intended simply to be downsized versions of the old institutions. As described in Dowdall's discussion of deinstitutionalization at the Buffalo State Hospital, the functions of the institution itself underwent significant change. Buffalo State Hospital, like similar facilities in other states, became Buffalo Psychiatric Center, with a new mission that entailed a new set of functions. As Dowdall (1996) notes, the new Buffalo Psychiatric Center reported to the Joint Commission that it offered the following services: inpatient care, rehabilitation services, day/continuing treatment, intensive psychiatric rehabilitation training, case management, intensive case management, psychosocial clubs, screening and evaluation services, family care, community residence, residential care centers for adults, and sheltered workshop. In so doing, the hospitals' administrators and those overseeing the community system sought to make the state hospital one of the foci of the local system of care – a function never envisioned in *Action for Mental Health* or by the designers of the community mental health movement.

These apparent changes in function are notwithstanding, there is evidence to suggest that public psychiatric hospitals continue to play a role in the mental health system that was not successfully transferred to a community setting. While general hospital psychiatric units see a significant number of persons with serious mental illnesses, a subset of individuals who are too violent, need a period of treatment extending beyond the limits of what can be provided in a small general hospital psychiatric unit, are involved with the courts or criminal justice system, or who may exhibit deviant behaviors that make general hospital admission difficult (Fisher, Barreira, Geller et al., 2000; Fisher et al., 2009).

None of this is to deny the fact that in the decades since deinstitutionalization began, state hospitals have seen numerous changes not only in numbers of patients served, but also in the ability to successfully treat patients. There have been major advancements in mental health treatment, including the development of highly effective and safer medications as well as the development of many widely used evidence-based therapies and practices. These developments have in turn led to shorter hospital stays with greater levels of symptom reduction than was seen in the past.

But while the mission statements and treatment options provided by the current state hospitals have certainly changed, these facilities continue to fill some of the same functions as in the pre-deinstitutionalization era. Stated simply, state hospitals still maintain the function of housing those people society would prefer not to see, does not know what else to do with, and for whom the existing mental health system has no other appropriate setting. Indeed, as has been the case since "unbundling" efforts began over 50 years ago, policy makers and community providers still struggle to provide effective services to "difficult populations" transitioning out of state hospital care.

A CASE EXAMPLE

To illustrate these policy dynamics, we offer the example of a contemporary public psychiatric hospital on the east coast of the United States, and consider its relationship with community providers in the area the hospital serves. This hospital has seen a marked increase in the number of forensically involved patients and patients with problematic sexual issues, a term previously described as the "forensification" of state hospitals (Fisher et al., 2009). Complicated court issues and the general unwillingness or inability of many community providers to accept the risk of providing services to this population greatly complicate discharge. This hospital is also seeing the effects of the aging "baby boomer" population. State systems and community service funding have not kept pace with the changing needs of the aging mental health population. There is a lack of community services and suitable nursing/long-term facilities for persons with co-occurring mental illness and chronic medical issues. Many long-term care facilities are unwilling to accept patients with a history of mental illness, violence, legal, or sexually problematic behaviors, leaving this population to age in the psychiatric hospital. At a time when the provider market for elder services has grown dramatically, the demand for those providers' services has as well. As was the case decades ago, nursing homes can and do decline to accept the problems associated with referrals of elders from state hospitals. This function – caring for mentally ill elders not manageable or wanted elsewhere – was in decline in the latter half of the 20th century, but appears to have been revived as one of the hospital's functions (Semke, Fisher, Goldman, & Hirad, 1996).

Patients who are admitted to a state facility because they require longer term care than private or more acute settings can provide are difficult to discharge. A shortage of housing options for people with mental illness, together with a decline in community support services, often leave stabilized patients stalled in the hospital waiting for a place to live. Given shrinkage in the bed supply, the dynamic that led to overcrowding in the past may have reemerged, but with broader consequences. Discharge barriers that state hospitals face today impact the number of admissions they are able to take, leaving many people who are in need of state hospital care hanging in the balance. Moreover, the difficulties associated with admitting patients to state hospitals have had a destabilizing system-wide effect. In this state, patients in general hospital psychiatric units cannot be directly transferred to state hospitals. As a result, some individuals seen in emergency departments are denied access to general hospital beds for fear that they will be unmanageable or difficult to discharge. In some areas served by this hospital, individuals remain untreated in general hospitals' psychiatric emergency settings waiting to access a general hospital bed. The optimistic view of the role of the general hospital outlined in *Action for Mental Health* would appear not to have come to fruition in this locale, thus defining its state hospital's function as the "setting of last resort" for a subset of the mentally ill population.

Dorothea Dix Returns

Were Dorothea Dix to return for a sesquicentennial inspection, she would likely be disappointed. The hospital growth she championed peaked and then declined, leaving very few behind. There is no longer an East Cambridge Jail, but if she were to visit the modern county jail that replaced it she might be dismayed to find many individuals exhibiting clear symptoms of severe mental illness – a pattern she would come to find ubiquitous. She might be heartened to find, however, that at least minimal mental health treatment while incarcerated has become recognized as a fundamental constitutional right. But she would surely argue that jail is the wrong place for those who need treatment. And she might also argue that recent efforts to improve services for criminally incarcerated persons with mental illness are a misplacement of time, energy and funds. Better to spend these resources providing treatment for mental illness in institutions built to treat mental illness.

Analyzing Major Social Interventions: The Value of Functional Analysis

In this chapter, we have attempted to provide a brief overview of functional changes in mental health systems derived from the process that has come to be called deinstitutionalization. As we have described, the process occurred against the backdrop of a range of other social movements – the growing antipathy toward institutions as solutions to social problems; advances in medical approaches for treating mental illnesses; and expanded concerns for civil liberties, among others. One can approach analyses of this kind by examining outcomes quantitatively, as many have done. Clearly, many of the references cited here have assessed beds closed, patients discharged, expenditures for community programs, attrition rates, and other measureable entities. We argue, though, that any assessment of a major social intervention, be it a change in law, spending, or in this case, the closure of institutions, begin with a careful analysis of the functions of the entities involved. The authors of *Action for Mental Health* came close to meeting this requirement (although they were overly optimistic regarding the total replacement of the state hospital). However, they failed to consider less obvious functions, such as incapacitation from criminal offending and public displays of deviance, problems that emerged slowly and progressed steadily throughout the decades to become major social issues.

Examining the "unbundling" processes associated with dismantling, the original state hospital system provides interesting insights into how systemic and institutional reforms proceed and how other forces in hospitals' social and resource environment shape functions displayed at any given time. Attention to these institutions, the evolution of their roles, and plans for both their closure and/or their future, offer interesting foci for study, particularly by sociologists interested in organizational and systemic change, and especially as applied to the care and treatment of persons with mental illness.

NOTES

1. The population we focus on here includes those persons who have serious mental illnesses, including psychotic disorders, major affective disorders, and certain personality disorders. This "case mix," which would likely be observable in contemporary public hospitals, was not that limited in the early days of state hospitals, as we note.

2. This chapter focuses on the deinstitutionalization process as it refers to the reduction in use of public mental hospitals. While the majority of these hospitals were operated by states, many were county operated. These were subject to the same policies and social forces. We use the term "state hospital" here generically to refer to the entire class of public hospitals, recognizing that some of these were not state operated.

3. The belief that individuals were admitted to public psychiatric hospitals throughout the first half of the 20th century but were never discharged is a common misperception. At Worcester State Hospital in the 1920s, for example, an important performance indicator for the staff psychiatrists was their discharge rate. What did happen is that each year a typical state hospital would admit about 500 patients and discharge 400. Thus, over a 10-year period, the hospital had increased its census by 1,000. A few decades of this admission to discharge ratio yields public psychiatric hospitals with censuses in the thousands (Geller, 2000a).

4. It is worth noting, perhaps, that today discoveries made through such a process would be unlikely. Testing drugs on institutionalized persons – psychiatric patients, prison inmates, and the like – is now considered unethical and illegal without strict oversight by an institutional review board, an entity that did not exist at the time for such purposes.

5. Some have disputed the primacy of chlorpromazine's effects on census reduction. It has been argued that the creation/expansion of nursing homes and a federal role in their funding, which occurred somewhat earlier, should be credited with at least a fattening of that trend from its previous continual upward rise. The desire to close state hospitals and the actions taken in pursuit of that goal were real, however, and the availability of a psychiatric wonder drug, in an era when polio vaccines and antibiotics were gaining attention in the public mind, certainly provided cover for the introduction of approaches that would not involve large mental hospitals.

Gronfein has argued, for example, that "drugs did not affect movement out of the hospital ... [but] encouraged policy changes that hastened the process of deinstitutionalization in the 1960s (1985a, p. 437)." It has also been argued that the availability of Medicaid, rather than the community mental health program, had the greater overall effect on deinstitutionalization process (Geller, 2000b; Gronfein, 1985b)

6. The reform of civil commitment laws was one of the major socio-legal interventions in the U.S. history. Beginning in 1969 with California's Lanterman-Petris-Short Act (see Warren, 1982), by the early 1970s every state in the union had changed their commitment laws in ways that limited who, where, for how long, and for what reasons persons could be detained and held in psychiatric hospitals. The legal and social factors that led to this outcome are numerous and significant, but excellent descriptions of these processes can be found in Appelbaum (1994), Warren (1982), Durham and La Fond (1985), Pierce, Durham, and Fisher (1986), Durham, Fisher, and Pierce (1986), and numerous others. An unintended consequence was the criminalization of behaviors of those with mental illness to gain access to state hospitals previously accomplished through civil commitment (Geller & Lister, 1978).

REFERENCES

Abramson, M. F. (1972). The criminalization of mentally disordered behavior: Possible side effect of a new mental health law. *Psychiatric Service*, *23*, 101–105.

Alverson, H., Alverson, M., & Drake, R. E. (2001). Social patterns of substance use among people with dual diagnoses. *Mental Health Services Research*, *3*, 3–14. Retrieved from http://link.springer.com/article/10.1023%2FA%3A1010104317348

Appelbaum, P. S. (1994). *Almost a revolution: Mental health law and the limits of change*. Oxford: Oxford University Press.

Chu, F. D., & Trotter, S. (1974). *The madness establishment: Ralph Nader's Study Group Report on the National Institute of Mental Health*. Oxford: Grossman.

Deutsch, A. (1948). *The shame of the states*. New York, NY: Harcourt, Brace & Company.

Dorwart, R. A., & Epstein, S. (1993). *Privatization and mental health care: A fragile balance*. Westport, CT: Auburn House.

Dowdall, G. (1996). *The eclipse of the state hospital: Policy, stigma and organization*. Albany, NY: State University of New York Press.

Drake, R. E., & Wallach, M. A. (1989). Substance abuse among the chronically mentally ill. *Psychiatric Services*, *40*, 1041–1046. doi:h10.1176/appi.ps.51.11.1397.1176/ps.40.10.41

Drake, R. E., Wallach, M. A., & McGovern, M. P. (2005). Future directions in preventing relapse to substance abuse among clients with severe mental illnesses. *Psychiatric Services*, *56*, 1297–1302. doi:10.1176/appi.ps.56.10.1297.

Durham, M. L., Fisher, W. H., & Pierce, G. L. (1986). The impact of legislative change, resource constraints and judicial decisions on length of stay of patients admitted to a state mental hospital. *Law, Medicine and Health Care*, *13*, 290–296.

Durham, M. L., & La Fond, J. (1985). *Back to the asylum: The future of mental health law and policy in the United States*. Oxford: Oxford University Press.

Fischer, P., & Breakey, W. J. (1991). The epidemiology of alcohol, drug and mental disorders among homeless persons. *American Psychologist*, *46*, 1115–1128. doi:10.1037/0003-066X.46.11.1115.

Fisher, W. H., Barreira, P. J., Geller, J. L., White, A., Lincoln, A. K., & Sudders, M. (2001). Long-stay state hospital patients at the end of the twentieth century. *Psychiatric Services*, *52*, 1051–1056. doi:10.1176/appi.ps.52.8.1051.

Fisher, W. H., Dorwart, R. A., Schlesinger, M., Epstein, S., & Davidson, H. (1992). The role of general hospitals in treating the severely mentally ill. *Psychiatric Services*, *43*, 1114–1119. doi:10.1176/ps.43.11.1114.

Fisher, W. H., Geller, J. L., & Pandiani, J. A. (2009). The changing role of the state psychiatric hospital. *Health Affairs*, *28*, 676–684. doi:10.1377/hlthaff.28.3.676

Fisher, W. H., & Phillips, B. F. (1990). Modeling the growth of long-stay populations in public mental hospitals. *Social Science and Medicine*, *30*, 1341–1347. Retrieved from http://www.sciencedirect.com/science/article/pii/027795369090314I

Fisher, W. H., Roy-Bujnowski, K., Grudzinskas, A. J., Banks, S. M., Crockett, E., & Wolff, N. (2011). Comparing risk of arrest among public mental health services recipients and the general public. *Psychiatric Services*, *62*, 67–72. Retrieved from http://ps.psychiatryonline.org/doi/10.1176/ps.62.1.pss6201_0067

Frank, R. G., & Gleid, S. A. (2006). *Better but not well: Mental health policy in the United States since 1950*. Baltimore, MD: Johns Hopkins.

Geller, J. L. (2000a). The last half-century of psychiatric services as reflected in psychiatric services. *Psychiatric Services*, *51*, 41–67. doi:10.1176/ps51.1.41.

Geller, J. L. (2000b). Excluding institutions for mental diseases from federal reimbursement for services: Strategy or tragedy. *Psychiatric Services*, *51*, 1397–1403. doi:10.1176/appi.ps.51.11.1397

Geller, J. L. (in press). The first step in health reform for those with serious mental illness: Integrating the dis-integrated mental health system. *Journal of Nervous and Mental Disease*, *203*, 909–918.

Geller, J. L., & Fisher, W. H. (1993). Transitional residences in the linear continuum: Debunking the myth. *American Journal of Psychiatry*, *150*, 1070–1076. Retrieved from http://search.proquest.com/openview/81401aeaf374f52f3e0ff9ce638f8fa7/1?pq-origsite=gscholar

Geller, J. L., Fisher, W. H., Simon, L. J., & Wirth-Cauchon, J. L. (1990). 'Second generation deinstitutionalization' II: *Brewster v. Dukakis*'s impact on community and hospital utilization. *American Journal of Psychiatry*, *147*, 988–993. PMID:2115750.

Geller, J. L., & Lister, E. (1978). The process of criminal commitment for pretrial psychiatric examination: An evaluation. *American Journal of Psychiatry*, *135*, 53–60. PMID:618529.

Goldman, H. H., Morrissey, J. P., & Ridgely, S. (1994). Evaluating the Robert Wood Johnson foundation program on chronic mental illness. *Milbank Quarterly*, *72*, 37–47. PMID: 8164611.

Gorman, M. (1956). *Every other bed*. Cleveland, OH: World Publishing Co.

Grob, G. N. (1966). *The state and the mentally ill: A history of Worcester State Hospital in Massachusetts 1830–1920*. Chapel Hill, NC: University of North Carolina Press.

Grob, G. N. (1973). *Mental institutions in America*. New York, NY: The Free Press.

Grob, G. N. (1991). *From asylum to community: Mental health policy in modern America*. Princeton, NJ: Princeton University Press.

Gronfein, W. (1985a). Psychotropic drugs and the origins of deinstitutionalization. *Social Problems*, *32*, 437–454. doi:10.2307/800774

Gronfein, W. (1985b). Incentives and intentions in mental health policy: A comparison of the Medicaid and community mental health programs. *Journal of Health and Social Behavior*, *26*, 192–206. PMID: 3905940.

Jacobs, P. E. (1974). Wither community mental health? *International Journal of Mental Health*, *3*, 35–43.

Johnson, A. B. (1992). *Out of Bedlam: The truth about deinstitutionalization*. New York, NY: Basic Books.

Joint Commission on Mental Health and Illness. (1961). *Action for mental health*. New York, NY: Basic Books.

Lutterman, T. (2015). *Tracking the history of state psychiatric hospital closures from 1997 to 2015*. Washington, DC: National Association of State Mental Health Program Directors Research Institute, Inc. Retrieved from http://media.wix.com/ugd/186708_ae5cd70d3f0049b88126ee224c7505ca.pdf

Maisel, A. Q. (1946). Most U.S. hospitals are a shame and a disgrace. *Life Magazine*, May 6.

Mechanic, D. (2008). *Mental health and social policy: Beyond managed care* (5th ed.). Boston, MA: Pearson.

Merton, R. K. (1968). *Social theory and social structure*. Glencoe, NY: The Free Press.

Morrissey, J. P., Cuddeback, G., & Meyer, P. (2007). Extending assertive community treatment to criminal justice settings: Origins, current evidence and future directions. *Community Mental Health Journal*, *43*, 527–545. doi:10.1007/s10597-007-9092-9

Morrissey, J. P., Goldman, H. H., & Klerman, L. (1980). *Theenduring asylum: Cycles of institutional reform at Worcester state hospital*. New York, NY: Grune & Stratton.

National Association of State Mental Health Program Directors Research Institute, Inc. (2013). Retrieved from http://www.nri-incdata.org/ProfilesReport.cfm?Variable=P_9c&State

National Governor's Association. (2002). *Strategies states can use to employ persons with mental illness*. National Governor's Association, Center for Best Practices. Retrieved from www.nga.org/cda/files/0703MENTALILLNESS.pdf

Parsons, T. (1950). *The social system*. Glencoe, NY: The Free Press.

Pierce, G. L., Durham, M. L., & Fisher, W. H. (1986). The impact of public policy and publicity on admissions to state mental hospitals. *Journal of Health Politics, Policy and Law*, *11*, 41–66. doi:10.1215/03616878-11-1-41

Rothbard, A., Hadley, T., & Richman, E. (1997). Unbundling of state hospital services in the community: The Philadelphia Hospital story. *Administration and Policy in Mental Health and Mental Health Services Research*, *24*, 391–398. PMID:9239943.

Rothman, D. J. (1971). *The discovery of the asylum*. Boston, MA: Little Brown.

Sampson, R. J., Raudenbush, S. W., & Earls, F. (1997). Neighborhoods and violent crime: A multilevel study of collective efficacy. *Science*, *227*, 918–923. doi:10.1126/science.277.5328.918

Semke, J., Fisher, W. H., Goldman, H. H., & Hirad, A. (1996). The evolving role of the state hospital for older adults: Across state trends, 1984–1993. *Psychiatric Services*, *47*, 1082–1087. PMID:8890335.

Silver, E., Mulvey, E. P., & Swanson, J. W. (2002). Neighborhood structural characteristics and mental disorder: Faris and Dunham revisited. *Social Science & Medicine*, *55*, 1457–1470. doi:10.1016/S0277-9536(01)00266-0

Steadman, H. J., Osher, F., Robbins, P. C., Case, B., & Samuels, S. (2010). Prevalence of serious mental illness among jail inmates. *Psychiatric Services*, *60*, 761–765. doi:10.1176/appl.ps.60.6.761

Superintendent of Worcester State Hospital. (1921). *Annual Report*. Worcester State Hospital. Retrieved from http://www.mass.gov/anf/research-and-tech/oversight-agencies/lib/worcester-state-hospital.html

Teplin, L. A. (1994). Psychiatric and substance abuse disorders among male urban jail detainees. *American Journal of Public Health*, *84*, 290–293. doi:10.2105/AJPH.80.6.663.

Torrey, E. F. (1995). Jails and prisons – America's new mental hospitals. *American Journal of Public Health*, *85*, 1611–1613.

Torrey, E. F. (1997). *Out of the shadows: Confronting America's mental illness crisis*. New York, NY: Wiley.

Warren, C. A. B. (1982). *The court of last resort: Mental illness and the law*. Chicago, IL: University of Chicago Press.

"FOREVER CHILDREN" AND AUTONOMOUS CITIZENS: COMPARING THE DEINSTITUTIONALIZATIONS OF PSYCHIATRIC PATIENTS AND DEVELOPMENTALLY DISABLED INDIVIDUALS IN THE UNITED STATES

Adrianna Bagnall and Gil Eyal

ABSTRACT

Purpose – *We compare the deinstitutionalization of psychiatric patients and the developmentally disabled in the United States and demonstrate that there were two path-dependent processes with significant qualitative and quantitative differences, ultimately leading to better outcomes for developmentally disabled individuals.*

50 Years after Deinstitutionalization: Mental Illness in Contemporary Communities
Advances in Medical Sociology, Volume 17, 27–61

ISSN: 1057-6290/doi:10.1108/S1057-629020160000017002

Design – *Using secondary literature, we construct a sustained comparison of the two processes in terms of outcomes, timing, tempo, extent, funding, demographic composition, and investment in community services. We then reconstruct the strategies of de-stigmatization and framings of moral worth deployed in the two cases, analyzing their effects on deinstitutionalization in terms of conceptions of risk, rights, and care.*

Findings – *Deinstitutionalization began later for developmentally disabled individuals than for psychiatric patients, and was a more gradual, protracted process. It was not driven by fiscal conservatism, discharges, and the trans-institutionalization of the senile aged, as was deinstitutionalization for psychiatric patients, but primarily by the prevention of institutionalization of young children, and increased investment in infrastructure. Consequently, the deinstitutionalization of the developmentally disabled was far more thorough and successful. The process was shaped by the framing of the developmentally disabled as "forever children" by parents' organizations that demanded a balance between autonomy, protection, and the provision of care. In contrast, the deinstitutionalization of psychiatric patients was shaped by their framing as autonomous citizens temporarily suffering from "mental health problems" that could be prevented, treated, and cured. This frame foregrounded the right to choose (and also refuse) treatment, while undervaluing the provision of care.*

Keywords: Deinstitutionalization; mental illness; mental retardation; developmental disability

INTRODUCTION

When researchers and commentators speak of "deinstitutionalization," they often have in mind the processes by which psychiatric patients[1] in the United States were moved out of institutions. Perhaps implicitly, the deinstitutionalization of psychiatric patients is taken as the prototype for a generic process taking place in several fields. In consequence, attitudes toward deinstitutionalization are strongly shaped by the prevailing image of the spectacular emptying and dismantling of mental institutions; the revolving door of short-term admissions; the suspected prevalence of psychiatric disorders among the homeless and the incarcerated; and the phenomenon of trans-institutionalization to nursing homes, hospitals and jails. This has contributed to an oft-repeated refrain that deinstitutionalization was a "stunning policy failure" (Durham, 1989; Mechanic & Rochefort, 1990), "re-institutionalization" (Bassuk & Gerson, 1978), "trans-institutionalization" (Fakhoury & Priebe, 2007), or a "transfer of care" (Brown, 1985) largely driven by economic considerations.

We would like to push back against what we believe to be the undue centrality of deinstitutionalization of psychiatric patients in the United States. If we would have taken the deinstitutionalization of the developmentally disabled as our prototype, we would have obtained a different image. Deinstitutionalization in this field has been far more gradual and deliberate, with sustained focus on creating residential and treatment arrangements in the community. Deinstitutionalization in the United States *does not* stand for a "single, unitary phenomenon" (Scull, 1984, p. 141), but for a loose agglomeration of different processes, resembling each other, but also diverging in fundamental respects. Researchers, commentators, and policy-makers should account for these differences and their underlying historical causes when they assess deinstitutionalization and debate future policy.

We offer the following rationale for the comparison of the deinstitutionalizations of psychiatric patients and the developmentally disabled:

(1) *They were formally initiated by the same piece of legislation, namely, the* Mental Retardation Facilities and Community Mental Health Centers Construction Act of 1963 (PL 88–164). Indeed, the struggle to deinstitutionalize psychiatric patients "rode on the back" of the parallel struggle to deinstitutionalize the "retarded," as they were called at the time. Advocates for psychiatric patients desperately sought to link the campaigns so they would enjoy the "popularity and noncontroversial nature" of the far better organized and politically legitimate retardation provisions (Grob, 1991, pp. 219–231).
(2) *Because of their common origins, the policies are financed by the same funding mechanisms*, namely, Federal welfare programs such as Medicaid, Medicare, SSI, and SSDI (Lerman, 1982, pp. xiv–xv).
(3) *The populations served by the policies are not completely distinct from one another*. A sub-group among residents of State Mental Hospitals had a dual diagnosis of mental illness and mental retardation. They were among the most difficult to deinstitutionalize and among the last to be moved out (Geller, Fisher, Wirth-Cauchon, & Simon, 1990). By the same token, many of the developmentally disabled, whether in

institutions or outside, suffer from emotional and mental health problems and are prescribed psychoactive medications.

While comparisons are rare, research that does distinguish between these groups agree that the deinstitutionalization of the developmentally disabled has been "far less controversial" than that of psychiatric patients (Bagenstos, 2012), and more successful in the long-run.

The main difference is residential placement or living circumstances. In 2010, 56.5% of individuals with intellectual disability were living with family members, 8% were receiving residential support services in their own homes, and 5.4% of individuals with intellectual disability resided in public and private institutions (with 16+ individuals). The rest (about 30%) were in group homes and similar settings with 15 or less residents.[2] People with DD/ID have never been a significant group among the homeless (Bagenstos, 2012, p. 13). A lack of similar data for psychiatric patients speaks volumes about the differences between the two processes of deinstitutionalization. Individuals with ID/DD, even outside institutions, are still integrated within a fairly cohesive institutional matrix of service delivery and supervision: they are counted and followed. Individuals with psychiatric diagnoses (PD), on the other hand, navigate a fractured and disconnected "patchwork system" where the proverbial "white spots" of *terra incognita* are much larger than the areas known and mapped. Few settings have the oversight to track people with PD (Davis, Fulginiti, Kriegel, & Brekke, 2012, p. 260) and lack of centralization makes it difficult to compile aggregate data (Wong & Stanhope, 2009, p. 1378). Hence, the residential location of about 71% of individuals with serious mental illness (SMI) is "unknown." From a libertarian point of view, this ignorance could be construed as a good outcome. *What is known*, however, is not encouraging: 13% are with family and friends, 6% are homeless, 4.4% in prisons and jails, 2% in nursing homes, 1.8% in mental hospitals, and 1.8% are in residential care facilities. Information on the composition of specific institutional settings is more enlightening: 9–20% of nursing home residents are estimated to have SMI. Nearly, 1 million people with PD are booked into jail every year but most are quickly released. Growth in the residential rolls of state hospitals is due almost entirely to transfers from correctional facilities. Stays at mental hospitals are short and 36% of those discharged become homeless within 6 months. Of the more than 2 million individuals who experience homelessness annually, roughly 25–33% have PD of some kind (Davis et al., 2012, pp. 260–262). The homeless, in turn, are likely to end up in a correctional facility, perpetuating a cycle in which many of the

70% whose location is unknown are likely stuck. In contrast, supportive housing for individuals with developmental disabilities (DDs) is more spatially dispersed, in less distressed, less unstable, and more secure neighborhoods than for people with psychiatric diagnoses (Wong & Stanhope, 2009).

These disparities translate to major differences in morbidity and mortality. People with SMI die, on average, 25 years earlier than the general population (30–40% is due to suicide and injury, the rest to chronic and acute medical conditions) (Parks, Svendsen, Singer, Foti, & Mauer, 2006). This is true for people with SMI living "in the community" as well as in institutions (Davis et al., 2012, p. 265). While there has been some debate whether deinstitutionalization in California increased the rate of mortality among DD individuals (Strauss & Kastner, 1996), the bulk of the research has documented increases in the life expectancy of people with ID. Improvements in medical care made a significant contribution to this increase, but life expectancy remains shorter among institutionalized individuals with ID/DD suggesting that community living also plays a role (Coppus, 2013, pp. 7, 13). This has contributed to an increase in the number of aging DD individuals who are at home with aging parents. We will return to this problem later.

Research has also documented better behavioral and psychological outcomes for individuals with DD than for individuals with PD in consequence of deinstitutionalization. Overall, outcomes on a variety of behavioral and psychological measures – interaction in group activities, degree of self-reliance, independence and exercise of choice, maladaptive behavior, language development, self-care, and skills acquisition – were superior in community placements for individuals with DD (Beadle-Brown, Mansell, & Kozma, 2007; Edgerton, 1993; Kim, Larson, & Lakin, 2001; Kozma, Mansell, & Beadle-Brown, 2009; O'Neill, Brown, Gordon, & Schonhorn, 1985; Stancliffe & Abery, 1997; Walsh & Walsh, 1982). In comparison, there seems to be no such consensus for people with PD. One study noted that "participants were well aware of, and quite articulate about, several serious drawbacks of community living," listing the benefits of inpatient care for the provision of basic needs even though they generally preferred the community (Davidson, Hoge, Godleski, Rakfeldt, & Griffith, 1996).

These different outcomes are a reflection of fundamental differences between the two *processes* of deinstitutionalization. As can be seen in Fig. 1,[3] the population of state mental hospitals peaked in 1955, and began to decline precipitously from then onwards. By 1975, resident patients at county and state mental hospitals numbered 193,436, a decline

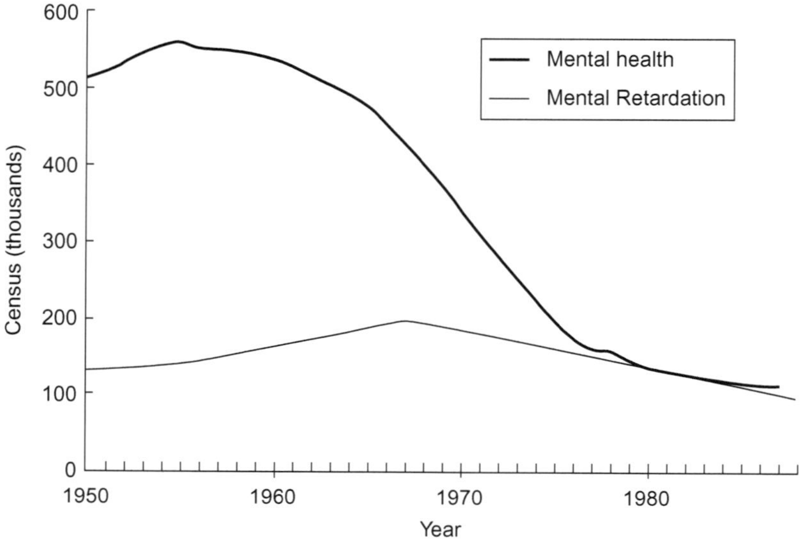

Fig. 1. Daily Census of State Mental Institutions: 1950–1988. *Source*: Mental health data from Witkin (1989); mental retardation data from Lakin (1980) for 1950–1976 and from Braddock et al. (1990) for 1977–1988.

of 65% from 1955. By 1985, they were 109,939, a decline of 81% (Davis et al., 2012, p. 259; Mechanic & Rochefort, 1990, p. 307). The rate of institutionalization of the developmentally disabled, on the other hand, peaked in 1967 (at 115.72 per 100,000). In 1977, there were still 167,056 individuals with MR/DD in large state MR or Psychiatric facilities, a reduction of 27% from 1967, and by 1986, they were 103,296, a decline of 55% (Braddock, 1992, pp. 175–176; Prouty, Smith, & Lakin, 2001, pp. 8–9).[4]

More revealing than numbers of residents are patterns of admissions, discharges, readmissions, average lengths of stay, and inpatients' episodes. While the number of residents in state and county mental hospitals in 1975 declined 65% from its peak in 1955, the number of admissions more than doubled, from 178,003 to 376,156. The number of total inpatient episodes declined 27% from 818,832 to 598,993 in the same time period. From 1969 to 1982, the average length of stay declined from 421 days to 143 days. These numbers demonstrate that the reduction in the population of institutionalized psychiatric patients was achieved primarily through a "revolving door" of readmissions (composed of massive discharges, short stays, discharges, and back again) (Mechanic & Rochefort, 1990, pp. 307–308). By comparison, the absolute number of admissions to large state MR facilities was much more modest, declining after 1974 from 18,075 to 6,535 in 1986 and 2,338 in 1995. The number of discharges also declined (Prouty et al., 2001, pp. 14–15). Thus, the gradual reduction in the institutionalized MR/DD population was achieved through the *prevention of institutionalization*, and thus of readmissions (Landesman & Butterfield, 1987, pp. 810–811).

Statistics about levels of funding and the creation of community services support these contrasting patterns of deinstitutionalization. Until the 1970s, spending on mental health dwarfed spending on MR – likely because the prevalence of SMI was much larger than the prevalence of DD; in 1955 the psychiatric institutionalized population was at least four times larger than the population of MR institutions. By 1983, spending by state programs was roughly equal in absolute terms, and so much larger per capita for DDs (Braddock, 1992, pp. 175–176). In the following years, expenditures on community services for individuals with DDs increased substantially more than for individuals with PD, and in 1987 funding for DD community services was 72% higher *in absolute terms* than for psychiatric community services. Half of all DD funding by state programs was for community services, while for PD it was only a third. The number of DD community facilities (excluding nursing homes) grew from 4,390 in 1977, serving 62,397 residents, to 28,000 in 1988, serving 174,000 residents. The comparable development of community services for people with PD lagged far behind (ibid. pp. 176–179). Yet states also invested large sums in renovating MR institutions and improving the quality of care – during 1978–1980 almost a billion dollars was spent on renovation and 1.2 billion was spent on improving quality of care. While deinstitutionalization of psychiatric patients in the United States was tied to reductions in state funding for institutions, deinstitutionalization of individuals with DD involved increased investment in both institutions and community alternatives, *inclusive of increases specifically in States' funding for community services from about half a Billion dollars in 1977 to 3.2 Billion in 1987!* (Braddock, 1981, 1992, p. 181). So while the evidence is overwhelming that financial incentives to states to shift the fiscal burden to Federal programs played a crucial role in the deinstitutionalization of psychiatric patients in the United States (Bassuk & Gerson, 1978; Estes & Harrington, 1981; Lerman, 1982; Mechanic & Rochefort, 1990), it would be much harder to make the same argument for the deinstitutionalization of DD individuals, where a vast funding increase has contributed to a 36% increase in total system capacity (Braddock, 1999).

These numbers do not fully capture the differences in deinstitutionalization. To put it bluntly, the prevention of institutionalization in DD was primarily prevention of the institutionalization of *children*, while the massive discharges of psychiatric patients were primarily trans-institutionalization of the *aged*. The proportion of children and youth (younger than 21) in state MR institutions peaked in 1965 at about 48.9%, declined to 35.8% in 1977 and 12.7% in 1987, while the mean age of first admission increased from 13.3 to 18 (Prouty, Smith, & Lakin, 2007, p. 41). At the same time, the largest category of first admissions to mental hospitals in 1962 was individuals aged 65 or older (163.7 per 100,000), while children under 15 were the smallest category (6 per 100,000). By 1972, the rate of first admissions of the aged decreased sharply to 69.2 per 100,000, while the 4 largest categories were now between the ages of 15 to 54, and the rate of first admissions for the young (0–24) actually increased (Grob, 1991, pp. 268–269).

The destinations for these groups were vastly different. Whereas the deinstitutionalization of adults with DD was a slow and protracted process, underlying it was a rapid transformation in the status of children who were kept at home rather than institutionalized. In 1987, 18.2% of all ID out-of-home placements were children and youth (under 21), declining to 7.6% in 1997, and to 6.2% in 2005 (Stancliffe, Lakin, & Prouty, 2005). DD children and adults staying at home are supported by a combination of Federal and State funds, with the latter increasing by a factor of 6 over the 1980s (Braddock, 1992, p. 181), a fact that reduces the significance of fiscal incentives in explaining the deinstitutionalization of DD individuals.[5] On the other hand, the number of aged psychiatric patients in nursing homes doubled from 187,675 in 1963 to 367,586 in 1969 (Grob, 1991, pp. 268–269). In 1977, the vast majority (1.15 out of 1.7 million) of chronic psychiatric patients resided in nursing homes or board-and-care facilities funded primarily through Medicaid. By 1985, nursing homes housed over 600,000 people diagnosed with PD, and Medicaid was the largest federal program funding the long-term care of psychiatric patients (Grob, 1995, p. 54). Thirty percent of the 1.3 million residents of nursing homes had a diagnosis of chronic MI, and 57% had a diagnosis of chronic senility (Shadish, Lurigio, & Lewis, 1989, p. 3). This clearly supports the fiscal explanation for the deinstitutionalization of psychiatric patients.

Framings of Social Worth

Most existing theories of deinstitutionalization are not sensitive to the profound differences between these two processes. Attempts to explain differences emphasize the role of advocacy groups in the progression of deinstitutionalization. Both Bagenstos (2012, pp. 18–19) and Braddock (1992, pp. 176–177) cite the superior clout of "consumer advocacy groups" such as the Association for Retarded Citizens (ARC) as an explanation for the better outcomes in this field. They attribute this clout not only to better organization and more experience, but also to the extensive involvement of family members, especially parents, in these organizations as compared to advocacy organizations for psychiatric patients.

With certain caveats, we agree that the role played by parents' organizations in the deinstitutionalization of DD is a crucial variable differentiating the two processes. Family advocacy organizations on behalf of psychiatric patients do exist, but their impact is unlikely to have been equivalent to the ARC and similar organizations. The first reason is timing. The National Alliance for the Mentally Ill (NAMI) was formed by family members of psychiatric patients in 1981, 30 years after the formation of the National Association for Retarded Children (NARC, later renamed ARC), and 26 years after deinstitutionalization of psychiatric patients began. Before its formation, researchers felt that families of psychiatric patients were "probably the least organized and vocal of those groups affected" by deinstitutionalization (Doll, 1976, p. 386). Given this late formation, the focus of NAMI and similar organizations was not on shaping the process of deinstitutionalization, but on influencing NIMH to turn away from psychosocial toward brain-based research.

One could argue that this difference is explained by the greater stigma of "mental illness"; the greater legitimacy of the cause of DD; or by the singularity of focus of the ARC on community solutions (Braddock, 1992, p. 181; Grob, 1991, pp. 219–231). None of these explanations is very convincing. To begin with the matter of legitimacy, the argument is that the public saw DD children as innocent, vulnerable, and in need of help, while the same public feared psychiatric patients, had less sympathy for them, and blamed them for their plight. Politicians responding to NIMBY sentiments would not direct resources at community services for psychiatric patients. While services for DD faced similar hurdles, they were able to garner more sympathy, partly because of the political clout of parents' organizations. If you take a freeze frame of the situation, let's say, in the late

1980s, and you do not look too deeply, you might believe this. But the story is more complicated.

To begin with the obvious point: most individuals with ID/DD *are not children*, but adults. They are not *naturally* more sympathetic, less stigmatized, and less threatening than psychiatric patients. If we go back to the earlier decades of the 20th century we find that the "feebleminded" and the "insane" were similarly stigmatized, feared, and shunned. Representing the same eugenic threat, they were placed in the same institutions. The prevailing image of the feebleminded was as *delinquent adolescents*. Before the 1950s, there were hardly any very young children (5 years of age or under) in state MR institutions. Superintendents rejected applications to institutionalize very young children except as a last resort (Metzel, 2004, pp. 431–433). From 1904 to 1945, more than half of first admissions to state institutions were *older children and adolescents* (10–19 years of age), typically lower-class, minority, or immigrant "morons" (i.e., slightly below "normal" IQ). Truancy, delinquency, epilepsy, alcoholism, sexual promiscuity, even masturbation, served as pretexts to commitment as "mentally deficient." The goal of institutionalization was social defense from "defective delinquents" and "morally imbecile" youth (Malzberg, 1952; Trent, 1994). The insane may have even attracted more sympathy and less stigma than the feebleminded, because the institutionalized insane increasingly included the senile aged. Before the 1890s, the aged – infirm, needy and senile – were typically cared for at local almshouses at the expense of municipalities and counties. During the first decades of the 20th century, however, local officials began to "redefine senility as a psychiatric problem" and transferred the aged to mental institutions and state budgets: 18% of first admissions to NYS mental hospitals in 1920 were of individuals 65 years or older; 31% in 1940; 33.3% in 1951. Growth was similar in other states (Grob, 1977, 1995). Yet, it was mostly the case that the insane, even the aged among them, were viewed with suspicion and fear, and were tainted with the stain of degeneracy, poverty, and immorality (especially as many of the aged patients were syphilitic).

Our contention, therefore, is that the difference between the deinstitutionalizations of psychiatric patients and of the developmentally disabled is not because one condition is naturally less stigmatizing, but because each process of deinstitutionalization was continuous with a different path out of stigma and moral taint. In each of the two spheres, a different strategy of de-stigmatization, moral cleansing and valorization – endowing a once despised existence with a form of social worth – was attempted, and while it did not necessarily begin with the intent of deinstitutionalization, it ultimately led to it and shaped its course. Our emphasis on the role played by framings of social worth is not a "culturalist" or "discursive" explanation. Framings of social worth are a crucial link between individuals and the distributive mechanisms of the welfare state, understood as a complex "economy of worth" (Boltanski & Thévenot, 2006). Welfare state categories-qua-framings of social worth determine not only how much gets distributed to whom, but also in what form, under which conditions, and to what purpose. Thus, the comparative analysis developed below is specific to the particular "world" of Anglo-American welfare capitalism (Esping-Andersen, 2013; Lerman, 1982).

The key to what happened in the sphere of DD is the framing of affected individuals as "forever children" in need of guardianship, education, and habilitation, a frame that dates back to at least 1950 and Pearl Buck's *The Child who Never Grew Up*. This frame, adopted as the explicit strategy of NARC, must be understood in the context of the larger post-WWII invention of the child-centered family – what others have called the "reproductive consensus" of the era (Castles, 2004, pp. 359–360; Fass, 2012; Trent, 1994, pp. 231–241). That the 1950s were the time of straight-laced, middle-class, suburban families is of course a myth, but it was a powerful myth operative at the time. More precisely, it was a formula for assigning social worth (and for redistributing state resources) on the basis of "normality": producing and raising healthy children as an ethical goal of middle class adulthood thereby making a "contribution" to society. Organizations of parents of "retarded" children formed during this time (Metzel, 2004, pp. 431–433) were mobilized to lay claim to services, but more generally to membership in this normality. Lee Marino, one of the founders of New Jersey's Parents Group for Retarded Children, explained the purpose of his organization in these terms: "parents in this era invested heavily in their children … but, for him and others like him, the investment did not carry the same dividends. Their families carried a special burden, one that seemed to put normal family relations out of reach, and they wanted to do something about it" (Jones, 2004, pp. 326–327). The term "dividends" used here should not be understood literally. The investment in children brought moral, not economic worth. The New Jersey parents lobbied for entitlements on the basis of being "exceptional families," but at the same time they claimed recognition and moral worth on the basis of being equivalent to "normal" families, since they too invested in their children.

This explains why parents initially lobbied *for* institutionalization as a way of reclaiming normality for the family. It is well-known that doctors in this period encouraged parents to commit their very young children to institutions for the mentally retarded. Surveys of parents in the late 1950s at MR clinics found that half were instructed by their doctors to institutionalize their retarded child (Castles, 2004, p. 363). Doctors, especially child psychiatrists, envisioned institutionalization as a crucial plank in a larger surveillance system for early childhood: a system that could detect abnormalities and assign children as early as possible to the right intervention – of which institutionalization was one possibility (Kanner, 1949; Schumacher, 1946). Consequently, there was a dramatic increase in the proportion of very young children (0–5) institutionalized: from 6% of first admissions in 1938 to 18% in 1951, while children 0–9 years of age became the largest group of first admissions: from 23% in 1938 to 42% in 1951 (Goldstein, 1959).

It is less well known, however, that often *the parents themselves* exerted strong pressure on (sometimes reluctant) pediatricians to institutionalize their children (Brockley, 2004, pp. 144–45; Castles, 2004, pp. 352–53, 361–63). Donald Jolly (1952, pp. 632–635), a physician in a state school for the mentally retarded, reported that in his experience the main reason for the large increase in the institutionalization of very young children was the strong pressure exerted by parents. Both doctors and parents, however, articulated the same rationale for institutionalization: no longer social defense, but *a concern for the well-being of the child and of the middle class family*. Regarding the child, Jolly explained that the positive features of institutional life were the fact that he or she were protected from the frustration of competition; that they received special training adjusted to their needs; and that they could rely on continued care after their parents' death. While benefits were dependent on the commitment being voluntary, Jolly was confident that parents eventually would see institutionalization as "proper positive action in planning for the future of the exceptional child." Institutionalization also benefited overburdened parents, neglected siblings, and marriages threatened by divorce. John and Lorraine Frank, who after much agonizing decided to institutionalize their young daughter, explained that they did not wish to sacrifice "the chance for a normal life for our expected [second] child" (Quoted in Jones, 2004, pp. 326). In short, doctors recommended institutionalization, and many parents concurred, in order to allow families to attain the middle-class normality that was the linchpin of the postwar social bargain (Brockley, 2004, p. 148–49; Castles, 2004, pp. 361–63).

Hence parents' organizations lobbied to repeal bans on the institutionalization of very young children, to shorten institutional waiting lists, to build new institutions, that is, to relieve middle-class families of the burden of caring for their disabled children and allow them to be "normal" (Malzberg, 1952, p. 30; Trent, 1994, pp. 236–41). The secretary of the local chapter at New Brunswick "used her position in the group to advance the cause of institutionalization and to urge greater support ... for the state system of institutions." She explained that she decided to institutionalize her own daughter "to preserve the family unit," but that her daughter was "still a valuable part of her family." Indeed, the quest for normalcy did not permit to "simply put children away and forget about them." On the contrary, the parents groups included institutionalized children in "scripts of togetherness": there were family bus trips to the state institutions; fathers organized a building and grounds committee to build a playground; mothers took turns in giving haircuts to institutionalized children; there were holiday parties and gift exchanges (Jones, 2004, pp. 331–33). Institutionalization thus allowed the family unit to become normal not simply by removing the disabled child, but also by serving as a focal point around which family rituals of domesticity and community rituals of civic activism were reenacted, thereby re-including the disabled child.

This was the background for the emergence of the "forever children" frame. Not only were there indeed many more children in state institutions for the mentally retarded, so the frame was anchored by a certain reality, but to cast the developmentally disabled as children accorded with the post-war formula for assigning social worth. The middle-class parents who formed advocacy organizations were demanding the chance to be "normal Americans" like everybody else, which meant being able to lead a normal family life centered on "investing" in their children, cultivating and maximizing their health and potential. It was in the name of this ideal that children were institutionalized – no longer to protect "society" from the danger represented by adolescent morons, but to provide "forever children" with a sheltering, nurturing environment that substituted as best as possible for the middle-class family, while protecting the family itself from the burden they represented.

The historical irony is that the very same values and energies that the "forever children" frame first mobilized in favor of institutionalization were ultimately a catalyst for deinstitutionalization. The aspirations for "normality" turned into the rhetoric of "normalization." It was against this frame of "forever children" and the ideal of middle-class normality, that the institution was criticized as "warehousing" and a form of social waste (Castles, 2004; Jones, 2004). The ideal of middle-class, "normal" parenting, and the activism to which it gave rise in NARC was not only in search of conformity (as it is often depicted in simplistic accounts), but also in pursuit of an ethical goal: through the activism of the parents, their child's existence would be valorized and transformed into a social contribution. Pearl Buck, for example, wrote that she decided against doctors' advice – not to institutionalize her daughter because "I resolved that … my child … was not to be wasted … her existence as it was and as it is today, must be of use to human beings" (quoted in Trent, p. 231). The same message was echoed by parent advocates such as Dale Evans Rogers or Maria Egg. The task was to valorize this existence; to turn it from a burden into something with social meaning and value. A family grows and matures spiritually by caring for the child. In turn, this care provides a beautiful and inspiring example to others, creating societal value (Brockley, 2004, pp. 154–156; Egg, 1964, pp. 38–40). The institution was found wanting not only because it failed to cultivate the child, but also because it was secretive, a place where children were hidden away instead of becoming a "blessing for others." Through the "forever children" frame, the retarded child was transformed from a destructive and disintegrative influence, into a factor of family strength and cohesion. Her presence represented a moral test through which the family could emerge stronger, more harmonious, having given their existence a more beautiful and authentic shape (Egg, 1964, p. 42).

There was thus a fundamental continuity between institutionalization and deinstitutionalization in how the "forever children" frame was mobilized to assign social worth to parents, their activism and their claims toward the state. By the same token, community treatment was not the opposite of the drive to create a comprehensive surveillance system for early childhood, but its continuation by other means. The main discontinuity was in the role of medical expertise. While at the height of the institutionalization wave, child psychiatry seemed to claim for itself the authority to diagnose the social destiny (and hence social worth) of very young children, deinstitutionalization, and the parent-led valorization of retarded existence repudiated this claim, and centered early detection and early intervention in the family, surrounded by various auxiliary agencies (Eyal et al., 2010, pp. 91–97).

So is it the case, as Braddock (1992, p. 181) suggested that the key difference between the deinstitutionalizations of these two groups was the singular focus of parents' organizations on community solutions? We think this is a serious misunderstanding. In reality, these organizations were never unified in uncompromising support for community solutions. As Gunnar Dybwad (1961), NARC's Executive Director from 1957 to 1963 argued, the frame of the "forever child," which NARC helped to disseminate, could be detrimental to the formation of community services for its "hesitancy to recognize the retarded as adults capable of sustained productive effort." We believe that what made the deinstitutionalization of DDs ultimately more successful was neither a single-minded focus on a community approach, nor an opposite reluctance and suspicion toward it, but this tension, this unique push-and-pull, stop-and-go process vacillating between the two.

While NARC and other parents' groups were among the most vocal supporters of deinstitutionalization, initiating the process through class action lawsuits, there were many other parents' organizations (sometimes the same organizations that initiated the lawsuits) that were opposed to institution closings, or who insisted that for some children residential placements were the more appropriate solution, or who wondered aloud what would become of the "children" when their parents pass away (Egg, 1964, p. 148; Sullivan, 1981). Bagenstos (2012, pp. 18–19) calls their opposition, in alliance with unions of state employees, "the most significant obstacle to further deinstitutionalization of people with DDs." This was especially true in States where the local ARC was itself a service provider, operating residential schools and nursing homes (Parish, 2005).

The key for explaining what happened to psychiatric patients is the framing of insanity as "mental illness" or even "mental health problem" continuous with less severe emotional problems and personality disorders. Unlike the taint of degeneracy, organic and moral defect associated with insanity, the post-war reformers depicted mental illness as something that could happen to anybody but that could be prevented, treated, and cured like any other illness (Grob, 1991, p. 263, 271, 303–304). This frame too is a formula for assigning social worth and should be understood in the post-WWII context. Earlier in the century, the British physician and eugenicist Alfred Frank Tredgold (1908) compared "mental disorder" and "mental deficiency"; thus, the mentally disordered were like a person in temporary financial embarrassment while the "mentally deficient" were like the poorest of the poor, who never possessed a bank account. The first have temporarily lost the means, the mental wherewithal, they previously possessed, but could hope to regain it; the second never had any means; they were literally "without a mind" ("amentia"). Along with the fiscal incentives discussed earlier, this point of view explains the massive institutionalization of the senile aged in the pre-WWII period, just as it justified the institutionalization of "morons" as social defense. The economic metaphor implies that it is worth society's while to invest resources in the intensive treatment and prevention of mental disorder, since the payoff – in terms of autonomous social contribution – will be several multiples larger upon recovery. Individuals who can no longer recover from their bankruptcy (because they were "mentally decayed," as Tredgold called the senile aged), however, or who were never able to care for themselves, should be provided enlightened custody.

This point of view became especially poignant during and after WWII (Grob, 1991, pp. 5–23). Young psychiatrists serving in the war were exposed to a much larger range of neuro-psychiatric disorders, presenting in a larger population than previously recognized. Moreover, many of the disorders were clearly the result of stress associated with combat situations. Having proven themselves "socially capable" of societal contribution, returning GIs were clearly deserving of treatment. They were socially worthy on condition that they could be successfully treated and cured. Destigmatization and valorization, therefore, went through a different route and a different image than in the field of DD: not the image of the "forever child," but the image of the self-reliant, autonomous citizen, temporarily hobbled by stress and illness, but ultimately capable of self-control and choice if assisted. At the heart of this frame, there was thus a paradox or catch-22: the only way to be treated as a rational and autonomous person, that is, not sick, is to admit that one is sick, since denying that one is sick is the most quintessential symptom of "mental illness." To admit that one is sick is to aspire to become a "person with an illness," a citizen fully possessed of the faculty of choice and the capacity for autonomy, who also happens to have a sick body. This frame is inherently unstable as it relies on a fictitious separation between the citizen and her body (Estroff, 1981; Luhrmann, 2000).

Nonetheless, on the basis of this image of a continuum of "mental health problems," a group of elite professionals (psychiatrists and psychologists) and health policy leaders (at NIMH, APA, etc.) embarked on a campaign to modernize treatment and destigmatize mental illness, integrating it more fully within a rational public health policy.[6] At the heart of the campaign was the claim that insanity was the last and most severe stage of mental illness, initiated and perpetuated (if untreated) by a combination of genetic, environmental and social factors. The instability at the heart of the concept of "mental illness," however, meant that the notion of a "continuum" worked best for the reformers when the focus was on identifying mild presentations early, among non-institutionalized populations, and acting to remediate their environmental and social causes. If applied to institutionalized populations, it merely led to paradoxes and often collapsed because a claim to be healthy was also a failure to rationally recognize illness. Thus, the reformers became champions of deinstitutionalization because institutionalization meant that treatment came doubly too late (Grob, 1991, p. 5, 302): too late to be effective and economic, and too late because the patient could no longer be stably construed on the model of the autonomous citizen with a sick body. It is understandable, therefore, why evidence emerged later that the reforms involved a shift of focus in mental health policy from the severely mentally ill to a more diffuse target population in the community with milder and more episodic presentations (ibid. pp. 251–261).

Finally, this framing also meant that the connection between "care" and "treatment" was severed. While the institution was supposed to provide both, the focus of Community Mental Health Clinics (CMHC) was to be on providing outpatient therapeutic services to a broad population. Their jurisdiction did not include most of the more quotidian care needs of recently released psychiatric patients – residential services, supervision, sheltered employment, etc. To put it in a nutshell: the senile aged, trans-institutionalized to nursing homes, were provided care, but not treatment; younger, mostly schizophrenic, patients discharged to CMHCs received treatment, but not care (Grob, 1991, pp. 303–304, 271).

While articulating a social mission for psychiatry and seeking to modernize its outlook and practices, young elite psychiatrists had to overcome both the resistance of older psychiatrists serving as superintendents of mental asylums and the skepticism of many of the rank-and-file who saw prevention as too ambitious, and a threat to their normal practice. For this reason, the reformers built an inter-professional coalition incorporating psychologists, advocacy organizations and foundations, legislators and their staffers and the administrative leadership of several Federal agencies. Mental health policy became a "hinge" issue linking the professional and state "ecologies." The "social psychiatry" articulated by the reformers, and with it deinstitutionalization, became linked to the "liberal" or "progressive" outlook that sought to shift responsibility for health and welfare policy from states to the Federal Government (Grob, 1991, pp. 93–123).

It would be tempting to say that the continuum model "medicalized" insanity, but this would be an oversimplification. Earlier constructions of insanity and degeneracy were integral parts of medical science in the early 20th century, and the "continuum model" was not necessarily medical, but relied on notions of environmental and social causation. More importantly, the mental illness frame was (and is) inherently unstable. The psychiatric patient with a merely medical diagnosis, the citizen with a sick body, frequently collapses back to a morally suspect and stigmatized individual, because the very means by which one demonstrates autonomy and self-possession – speech, communication, self-descriptions, reports, sureties provided, choices made – are suspect. Indeed, it was this very suspicion that initially made one's illness or complaint "mental" rather than physical (Foucault, 2006). Consequently, morality and stigma are always around the corner, contaminating the medical means and symbolisms that were meant to chase them away. The individual who fails to act with self-control and autonomy when discharged becomes morally culpable for failing to adhere to his/her treatment schedule for reasons understood at one and the same time as symptoms of illness and as moral faults.

We can return now to the role played by psychoactive medications in the deinstitutionalization of psychiatric patients. To attribute deinstitutionalization to their discovery is no doubt a fallacy. More precisely, it was a story told in order to accelerate reform (Grob, 1991; Scull, 1984). Great enthusiasm for the drugs stemmed less from their demonstrated effects than from the fact that they fit within the rational frame of mental illness, holding the promise of proving that insanity was nothing but illness – treatable, preventable, and curable – and that psychiatric patients were simply citizens with a sick body. Yet, for all their utility, the side-effects of the drugs soon became contaminated with the stigma they sought to exorcise. By the late 1960s, side-effects, namely, tardive dyskinesia, were effectively stigmata of mental illness. Even as the "meds" were improved and their side-effects minimized or made less visible, it was also acknowledged that they do not "cure" mental illness so much as imperfectly control its symptoms. And if patients failed to take their meds, was it due to willfulness or a symptom of their illness? Soon, "taking your meds," was a moral act, intermittently mixed with, substituted by or for, forms of substance abuse: evidence simultaneously of mental illness and moral fault.

In what remains of this chapter, we would like to spell out the implications of these framings of social worth in terms of shaping divergent processes of deinstitutionalization. The main difference we identified earlier between the two processes was the fact that community services for DD individuals were far more developed and much better funded than community services for psychiatric patients, who tend to circulate between short-term hospitalizations, incarceration, substance abuse, and homelessness. Our argument is that this difference follows from how each frame configures the moral worth of "care" and of being cared for. The divergent worth of "care," however, is itself partly dependent on whether it is understood to impinge, or not, on the rights of the affected individuals; and on whether it is understood to be necessary in order to protect vulnerable individuals from risk, or on the contrary to protect others from the threat they pose. Hence, we organize the discussion below beginning with how each frame configures who is risky and to whom, proceeding to how it construes the rights of disabled individuals, and finally ending with the moral worth of "care" within each frame.

Risk

To put it simply from the outset: the frame of "forever children" foregrounded the risks that the community environment posed to the DD. In comparison, the frame of "mental health problems" minimized both the risk to psychiatric patients and the risk they posed to others, presenting deinstitutionalization as safe. Yet, it also led to other processes that accentuated perceptions of the risk psychiatric patients posed to others.

The institution embodied this tension between risk and protection. (Fakhoury & Priebe, 2007). Earlier in the 19th century, residential schools for the feebleminded and asylums for the insane were justified as providing protective custody for individuals who could not fend for themselves. Later, during the first decades of the 20th century, the justification shifted to focus on the risks that the insane or the feebleminded posed to society. The theory of degeneration cast both as representing a eugenic threat to the long-term viability of the (white) race, while theories of social defense attributed to them a disproportionate share of crime, sexual promiscuity, idleness, poverty, etc.

This tension between risk and protection has resolved itself in two ways. To begin with psychiatric patients, the frame of "mental health problems" de-emphasized their need for protection as well as the risk they posed to others. Yet, the separation of "treatment" from "care" ultimately led to increased worries about the risk they represented to the communities into which they were discharged. As we saw earlier, deinstitutionalization involved a massive trans-institutionalization of the aged in need of care to nursing homes. Individuals with both DD and organic (as opposed to functional) illnesses were also discharged to nursing homes and ICF-MRs. In short, those most obviously in need of *protection* were trans-institutionalized to various care facilities. By the same token, the bulk of those who were discharged to be treated in CMHCs were individuals more likely to be perceived as posing some level of risk to those around them: young schizophrenics and what came to be known as "borderline personality disorder." Moreover, the first generation of psychiatric patients to reach adulthood in the community was baby boomers. Like their "normal" age peers they questioned authority and experimented with new life styles. Consequently, they were characterized by higher levels of substance abuse and homelessness, aggressiveness, and noncompliance (Geller et al., 1990; Grob, 1995).

As a result, commentators have paid a great deal of attention to the risky behaviors of former psychiatric patients and to the risks they posed to others. While some researchers pointed out that those who pose a risk to society were a minority and that most should be understood as vulnerable (Allen & Nairn, 1997; Laws & Dear, 1988), many researchers and commentators, highlighted the overlap between psychiatric diagnosis, homelessness, substance abuse, and crime which served as strong evidence of the failure of community-based care (Durham, 1989; Steadman, Monahan, Duffee, & Hartstone, 1984).

The opposite is true of the DD. Given their framing as "forever children," the focus of advocates, lawmakers, service providers, and especially of parents' organizations was on risks they faced outside the institution. Under the Willowbrook consent decree, for example, residents were not released until there was an adequate residential alternative available. In fact, precisely because of the previous experience with the deinstitutionalization of psychiatric patients, reformers were concerned that the state would attempt to simply "dump" Willowbrook residents, which it tried to do before the consent decree was signed. After it was signed, the court-appointed review panel had to overcome the resistance of parents' organizations, who preferred trans-institutionalization to borough "developmental centers." Throughout the process, the governing language was one of concerns to prevent "harm." Similar precautions were taken during the mandated deinstitutionalization of Pennhurst and other institutions. Reformers articulated a theory according to which institutional environments caused "intellectual, social, and emotional harms," while parents emphasized the potential for harm outside a protective environment (Carey, 2009; Rothman & Rothman, 2005, pp. 70, 90–93, 102–103, 106–111, 127–141, 151–174, 200). The most poignant commentary and critique came from *Voice of the Retarded* (VOR), a parents' group. They drew on the "forever children" frame to accentuate the risks to the DD, and to ridicule the discourse of "rights." VOR quipped that the insistence on the civil rights and freedom of choice of the DD would merely become "the rights of people with DDs to eat too many doughnuts and take a nap" (Bannerman, Sheldon, Sherman, & Harchik, 1990). If the DD needed rights at all, said VOR activists, it was a "right to be retarded," namely, a right not to be placed at risk because of a misguided insistence on autonomy (Bagenstos, 2012).

The leadership of NARC, on the other hand, while firmly in favor of deinstitutionalization, searched for the right balance between protection and autonomy, the right level of "acceptable risk." Perske (1972) argued that protecting the disabled person from all types of risk limited their access to a "normal life" and violated the main principle of normalization theory – "letting the mentally retarded obtain an existence as close to the normal as possible." A certain level of risk was normal and endowed those exposed to it with social worth, what Perske called the "dignity of risk." Ultimately, the 1975 Developmentally Disabled Assistance and Bill of Rights Act reflected this balanced stance on risk in their mandated selective deinstitutionalization of developmentally disabled individuals "who have been prepared through programs of habilitation and training to function adequately in appropriate local settings" (Landesman & Butterfield, 1987, pp. 810–811). While there was fierce debate among parent activists and advocates about how to balance risk, there did not seem to be similar levels of worry about the risk that DD individuals posed to others.

These differentials focus on risk no doubt shaped decisions about the location of residences for psychiatric patients and DD individuals. While survey research found that citizens were in theory supportive of having both psychiatric patients and DD individuals live in the community (Gallup, 1976; Gottwald, 1970), the actual placement of community residences in neighborhoods typically led to protests based on the anticipated impact on property values, safety, and health risks to the community (Kastner, Reppucci, & Pezzoli, 1979; Piat, 2000). Once DD individuals actually moved into a neighborhood and became a regular presence, the opposition typically subsided. Concerns about the risk psychiatric patients posed remained more entrenched (Lubin, Schwartz, Zigman, & Janicki, 1982). Moreover, concern about risks posed to the developmentally disabled by community placement dictated a great deal of care in choosing "safe" community settings for permanent residences while psychiatric patients tended to be pushed toward dilapidated urban areas, welfare hotels, and similar temporary residences that house also former convicts, people in substance abuse programs, etc. (Wong & Stanhope, 2009). This has reinforced the perception of psychiatric patients as "risky," and contributed to a vicious cycle in which various forms of confinement and "secure accommodations" become a preferred residential placement for "mentally disordered offenders" (Moon, 2000).

Rights

In both fields, deinstitutionalization was driven in large part by concern for the civil rights of inmates (Accordino, Porter, & Morse, 2001; Estes & Harrington, 1981). Exposes of abuse, maltreatment, and coercion at institutions highlighted that people were being held against their will without treatment or care (Kugel & Wolfensberger, 1969; Blatt & Kaplan, 1974). Legal activists, reformers, and civil libertarians, inspired by the larger civil rights movement of the 1960s, drew on these reports to launch a wide-ranging legal attack on institutions (Mechanic & Rochefort, 1990).

Despite similarities, there were also important and telltale differences in the legal argumentation and rhetoric of rights deployed in the two fields. Bagenstos (2012) introduces a useful distinction between two lines of due process doctrine used in early litigation. One was an argument for "negative rights": a "right against treatment" which targeted involuntary commitment (and involuntary medication) and attempted to impose procedural limitations so individuals could not be held against their will unless they were dangerous to themselves or others. This strategy was prominent in litigation regarding psychiatric patients. It was articulated by civil libertarian lawyers, who saw "institutionalization as an end run around the criminal procedure revolution" (Bagenstos, 2012, pp. 24–25). For this reason, they were highly suspicious of the expert opinion of professionals and sought to limit the authority psychiatrists exercised as public health officials. Autonomous citizens are not compelled to be treated; they choose whether to follow a doctor's advice regarding course of treatment. Hence, the rights of psychiatric patients were framed as civil rights: the right to choice and the right to be free from coercion. Denied in the institution, movement to the community was the only way to restore them. While this reasoning leads naturally to closing institutions and fairly rapidly moving individuals into the community, it is silent about how individuals should be assisted to cope and thrive in the community[7] (Bagenstos, 2012, p. 15, n. 61).

The other litigation strategy articulated a positive "right to treatment".[8] This strategy did not target involuntary commitment but the substantive *quid pro quo* underlying it: if you confine somebody with the justification of providing treatment, then you must indeed provide treatment that aligns with professional standards: "only the fulfillment of the therapeutic promise in fact can justify the deprivation of fundamental human liberties" (Schwitzgebel, 1973, p. 535). Moreover, treatment must provide "minimally adequate habilitation" and should "be designed to promote the acquisition of skills necessary to live outside of an institution." This strategy was far more effective than the "right against treatment." DD claimants and their families were able to win compensation for harm because of failure to provide habilitation (*Halderman v. Pennhurst State School & Hospital*). There are three points we would like to make about this strategy: first, note that its implications are more ambiguous than the "right against treatment." It could be used either to close institutions or to improve them. Unlike the "right against treatment," the right to treatment cannot be interpreted as providing license to disinvest in services – institutional or community – for the DD. Second, instead of sidelining expert opinion as the right against treatment does, what qualifies as "minimally adequate habilitation" depends on "accepted professional judgment, practice, or standards" (Bagenstos, 2012, pp. 25–26), around which legal activists, patients, parents, *and* professionals can form an enduring coalition.

Finally, whereas the world conjured by the right against treatment is binary, the terms in which the right to treatment are phrased construct a continuum between the institution and the community. The key development was the switch to a "right to habilitation." Early commentary pointed out that the right to treatment was phrased in medical terms that were irrelevant and unrealistic for DD individuals because they assumed cure as an end goal. Habilitation, on the other hand, would assist the DD individual in acquiring and maintaining skills to cope with the demands of life in the community (Mason, Menolascino, & Galvin, 1976). This right to habilitation was further expanded by *Welsch v. Likins*, which established the right to habilitation in the *Least Restrictive Environment* (LRE), incorporating the right against treatment in a less destructive way. Not only was it possible to sue institutions because they did not provide adequate habilitation, it was also possible to sue them if – according to professional opinion – the same habilitation could be provided in a more "normal" setting (*Horacek v. Exon*). Unlike "cure" or "recovery," "habilitation" – namely, "making able" – is potentially never-ending and consonant with the "forever children" frame. We educate and train children so they acquire self-care skills, extending their sphere of autonomy slowly and cautiously, with an adult always close by. "Making able" to live and work outside the institution would happen through supportive services that mirrored this care of children. This is poignantly captured in the concept of the "prosthetic environment" coined by the Director of the Eden School for Autistic Children (Holmes, 1990), which indicates that between protective custody and full-fledged autonomy stretches a whole range of hybrid and ambivalent arrangements: "supports" in the double sense of protecting incomplete beings (the developmentally disabled-as-children) and making them able, allowing them to develop.

These litigation strategies had a profound impact on the process of deinstitutionalization. The greater emphasis on due process and the right of psychiatric patients to refuse treatment reinforced the distinction between treatment and care and created a binary opposition between coerced institutionalization and voluntary community treatment. It thus inhibited the development of hybrid services that – because they focus on care and continuous habilitation – appear paternalistic. Additionally, many hospitals were cautious about admitting people with psychiatric diagnosis lest they be accused of violating the rights of patients who may not be able to fully consent to commitment (Mason et al., 1976; Teplin, 1984).

In contrast, emphasis on positive rights to habilitation for DD individuals required attention to support services in the community as part of providing adequate care into and through adulthood. To habilitate the developmentally disabled is not to "cure" them, restoring a sanity or normalcy they once possessed, but is to move along an ascending gradient of acquiring new skills and abilities through therapies that are often much closer to training and education than to medical treatment. Pressing for the right of the developmentally disabled for "minimally adequate habilitation" was to press for arrangements that combined treatment, care, and everything in between.

Litigation in the name of a right to habilitation, in which positive and negative rights clashed, acted as a brake on deinstitutionalization for the developmentally disabled (Carey, 2009). For psychiatric patients, the strong emphasis on negative rights emptied positive rights of their content. By the same token, for the developmentally disabled, the pursuit of positive rights often limited and even completely eliminated negative rights. If adequate habilitation could not be provided in the community with family, DD adults were kept in the institution until an appropriate placement was available (Rothman & Rothman, 2005). The very same advocates who litigated in the name of a right to habilitation, would sometimes contest the extension of civil rights for the developmentally disabled (Landesman & Butterfield, 1987). For example, while parents fought for the right to habilitation for their children, they also fought for guardianship rights and in some cases, for the right to keep their child in the institution (Rothman & Rothman, 2005). Normalization theory could be understood as an (only partly successful) attempt to mediate this tension, since it implies that limitations on negative rights could also be injurious to the positive right to habilitation, while the closest possible approximation to full civil rights has therapeutic value. This middle-way argument never satisfied all the sides in the debate, yet was able to facilitate the formation of workable coalitions in favor of a "continuum of care."

Care

As we saw earlier, the framing of psychiatric patients as autonomous citizens temporarily hobbled by "mental health problems" meant that their deinstitutionalization led to a separation between "treatment" and "care" (Grob, 1991). The senile aged, those with complex disabilities, or those who required follow-up after hospitalization, were transferred to nursing homes, where they received care, but little by way of treatment. The relatively younger schizophrenics, who were discharged into the "community," received only treatment, but no care (Scull, 1984; Bachrach, 1976; Bassuk & Gerson, 1978). This model worked for some, if their problems were not too severe; if their illness was episodic; and if they had medical insurance, since Federal funding for the CMHCs dried up over time (Davis et al., 2012). For the large group of poor, chronic, severely disabled, however, this model proved a vicious circle. Condemned to a precarious and stigmatized existence, they are perceived as complicit in their own situation (on account of their right to refuse treatment and because of high rates of substance abuse, incarceration, and welfare dependence) and as a public nuisance (because of high rates of homelessness, poverty, and unemployment). This has resulted in less public support for comprehensive care, and the segregation of individuals in areas where the care infrastructure is nonexistent (Durham, 1989; Grob, 1995).

Care without treatment; treatment without care; this seems to be the fate of psychiatric patients; their Scylla and Charybdis. Yet, the comparison with the deinstitutionalization of DD demonstrates that this predicament is historically contingent.

One could object and say that the real difference lies in the fact that unlike psychiatric patients, DD individuals discharged from institutions often had family homes waiting for them (Braddock, Emerson, Felce, & Stancliffe, 2001). This is partly true. In many cases, the families of psychiatric patients did not assume responsibility for their discharged kin. In contrast, as we saw, the deinstitutionalization of DD individuals began with parents who took the public stance of keeping their children home, while the first to be discharged from institutions were typically children and younger adults who were reabsorbed at home (Best-Sigford, Bruininks,

Lakin, K.C., Hill & Heal, 1982). Contemporary research on mentally ill and developmentally disabled living at home has shown that parents of the developmentally disabled report more satisfaction social support in doing so, even into old age (Seltzer, Greenberg, Krauss, & Hong, 1997). Indeed, the problem of DD individuals living at home with aging parents has become a serious policy concern. In 2010, 56.5% of individuals with intellectual disability were living with family members at home (RISP, 2010). About a quarter and perhaps more were living with family members over 60 years old. This phenomenon of aging parents with continuing caregiving responsibilities for their disabled children has been attributed to an increased lifespan for the disabled, the consequences of deinstitutionalization, and a shortage of residential options for adults with DDs (Braddock, 1999; Eyman & Borthwick-Duffy, 1994; Lefley, 1987). While psychiatric patients certainly face similar barriers to securing services and moving out of the family home, it is striking that both families and government programs assume that the housing needs of the developmentally disabled should be explicitly planned for and that families should take a leading role.

Ultimately, however, the differences in how care is conceived and organized are not simply a function of DD individuals being absorbed at home, while psychiatric patients are not, but of the framing of developmentally disabled individuals as "forever children," where treatment is construed as habilitation and modeled upon the care and cultivation that the "normal" family provides. In this frame, treatment-qua-habilitation and care are not easily distinguished, and certainly not easily separated. Courts interpreted the right to habilitation as a requirement that States develop comprehensive community-based services, because the developmentally disabled were perceived as in need of care. At the same time, there was an effort to balance this need for care with the presumed therapeutic effects of genuine (even if somewhat risky) integration. When it became clear that the mere location of services in the community did not guarantee integration (e.g., the continued segregation of special education within public schools, or the fact that many group homes did not provide community experiences), the 1984 Developmental Disabilities Assistance and Bill of Rights Act redefined community integration as residence in proximity to community resources, in home-like settings, regular contacts with non-handicapped, use of all community resources and participation in all community activities. The legislation was guided by the ideal of a "continuum of care," a continuum of residential settings and services with varying combinations and levels of care and treatment, protection and integration, supervision and autonomy (Wolfensberger & Nirje, 1972).

We can state the difference between how "care" is configured by the two processes of deinstitutionalization in the terms we suggested earlier. The strategy by which reformers and advocates sought to endow stigmatized psychiatric patients with social worth belongs to an economy of worth (Boltanski & Thévenot, 2006), in which "care" stands for lack of worth. Those who are cared for are unworthy beings because they are not autonomous. They are "dependent" and consequently their capacity to exercise "control, command, choices, self-determination … aspects of competent selfhood in our society" is diminished even in the framework of community treatment (Estroff, 1981, p. 175). The charge of the reformers against mental hospitals was that they "promote weakness and dependency … Patients become unable to trust their own judgement, become indecisive, overly submissive to authority, frightened of the outside world" (Chamberlin, 1978, p. 6). As these patients moved outside institutions, the opposition between care and autonomy remained. CMHC clients were strongly discouraged by the staff from receiving anything from their parents, since this would reinforce their dependency, their unworthy status as semi-"minors." (Estroff, 1981, p. 161). The similarity to the critique of "welfare dependency" is not accidental. The point is not that deinstitutionalization was motivated by libertarian or neo-conservative ideology (though there were definitely significant influences between the two), but that both were articulated within the same economy of worth, within the same "world" of Anglo-American welfare capitalism, where redistribution takes place through the stigmatizing mechanism of means-testing and is understood as "assistance" or "relief" (Esping-Andersen, 2013; Lerman, 1982). The characteristic catch-22 of this world applies in this case as well: if you are worthy (i.e., working or sane), you do not need assistance or care; if you need assistance or care (you are poor, unemployed, insane, homeless), you are unworthy, because you are no longer autonomous, and therefore you are only deserving of paltry assistance (e.g., SSI, sheltered employment), which will be immediately withdrawn if you attempt to regain your worth (by working, by being discharged) – unless this assistance could be construed strictly on the model of "medical treatment" (e.g., "meds," preferably self-administered and self-monitored) (Estroff, 1981, pp. 169–173). By the same token, moreover, those who care for dependents are also liable to be seen as unworthy to the extent that they are perceived as illegitimately encroaching upon the autonomy of others. The accusation of "tyranny" has been leveled at institutions' staff, CMHC's staff, board-and-care homes' operators, group homes' attendants, and welfare bureaucrats.

What from one side appears as the necessary supervision and guardianship involved in providing care, appears from the other side as tyranny and "social control."

The strategy by which parents and advocates sought to endow stigmatized DD individuals with social worth belongs to a completely different economy of worth, wherein "care" transmits and augments worth. Those who care for weaker beings are worthy because they contribute to a greater good – whether this good is understood in the secular frame of societal well-being and cohesion, or in the religious frame of *caritas*. NARC parents were told that "a fine and beautiful mission awaits you, [because] the cross we bear can become a blessing for others" (Egg, 1964, pp. 38–42). Those who are cared for are valorized because their lives, their struggles, their experiences, and the very care they received become a moral example – in Pearl Buck's words, "of use to human beings." In NARC literature, as well as in on-line postings of parents of autistic children (Fleischmann, 2005), disabled children are depicted as "teachers" from whom their parents, the whole family, or even others learn the true meaning of life, or discover powers and abilities they did not know they possess. This economy of worth developed, as we have argued, on the basis of the "reproductive consensus" of the postwar years and by framing the developmentally disabled as children.

CONCLUSIONS

We have demonstrated that the processes of deinstitutionalization of psychiatric patients and of DD individuals have unfolded in drastically different ways depending on framings of social worth and strategies of destigmatization. While it is indisputable that financial incentives played a crucial role in shaping the deinstitutionalization of psychiatric patients, they did not have the same effect in the case of DD individuals, where the framing was different. This contrast allows us to see that the framing of psychiatric patients as autonomous individuals temporarily suffering from "mental health problems" served as a precondition for the alignment of interests between advocates, experts, and fiscal conservatives. Deinstitutionalization was fought on the basis of the right to decline treatment, and an opposition between autonomy and care. It led to a process that was swift and concentrated on discharging patients, rather than arranging for care in the community. The deinstitutionalization of psychiatric patients is largely considered a failure because of this lack of supportive services in the community and because it has created a system in which psychiatric patients are moved through a "revolving door" of incomprehensive services.

Deinstitutionalization of DD individuals, on the other hand, has been considered a qualified success because alongside gradual and careful discharges it involved also significant investment in and the concurrent development of community-based services. The framing of DD individuals as "forever children," however paternalistic, meant that deinstitutionalization was fought on the basis of a right to habilitation, which did not oppose care to autonomy or separate it from treatment. It also meant that the alignment of interests behind deinstitutionalization was only partial, and the process was characterized by a constant push-and-pull which made it far more gradual. This has laid the groundwork for the creation of a continuum of both institution-based *and* community services at varying levels of support. We believe that this expanded picture of deinstitutionalization should inform discussion of civil rights, entitlements, and responsibilities as we continue to develop community-based services for both psychiatric patients and the developmentally disabled.

NOTES

1. We use the terms "psychiatric patients" and "developmentally disabled" to refer to the broadest possible groups of individuals who would have been institutionalized in the past on the basis of a diagnosis respectively of "mental illness" or "mental retardation" (MR). The 1969 legislation that created the category of "developmental disability" (DD) included three groups – those diagnosed with mental retardation, epilepsy and/or cerebral palsy. In 1977, autism was added. We occasionally use the terms "insanity", "mental illness," "mental retardation" or "feeblemindedness" when it is historically accurate to do so, namely when we need to refer to the categories and terminology used by people at the time that we are discussing. Finally, we use the term "intellectual disability" (ID) to refer specifically to individuals who currently are diagnosed with such disability on the basis of a lower score on an IQ test, and who are counted as such in official statistics.
2. Figures are based on the data collected by the National Residential Information Systems Project (RISP, 2010) at the Research and Training Center on Community Living at the University of Minnesota. http://rtc3.umn.edu/risp/build/index.asp (Last accessed 5.20.2015).
3. Taken from Braddock (1992)

4. An additional illustration of the differences between the two processes of deinstitutionalization could be provided by comparing the numbers of individuals with MR diagnosis in state MR and psychiatric facilities. The bulk of residents with MR diagnosis were housed in state MR facilities and the trend there tracks closely the numbers presented above. Some, however, were housed in state *psychiatric* facilities, i.e. together with psychiatric patients, and were discharged earlier and faster than those in state MR facilities. The number of individuals with MR diagnosis at state psychiatric facilities peaked in 1960, and declined rather quickly to 15,524 in 1977, a 59% decrease from the peak. By 1986 there were only 3,106, a 91% decrease. The corresponding decreases for individuals with in state MR facilities were 22% and 49% respectively (Prouty et al., 2001, pp. 8–9). It is quite possible that many of the individuals who resided in state psychiatric facilities were transferred to state MR facilities.

5. An important caveat is that there was huge variation between states in levels of funding (Braddock, 1992, p. 178), suggesting that the fiscal explanation is perhaps more valid in some states, but much less so in others. We would expect, however, that states with low levels of funding for community services also had lower levels of funding for institutions and a lower rate of institutionalization in the past. On state differences in rates of institutionalization, and their relationship to deinstitutionalization, see Eyal, Hart, Onculer, Oren, and Rossi (2010, pp. 64–67)

6. Grob's otherwise excellent and thorough account ignores, however, another source of this focus on prevention and understanding of mental illness as caused by early emotional problems, namely, the mental hygiene and child guidance movements. While child guidance began with a focus on "saving" immigrant and lower-class children from the risk of delinquency, by the time of WWII it was thoroughly focused on early identification of emotional problems before they turned into adult forms of mental illness. (Kanner 1941/1964, pp. 171–172; Nadesan, 2005, pp. 44–45, 58–73; Nehring, 2004, pp. 371–372)

7. Incidentally, this suggests that Scull's claim that deinstitutionalization constituted a single, unified phenomenon is better understood not as an explanation or hypothesis that could be verified or refuted, but as an "account" in the ethnomethodological sense, a narrative articulated by some of the key actors, namely civil libertarian lawyers. From their point of view there was a formal analogy between commitment procedures in all the distinct spheres of "social control". Their litigation strategy was based on an analogy between commitment and "arrest". Whether deinstitutionalization was a unified phenomenon or not depends on whether they managed to prevail, and whether this account could translate the interests of all the other parties involved and could hold the deinstitutionalization coalition together. As already indicated above, clearly it could not do so in the field of developmental disabilities.

8. Rothman and Rothman (2005, pp. 87–88, 106–111), however, explain that since the "right to treatment" was not accepted by the judge presiding over the Willowbrook case, the reformers' strategy was to extend "the right of protection from harm…until it was the equivalent of a right to treatment." Tellingly, this was done through an analogy to children's right to education – without which they are harmed because their development is stymied.

REFERENCES

Accordino, M. P., Porter, D. F., & Morse, T. (2001). Deinstitutionalization of persons with severe mental illness: Context and consequences. *The Journal of Rehabilitation, 67*(2), 16–21.

Allen, R., & Nairn, R. G. (1997). Media depictions of mental illness: An analysis of the use of dangerousness. *Australian and New Zealand Journal of Psychiatry, 31*(3), 375–381.

Bachrach, L. L. (1976). *Deinstitutionalization: An analytical review and sociological perspective.* Rockville, MD: National Institute of Mental Health.

Bagenstos, S. R. (2012). The past and future of deinstitutionalization litigation. *Cardozo Law Review, 34*(1), 1–52.

Bannerman, D. J., Sheldon, J. B., Sherman, J. A., & Harchik, A. E. (1990). Balancing the right to habilitation with the right to personal liberties: The rights of people with developmental disabilities to eat too many doughnuts and take a nap. *Journal of Applied Behavior Analysis, 23*(1), 79–89.

Bassuk, E. L., & Gerson, S. (1978). Deinstitutionalization and mental health services. *Scientific American, 238*(2), 46–53.

Beadle-Brown, J., Mansell, J., & Kozma, A. (2007). Deinstitutionalization in intellectual disabilities. *Current Opinion in Psychiatry, 20*(5), 437–442.

Best-Sigford, B., Bruininks, R. H., Lakin, K. C., Hill, B. K., & Heal, L. W. (1982). Resident release patterns in a national sample of public residential facilities. *American Journal of Mental Deficiency, 87*(2), 130–140.

Blatt, B., & Kaplan, F. (1974). *Christmas in purgatory: A photographic essay on mental retardation.* Syracuse, NY: Human Policy Press.

Boltanski, L., & Thévenot, L. (2006). *On justification: Economies of worth.* Princeton, NJ: Princeton University Press.

Braddock, D. (1981). Deinstitutionalization of the retarded: Trends in public policy. *Hospital and Community Psychiatry, 32*(9), 607–615.

Braddock, D. (1992). Community mental health and mental retardation services in the United States: A comparative study of resource allocation. *American Journal of Psychiatry, 149*(2), 175–183.

Braddock, D. (1999). Aging and developmental disabilities: Demographic and policy issues affecting American families. *Mental Retardation, 37*(2), 155–161.

Braddock, D., Emerson, E., Felce, D., & Stancliffe, R. J. (2001). Living circumstances of children and adults with mental retardation or developmental disabilities in the United States, Canada, England and Wales, and Australia. *Mental Retardation and Developmental Disabilities Research Reviews, 7*(2), 115–121.

Braddock, D., Hemp, R., Fujiura, G., Bachelder, L., & Mitchell, D. (1990). *The state of the states in developmental disabilities.* Baltimore, MD: Brooks Publishing.

Brockley, J. (2004). Rearing the child who never grew: Ideologies of parenting and intellectual disability in American history. In S. Noll & J. W. Trent (Eds.), *Mental retardation in America: A historical reader* (pp. 130–164). New York, NY: New York University Press.

Brown, P. (1985). *The transfer of care: Psychiatric deinstitutionalization and its aftermath.* Boston, MA: Routledge & Kegan Paul.

Carey, A. C. (2009). *On the margins of citizenship: Intellectual disability and civil rights in twentieth-century America.* Philadelphia, PA: Temple University Press.

Castles, K. (2004). Nice, average, Americans: Postwar parents' groups and the defense of the normal family. In S. Noll & J. Trent (Eds.), *Mental retardation in America: A historical reader* (pp. 351–370). New York, NY: New York University Press.
Chamberlin, J. (1978). *On our own: Patient-controlled alternatives to the mental health system.* New York, NY: McGraw-Hill.
Coppus, A. (2013). People with intellectual disability: What do we know about adulthood and life expectancy? *Developmental Disabilities Research Reviews, 18*(1), 6–16.
Davidson, L., Hoge, M. A., Godleski, L., Rakfeldt, J., & Griffith, E. E. H. (1996). Hospital or community living? Examining consumer perspectives on deinstitutionalization. *Psychiatric Rehabilitation Journal, 19*(3), 49–58.
Davis, L., Fulginiti, A., Kriegel, L., & Brekke, J. S. (2012). Deinstitutionalization? Where have all the people gone? *Current Psychiatry Reports, 14*(3), 259–269.
Doll, W. (1976). Family coping with the mentally ill: An unanticipated problem of deinstitutionalization. *Psychiatric Services, 27*(3), 183–185.
Durham, M. L. (1989). The impact of deinstitutionalization on the current treatment of the mentally ill. *International Journal of Law and Psychiatry, 12*(2), 117–131.
Dybwad, G. (1961). Rehabilitation for the adult retardate. *American Journal of Public Health and the Nation's Health, 51*(7), 998–1004.
Edgerton, R. B. (1993). *The cloak of competence* (Second.). Berkely, CA: University of California Press.
Egg, M. (1964). *When a child is different: A basic guide for the parents and friends of mentally retarded children.* New York, NY: The John Day Company.
Esping-Andersen, G. (2013). *The three worlds of welfare capitalism.* Hoboken, NJ: Wiley.
Estes, C. L., & Harrington, C. A. (1981). Fiscal crisis, deinstitutionalization, and the elderly. *American Behavioral Scientist, 24*(6), 811–826.
Estroff, S. E. (1981). *Making it crazy: An ethnography of psychiatric clients in an American community.* Los Angeles, CA: University of California Press.
Eyal, G., Hart, B., Onculer, E., Oren, N., & Rossi, N. (2010). *The autism matrix: The social origins of the autism epidemic.* Malden, MA: Polity Press.
Eyman, R. K., & Borthwick-Duffy, S. A. (1994). Trends in mortality rates and predictors of mortality. In Seltzer, M., Krauss, M., & Janicki, M. (Eds.). *Life Course Perspectives on Adulthood and Old Age* (pp. 93–105). Washington, DC: American Association on Mental Retardation.
Fakhoury, W., & Priebe, S. (2007). Deinstitutionalization and reinstitutionalization: Major changes in the provision of mental healthcare. *Psychiatry, 6*(8), 313–316.
Fass, P. (2012). *The child-centered family?: New rules in postwar America.* Philadelphia, PA: University of Pennsylvania Press.
Fleischmann, A. (2005). The hero's story and autism: Grounded theory study of websites for parents of children with autism. *Autism, 9*(3), 299–316.
Foucault, M. (2006). *History of madness.* London: Routledge.
Gallup, O. (1976). *Gallup organization report for the President's Committee on mental retardation: Public attitudes regarding mental retardation.* Washington, DC: President's Committee.
Geller, J. L., Fisher, W. H., Wirth-Cauchon, J. L., & Simon, L. J. (1990). Second-generation deinstitutionalization, I: The impact of Brewster v. Dukakis on state hospital case mix. *American Journal of Psychiatry, 147*(8), 982–987.
Goldstein, H. (1959). Population trends in US public institutions for the mentally deficient. *American Journal of Mental Deficiency, 63*(4), 599–604.

Gottwald, H. (1970). *Public awareness about mental retardation.* Arlington, VA: Council for Exceptional Children.

Grob, G. N. (1977). Rediscovering asylums: The unhistorical history of the mental hospital. *Hastings Center Report*, *7*(4), 33–41.

Grob, G. N. (1991). *From asylum to community*. Princeton, NJ: Princeton University Press.

Grob, G. N. (1995). The paradox of deinstitutionalization. *Society*, *32*(5), 51–59.

Holmes, D. L. (1990). Community-based services for children and adults with autism: The Eden family of programs. *Journal of Autism and Developmental Disorders*, *20*(3), 339–351.

Jolly, D. (1952). When should the seriously retarded infant be institutionalized? *American Journal of Mental Deficiency*, *58*, 632–636.

Jones, K. W. (2004). Education for children with mental retardation: Parent activism, public policy, and family ideology in the 1950s. In S. Noll & J. W. Trent (Eds.), *Mental retardation in America: A historical reader* (pp. 322–350). New York, NY: New York University Press.

Kanner, L. (1941/1964). *In defense of mothers: How to bring up children in spite of the more zealous psychologists.* Springfield, IL: Charles C. Thomas Publisher.

Kanner, L. (1949). Feeblemindedness: Absolute, relative and apparent. In *Childcare monographs.* New York, NY: Child Care Publications.

Kastner, L. S., Reppucci, N. D., & Pezzoli, J. J. (1979). Assessing community attitudes toward mentally retarded persons. *American Journal of Mental Deficiency*, *84*(2), 137–144.

Kim, S., Larson, S. A., & Lakin, K. C. (2001). Behavioural outcomes of deinstitutionalisation for people with intellectual disability: A review of US studies conducted between 1980 and 1999. *Journal of Intellectual and Developmental Disability*, *26*(1), 35–50.

Kozma, A., Mansell, J., & Beadle-Brown, J. (2009). Outcomes in different residential settings for people with intellectual disability: A systematic review. *American Journal on Intellectual and Developmental Disabilities*, *114*(3): 193–222

Kugel, R., & Wolfensberger, W. (1969). *Changing patterns in residential services for the mentally retarded.* Washington, DC: President's Committee on Mental Retardation.

Lakin, K. C. (1980). *Demographic studeis of residential facilities for the mentally retarded.* Minneapolis, MN: University of Minnesota: Department of Psychoeducational Studies.

Landesman, S., & Butterfield, E. C. (1987). Normalization and deinstitutionalization of mentally retarded individuals: Controversy and facts. *American Psychologist*, *42*(8), 809.

Laws, G., & Dear, M. (1988). Coping in the community: A review of factors influencing the lives of deinstitutionalized ex-psychiatric patients. In Smith, C., & Giggs, J. (Eds.), *Location and Stigma: Contemporary Perspectives on Mental Health and Mental Health Care* (pp. 83–102). Boston, MA: Unwin Hyman.

Lefley, H. (1987). Aging parents as caregivers of mentally ill adult children: An emerging social problem. *Psychiatric Services*, *38*(10), 1063–1070.

Lerman, P. (1982). *Deinstitutionalization and the welfare state.* Rutgers: Rutgers University Press.

Lubin, R. A., Schwartz, A. A., Zigman, W. B., & Janicki, M. P. (1982). Community acceptance of residential programs for developmentally disabled persons. *Applied Research in Mental Retardation*, *3*(2), 191–200.

Luhrmann, T. M. (2000). *Of two minds: The growing disorder in American psychiatry.* New York, NY: Alfred A. Knopf.

Malzberg, B. (1952). Some statistical aspects of first admissions to the New York State schools for mental defectives. *American Journal of Mental Deficiency*, *57*(1), 27–37.

Mason, B. G., Menolascino, F. J., & Galvin, L. (1976). Mental health-the right to treatment for mentally retarded citizens: An evolving legal and scientific interface. *Creighton Law Review, 10*, 124–166.

Mechanic, D., & Rochefort, D. A. (1990). Deinstitutionalization: An appraisal of reform. *Annual Review of Sociology, 16*, 301–327.

Mental Retardation Facilities and Community Mental Health Centers Construction Act of 1963. (1963). Pub. L. No. 77. United States of America.

Metzel, D. S. (2004). Historical social geography. In S. Noll & J. W. Trent (Eds.), *Mental retardation in America: A historical reader* (pp. 420–444). New York, NY: New York University Press.

Moon, G. (2000). Risk and protection: The discourse of confinement in contemporary mental health policy. *Health & Place, 6*(3), 239–250.

Nadesan, M. H. (2005). *Constructing autism: Unravelling the 'truth' and understanding the social.* New York, NY: Routledge.

National Residential Information Systems Project (RISP). (2010). *Research and training center on community living at the University of Minnesota.* Retrieved from http://rtc3.umn.edu/risp/build/index.asp. Accessed on May 20, 2015.

Nehring, W. (2004). Formal health care at the community level: The child development clinics of the 1950s and 1960s. In S. Noll & J. W. Trent (Eds.), *Mental retardation in America: A historical reader* (pp. 371–383). New York, NY: New York University Press.

O'Neill, J., Brown, M., Gordon, W., & Schonhorn, R. (1985). The impact of deinstitutionalization on activities and skills of severely/profoundly mentally retarded multiply-handicapped adults. *Applied Research in Mental Retardation, 6*(3), 361–371.

Parish, S. L. (2005). Deinstitutionalization in two states: The impact of advocacy, policy, and other social forces on services for people with developmental disabilities. *Research and Practice for Persons with Severe Disabilities, 30*(4), 219–231.

Parks, J., Svendsen, D., Singer, P., Foti, M. E., & Mauer, B. (2006). *Morbidity and mortality in people with serious mental illness.* Alexandria, VA: National Association of State Mental Health Program Directors (NASMHPD) Medical Directors Council.

Perske, R. (1972). The dignity of risk and the mentally retarded. *Mental Retardation, 10*(1), 24–27.

Piat, M. (2000). The NIMBY phenomenon: Community residents' concerns about housing for deinstitutionalized people. *Health & Social Work, 25*(2), 127–138.

Prouty, R. W., Smith, J., & Lakin, C. K. (2001). *Residential services for persons with developmental disabilities: Status and trends through 2000.* Minneapolis: University of Minnesota.

Prouty, R. W., Smith, J., & Lakin, C. K. (2007). *Residential services for persons with developmental disabilities: Status and trends through 2006.* Minneapolis: University of Minnesota.

Rothman, D. J., & Rothman, S. M. (2005). *The Willowbrook Wars: Bringing the mentally disabled into the community* (2nd ed.). New Brunswick, NJ: Transaction Publishers.

Schumacher, H. C. (1946). A program for dealing with mental deficiency in children up to six years of age. *American Journal of Mental Deficiency, 51*(1), 52–56.

Schwitzgebel, R. K. (1973). Right to treatment for the mentally disabled: The need for realistic standards and objective criteria. *Harvard Civil Rights-Civil Liberties Law Review, 8*, 513–535.

Scull, A. T. (1984). *Decarceration: Community treatment and the deviant – A radical view.* New Brunswick, NJ: Rutgers University Press.

Seltzer, M. M., Greenberg, J. S., Krauss, M. W., & Hong, J. (1997). Predictors and outcomes of the end of co-resident caregiving in aging families of adults with mental retardation or mental illness. *Family Relations*, 13–22.

Shadish, W. R., Lurigio, A. J., & Lewis, D. A. (1989). After deinstitutionalization: The present and future of mental health long-term care policy. *Journal of Social Issues*, *45*(3), 1–15.

Stancliffe, R. J., & Abery, B. H. (1997). Longitudinal study of deinstitutionalization and the exercise of choice. *Mental Retardation*, *35*(3), 159–169.

Stancliffe, R. J., Lakin, C. K., & Prouty, R. W. (2005). Growth in residential services in Australia and the United States: 1997–2002. *Journal of Intellectual and Developmental Disability*, *30*(3), 181–184.

Steadman, H. J., Monahan, J., Duffee, B., & Hartstone, E. (1984). Impact of state mental hospital deinstitutionalization on United States prison populations. 1968–1978. *The Journal of Criminal Law and Criminology*, *75*, 474.

Strauss, D., & Kastner, T. A. (1996). Comparative mortality of people with mental retardation in institutions and the community. *AJMR – American Journal on Mental Retardation*, *101*(1), 26–40.

Sullivan, R. C. (1981). What does deinstitutionalization mean for our children? *Journal of Autism and Developmental Disorders*, *11*(3), 347–356.

Teplin, L. A. (1984). Criminalizing mental disorder: The comparative arrest rate of the mentally ill. *American Psychologist*, *39*(7), 794–803.

Tredgold, A. F. (1908). *A textbook of mental deficiency*. Baltimore, MD: The Williams and Wilkins Company.

Trent, J. W. (1994). *Inventing the feeble mind: A history of mental retardation in the United States*. Berkeley, CA: University of California Press.

Walsh, J. A., & Walsh, R. A. (1982). Behavioral evaluation of a state program of deinstitutionalization of the developmentally disabled. *Evaluation and Program Planning*, *5*(1), 59–67.

Witkin, M. (1989). *Special analysis of the number of resident patients, total admissions, net releases, and deaths, state and county mental hospitals: United States, 1950–1987*. Rockville, MD: National Institute of Health.

Wolfensberger, W., & Nirje, B. (1972). *The principle of normalization in human services*. Toronto, ON: National Institute on Mental Retardation.

Wong, Y.-L. I., & Stanhope, V. (2009). Conceptualizing community: A comparison of neighborhood characteristics of supportive housing for persons with psychiatric and developmental disabilities. *Social Science & Medicine*, *68*(8), 1376–1387.

AN INSTITUTIONAL ANALYSIS OF PUBLIC SECTOR MENTAL HEALTH IN THE POST-DEINSTITUTIONALIZATION ERA

Teresa L. Scheid

ABSTRACT

Purpose – *In this chapter, I develop an analysis of the institutional logics which have shaped the organizational field of public sector mental health and which provide a framework for understanding the complexities facing policy makers, providers, researchers, and community mental health advocates.*

Approach – *I first assess the current state of public sector mental health care. I then describe institutional theory, which focuses our attention on the wider social values and priorities (i.e., institutional logics) which shape mental health care. In the current post-deinstitutionalization era, there are three competing institutional logics: recovery and community integration, cost containment and commodification, and increased social control over those with severe mental disorders. Each of these logics, and*

50 Years after Deinstitutionalization: Mental Illness in Contemporary Communities
Advances in Medical Sociology, Volume 17, 63–87

ISSN: 1057-6290/doi:10.1108/S1057-629020160000017003

the conflict between them, is explicated and analyzed. I then develop a theoretical framework for understanding how conflicting institutional logics are resolved. In the concluding section of this chapter, I offer some guidance to both researchers and advocates seeking meaningful system level reform.

Research implications – *Researchers studying mental health policy need to understand how competing institutional logics work to shape the political climate, economic priorities, and types of services available.*

Social implications – *Advocacy is critical for meaningful reform, and a fourth institutional logic – that of social justice – needs to be developed by which to evaluate policy reforms and service offerings.*

Keywords: Public sector mental health; institutional logics; social control; community care; recovery; advocacy

INTRODUCTION

In this chapter, I develop an analysis of the institutional logics which have shaped the organizational field of public sector mental health and which provide a framework for understanding the complexities facing policy makers, providers, researchers, and community mental health advocates. As defined by Mendal and Scott (2010, p. 249), "institutional logics are the cultural frames and belief systems that define and justify the roles of certain actors, help actors within the field to interpret events, and provide routines and rationales defining appropriate ways to carry on work." Put more simply, the care of and treatment provided to individuals with mental health problems reflect wider social values and priorities which are referred to as normative demands in institutional theory. These normative demands both reflect and shape the political climate, economic priorities, and types of services available and constitute prevailing institutional logics (as opposed to mere preferences for care). In the past, services for those with severe mental disabilities have gone through a series of cycles, from institutionalized care to deinstitutionalization, and from community-based care to managed care, reflecting competing institutional logics for care and treatment. The current system of care (post-deinstitutionalization) is characterized by a great deal of ambiguity and conflict, with competing normative demands for recovery and community integration and at the same time, increased institutionalization of those with severe mental illnesses (as reflected in the high rates of incarceration of those with mental illnesses and calls for expanded commitment criteria). Behind these competing normative demands is an overwhelming concern to contain costs – an institutional logic that has always pervaded public sector mental health care. Funding has never been adequate, and systems of care have never fully met the needs of those with severe mental illness. Researchers studying mental health policy need to understand how competing normative demands and institutional logics work against viable reforms, and this chapter provides a theoretical framework to not only understand our current policy impasse, but offers directions for future research.

BACKGROUND AND SIGNIFICANCE

Historically, there have been two systems of mental health care in the United States: the private and the public. Private mental health care is funded either out of pocket or by insurance and typically serves the "worried well." Public mental health care is funded by federal, state, and local monies and provides services to those with severe and chronic mental health problems. Funding for such care is not solely market driven, it results from government policies which affect not only health care, but also housing and welfare – the public sector.

In terms of public policy, the most critical group is those with severe and persistent mental disorders which results in substantial functional limitations. According to the Substance Abuse Mental Health Services Administration (SAMHSA) based on 2011 and 2012 state-level data, nationally about 4.0 percent of adults experience a serious mental illness (Substance Abuse Mental Health Services Administration [SAMHA], 2014). In addition to the severity of their illness, individuals served in the public mental health sector are poor and depend on public monies for sustenance as well as medical care. Rather than the short-term therapy, these individuals require long-term care, integrated services and social supports.[1] In the past, this care was provided in psychiatric hospitals, which with deinstitutionalization were replaced community mental health centers (CMHCs) under the Community Mental Health Centers Act of 1963. However, as has been well documented, CMHCs failed to provide or coordinate the necessary social supports needed by individuals with serious mental illness (Mechanic & Rochefort, 1990).

In the current post-deinstitutionalization era, we are still unable to provide and coordinate the many medical and supportive services needed by clients served by the public mental health sector including but not limited to: treatment and counseling, vocational rehabilitation, income maintenance, transportation, housing, emergency hospitalization, and crisis intervention. While most "care" is now provided in the community, with the constraints of managed care, much of this treatment is limited to medication maintenance. In 2008, 58.7 percent of those with a serious mental illness received treatment for their mental health problems, most of this involving prescription drug use (52.6 percent); 40.5 percent received care in an outpatient setting and only 7.5 percent in an inpatient setting (National Institute of Mental Health, 2008). In addition, public sector mental health care has increasingly become privatized, with private-managed care companies either managing or providing critical mental health services. While one could argue that the historic divide between private and public care is crumbling, in fact, public dollars are simply being funneled through private companies with little public oversight or accountability. A direct consequence of the loss of public sector community-based care has been that the criminal justice system has become the "de facto" system of care in many localities. While rates of inpatient hospitalization have dropped significantly, the percent of individuals with mental health problems who are incarcerated has increased (Harcourt, 2011). The U.S. Department of Justice reported that halfway through 2005 more than half of inmates had a mental health problem; with 15 percent of State prisoners and 24 percent of jail inmates exhibiting symptoms of a psychotic disorder (US Department of Justice [USDJ], 2006). Finally, there is no clear-cut federal policy governing mental health care, and consequently there is tremendous state-by-state variation. Institutional theory provides an excellent framework for understanding not only our current mental health care system, but also the public policies which shape mental health delivery systems.

CONTRADICTORY INSTITUTIONAL LOGICS AND PUBLIC SECTOR MENTAL HEALTH

Institutional theory directs our attention to the environment surrounding health care, specifically normative demands and societal preferences for mental health care. Referred to as institutional logics, competing normative demands exert influence on stakeholders, providers, and consumers in the mental health care sector. In their seminal work, Meyer and Scott (1983) distinguished between technical and institutional environments. In order to attain or maintain legitimacy, which is critical to survival and resource acquisition, organizations operating in technical environments must demonstrate technical competence (i.e., does a given drug reduce psychiatric symptoms?). Organizations operating in institutional environments must conform to normative demands and societal preferences for mental health care (i.e., providing community-based care as opposed to institutionalized care). For organizations facing institutional constraints, legitimacy is based upon evaluations by stakeholders that the organization is doing what it ought to be doing, as defined by normative demands and societal preferences which are often difficult if not impossible to operationalize (i.e., do CMHCs reduce stigma?).

Mental health organizations operate in institutional environments (Schlesinger & Gray, 1999) in part because there is no clear, unambiguous treatment technology by which to assess mental health care. The etiology of mental illness is not fully understood, and drug therapy often produces worse outcomes (Whitaker, 2010). For those with chronic and serious mental illnesses, even excellent programs may not produce notable signs of improvement (Mechanic, Schlesinger, & McAlpine, 1995). The course of serious mental illness is generally episodic and cyclical, with periods of stability and exacerbation of symptoms (Karp, 2001). Stern and Minkoff (1979) argued that community re-integration may be unattainable for those with chronic mental illness as the illness itself can prevent a return to normal life. However, another reason that public sector mental health care fits into the institutional model of organizational behavior is that government policies and funding constitute an important institutional force that affects the availability of mental health services. Mental health policy is framed at the state level and there is tremendous variation from state to state (Wolff, 2002). There are 50 different state mental health systems and even within states several different models of care may operate. Decisions about mental health care have not been made on the basis of rational or technical criteria, but on the basis of views about what constitutes appropriate mental health care, and there is disagreement among professionals, advocates, and other stakeholders about priorities for mental health care. The stigma of mental illness has also contributed to inertia in mental health policy (McSween, 2002).

Institutional demands can also be in conflict, producing what has been referred to as a turbulent institutional environment which will experience "cyclical legitimacy crises" (Hasenfeld, 1992, p. 1) or institutional fragmentation (Dobransky, 2014). There are two central sources for conflicting institutional demands: conflict between different normative demands and conflict between technical and normative demands. In terms of conflict between normative demands, there continues to be conflict between preferences for consumer empowerment and recovery and the desire to protect the public from those who due to their mental illness constitute a threat which leads to calls for more control over individuals with mental health disabilities. The conflict between technical demands for efficient, affordable treatment with normative demands for effective, quality services is also obvious. The movement toward evidence-based practices (EBPs) is clearly an attempt to instill technical criteria for evaluations of organizational performance. Schlesinger and Gray (1999) argue that the rise of managed care and propriety ownership of psychiatric hospitals constituted a fundamental shift toward technical considerations in the mental health field. However, technical demands for efficiency are more than considerations of how best to provide care – they reflect a larger process of commodification of care which includes an emphasis upon cost containment as well as privatization.

The Logic of Cost Containment and Commodification

Efficiency is the use of fewer resources and lower costs (Sullivan, 2000), and it is achieved through cost containment. Effectiveness involves assessments about the quality of care (Campbell, Roland, & Buetow, 2000; Flood, 1994). There is considerable agreement that health care has become commodified (Mechanic, 1999). What has been less commonly analyzed is the source of this commodification. Why are efficiency demands so widely accepted as appropriate? Meyer (1990) presents us with an interesting answer in his development of the commodity (as opposed to the bureaucratic) model of organizations. Meyer (1990) begins by extending the traditional bureaucratic model to include power; the efficiency of traditional bureaucratic organizations is the source of their power. However, powerful organizations are not necessarily more efficient – they can even be inefficient (witness banks and their role in the recent financial crises). Because of this potential for inefficiency to result from bureaucratic organizations, new organizational forms are increasingly governed by financial controls. Organizational structures have changed to maximize financial goals, and the commodity model is now dominant. Under the commodity model, selecting the best mean to a given end (i.e., rational action or efficiency) is replaced by a focus on the ends themselves – the accumulation of wealth or cost containment. In health care, commodification is apparent in the growth of managed care arrangements to control costs. However, the institutional logic of commodification is in conflict with the logic of community-based mental health care. A major dilemma faced by mental health care organizations and providers is to resolve the conflicts posed by the contradictory logics of commodification and professional-based logics for community care.

Conflict between the Logics of Commodification and Community-Based Care

Community-based care has been the preferred treatment for individuals with serious and chronic mental illness since the 1960s. As a treatment ideology, community-based care is based on a social rather than a medical model. While serious mental illness is widely accepted to be a disease requiring medication, psychosocial rehabilitation is the primary treatment modality. Medication allows for a reduction in the overt symptoms of mental illness, while psychosocial rehabilitation helps prepare an individual to live in the community by developing their adaptive capabilities and social skills, helping them to find social supports, and coordinating the continuum of care needed for successful community integration. Individuals with serious mental disability need long-term rehabilitation if they are to achieve optimal mental health and functional ability.

In contrast, managed care is based upon a medical model of illness; decisions to reimburse services are based upon external determinations of medical necessity. Mental health problems must meet established diagnostic criteria (now DSM-V); they must result in impaired social functioning, and the treatment must be clinically efficacious. Efficacy refers to the capacity of a treatment or intervention to improve a patient's condition in a controlled environment, while effectiveness focuses on the consequences of a treatment or intervention under normal conditions (Flood, 1994). Furthermore, efficiency constraints also mandate that mental health care must focus on measurable outcomes and utilize EBPs. As noted above, the course of serious and chronic mental illness is cyclical with often few signs of sustained progress. Dobransky (2014) describes the dilemmas posed by clients who will always need some level of services and social supports.

Minkoff (1997, p. 13) has described the concerns among mental health providers over the "perceived incompatibility of managed care with community mental health ideology, and with their own deeply held principles and ideals regarding public health service." Scheid (2004) describes how mental health care organizations and providers have responded to the competing demands of the commodity and the community logics of care, and has also analyzed the ability of one public sector mental health care system to incorporate the principles of managed care into a community-based system of care (Scheid, 2003). She found that despite a deliberate, carefully planned attempt to develop a system of managed care that preserved the principles of community care, the efficiency imperatives of the commodity model dominated changes in organizational structure. The organization implemented new measures of client level outcomes in response to standards for accreditation set by the National Committee for Quality Assurance. The outcomes emphasized reduced hospitalization and community stability as measured by employment and housing. However, measures of individual functioning were eliminated, and the new outcomes did not access continuity of care or quality of life – which are basic components to the philosophy of community-based care. Changes in the specific services offered indicated a declining commitment to community-based care. Scheid (2003) concludes that professional-based standards for effective, quality care had been displaced by technocratic standards for efficiency and efficacy.

More recently, Dobransky (2014) has examined how two community mental health organizations attempted to meet demands for bureaucratic accountability while also providing for community-based care and client empowerment and recovery. Dobransky (2014) provides a very nice analysis of institutional fragmentation, where various institutional logics conflict and pull both providers and clients in different directions. Resolution of these conflicts had as much to do with how the logic was institutionalized. Bureaucratic accountability was institutionalized in the rules and regulations which governed these two organizations, while the empowerment and community logics were institutionalized in the normative belief systems of providers. Violations of the bureaucratic rules could result in a loss of funding (i.e., legitimacy), whereas there were few mechanisms to support client empowerment or community logics. Dobransky (2014) separates demands for client empowerment and recovery from the community logic, and since recovery has been a guiding principle to mental health reform (US Department of Health and Human Services, 1999) I turn to a consideration of how calls for recovery have influenced the current system of public sector mental health.

Institutional Demands for Recovery

Recovery builds on the ideals of consumer empowerment, and is based on an advocacy model first introduced by Rose and Black (1985). While a focus on patient rights was certainly important to the original community care movement, empowerment pushed the idea of client autonomy to emphasize the individual's right to advocate for their own care and assume control over the direction of their own treatment. Some advocates of empowerment even rejected professional intervention, building upon critiques of both biomedical and psychosocial rehabilitation models which ultimately wanted clients to conform to professional definitions of mental health (Paulson, 1992). The concept of empowerment has evolved from independence from the system to choice within the system (McLean, 2000, p. 837). While recovery is certainly not essential for empowerment (one can advocate for one's services and not seek recovery), recovery has become the dominant normative demand – used by stakeholders, advocates, and consumers.

Recovery involves both a reduction in psychiatric symptoms (recovery from illness) as well as recovery within illness with client level determined quality of life (Dobransky, 2014). The development of psychosocial conditions for leading a fulfilling life (hope, connection, empowerment) as well as the external conditions which allow individuals to lead a productive life are necessary for recovery (Jacobson, 2004; Jacobson & Greenley, 2001). As such recovery is a fairly broad and ambiguous term that can serve as an umbrella for many different kinds of services. Jacobson (2004) describes how recovery has been used as a slogan by diverse groups promoting different ideological positions; as such it can serve as an "optimistic rhetorical devise" (Spandler & Stickley, 2011, p. 560). Recovery can mean an expanded service model as once an individual's symptoms are stabilized they will have an increased need for the social supports and skills building programs (Neugeboren, 1999). However, when defined as meeting certain limited functional goals recovery can also mean reduced reliance (and cost savings) on service systems. Recovery can be used as a yardstick for improved client outcomes (Spandler, 2014), with little commitment to creating the kind of therapeutic environments where recovery can be fostered (Spandler & Stickley, 2011).

The apparent political consensus over recovery is noteworthy, given the many debates over treatment for mental health problems. Federal level initiatives such as the 1999 Surgeon General's Report on Mental Health and the 2003 President's New Freedom Commission on Mental Health have set recovery as a standard for mental health reform. The National Consensus Conference on Mental Health Recovery was convened in 2005 by the Center for Mental Health Services involving over 100 consumers, advocates, providers, and researchers who developed a definition of recovery and articulated 10 principles of recovery (Anthony & Ashcraft, 2010). The components of recovery include self-direction, individualized treatment, empowerment, holistic, nonlinear, strengths-based, peer support, respect, responsibility, and hope (Anthony & Ashcraft, 2010, p. 467). It is not surprising that so many espouse recovery as a worthy aspiration; the issue is whether recovery can actually be fostered within our current system of mental health care, or in those communities where individuals with serious mental disabilities would like to reside.

Recovery is fundamentally a social process, not a clinical outcome and involves improved quality of life (Keith & Keith, 2013). Yanos, Knight, and Roe (2007) provide a nice theoretical framework for understanding recovery – emphasizing the role of social structure and individual agency rather than biological explanations. They argue that the personal agency of those with severe mental illnesses (such as coping mechanisms and the ability to set and strive for goals) is constrained by current social structures, including poverty, legal restrictions, a lack of affordable housing, distressed neighborhoods and the routinized practices of stigma and discrimination which in turn create further stress, hopelessness and anomie. Many individuals with severe mental illnesses are isolated in the external social community, with few friends or social supports (Keith & Keith, 2013). Given the realities of the larger external environment, clients may choose dependence on the service system where they are accepted and provided with scarce resources (Dobransky, 2014; Schutt & Goldfinger, 2011). However, such choices are not welcome when services and resources are limited or constrained.

Conflicting Logics of Recovery and the Efficiency Demands of Commodification

A key question is whether recovery can really be implemented within the now dominant managed care framework which is driven by the logic of commodification. Specifically, the standards described above to meet efficiency standards (medical necessity, short-term gains in functioning, and outcome assessment) are difficult to meet given the fairly diffuse, individualist, patient centered recovery model. Markowitz (2001) has raised concerns about limits to the nonclinical services central to recovery imposed by managed care entities McLean (2000) argues that both traditional and consumer alternatives are being curtailed by the cost-saving logic of managed care. Dobransky (2014) also finds that the logic of empowerment as it is currently practiced in the two organizations he studied is infused with market mechanisms (clients are now consumers). Bureaucratic constraints on reimbursement limited the use of many programs which would lead to recovery or facilitate consumer empowerment; recreation is not a billable service, even if it does build client capacity and self-esteem.

Scheid (2008) compared two state mental health reform initiatives (Wisconsin and North Carolina) in terms of their ability to incorporate principles of recovery. In 1995 Wisconsin reorganized its mental health care system around the principles of recovery following the recommendations of a specially formed commission (Blue Ribbon Commission of Mental Health Care, 1997) and attempted to reconcile conflicts between the ideological principles of recovery with technical demands for efficiency. The state (via the Blue Ribbon Commission which was comprised of a large and diverse group of stakeholders) moved to implement managed care via county run demonstration projects. However, these demonstration projects focused almost entirely on recovery as they were not able to determine a capitation rate compatible with recovery (Jacobson, 2004).

North Carolina moved much later in its reform initiative, with the State Auditor and two private consulting plans conducting research and preparing a report. Subsequently, a Legislative Oversight Committee was formed in 2000 to develop a plan to redesign mental health services in the state. This plan privatized all mental health services, mandating that local mental health authorities needed to contract out all direct care services to a qualified provider network. Local mental health authorities were furthermore to operate as managed behavioral health care organizations. The legislation was passed in 2002 and implemented beginning July 1, 2003. While the legislation referred to the principles of recovery, it mandated that programs had to implement evidence-based treatment programs (with no funding for such programs). The result was the elimination of public sector mental health and a period of what can only be described as chaos (Scheid, 2008). In 2010, the U.S. Justice Department opened a formal investigation into North Carolina's mental health system in response to complaints raised by advocacy groups about the effects of the reform.

A key question is whether recovery can indeed be operationalized in such a way as to meet standards for efficiency and outcome assessment. There are numerous treatment programs and modalities for recovery (Neugeboren, 1999) as well as attempts to establish "best practices" and standards for recovery (Jacobson, 2004) along with research on the effectiveness of programs-based on recovery. Markowitz (2001) found that recovery-based treatment programs did increase the individual's self-esteem and mastery, which then resulted in decreased symptomatology. Tew (2012) has linked social factors to successful recovery; yet "the social structures that restrict personal agency are seldom discussed in detail" (Yates, Holmes, & Priest, 2012, p. 111). These researchers point to housing and other conditions of poverty which create stress. Yet others see the major barrier to recovery as the failure of mental health organizations and providers to either be aware of, or to properly implement, EBPs (Doub, Morrison, & Goodson, 2010). However, the promise of "recovery" actually directs attention away from the need to provide comprehensive mental health care and social supports; instead, consumers can be held accountable for their own recovery, or lack thereof. A more fundamental issue is whether the ideals of recovery (empowerment) can be achieved in what is an "inherently coercive legal framework" (Spandler & Stickley, 2011, p. 561).

The Resurgence of the Logic of Social Control

The issue of social control has been a long-standing theme in medical sociology, and has been a particularly salient construct in understanding the treatment of those with mental illnesses. The criminalization of those with mental illness, and the reality that our criminal justice has become a major provider of mental health services, is certainly a testament to the persistence of social control imperatives. The power asymmetry between patient and provider is heightened by the association of mental illness with incomprehensibility, unintelligibility, irrationality or incompetence. Central is continued debate over the social control of those with alleged mental illnesses is the role of mandated community treatment (Bonnie & Monahan, 2005; Test & West, 2010). Also referred to as outpatient commitment, or assisted outpatient treatment, mandated community treatment involves the use of leverage (or hidden coercion) to elicit compliance with treatment from those with serious mental illness. In exchange for compliance with treatment demands in the community, various forms of leverage are used to avoid negative events such as hospitalization or incarceration, or to gain access to positive benefits such as the provision of housing or transportation. Both positive and negative forms of leverage are fairly common (Bonnie & Monahan, 2005) with some arguing that such leverage should be rare (Swanson, Van Dorn, Monahan, & Swartz, 2006) and used to expand, rather than constrict patient choice (Bonnie & Monahan, 2005).

Currently, far too many people with mental illnesses are receiving inadequate or no care, or are receiving care in the criminal justice system (Sederer & Sharfstein, 2014). Individuals with mental illnesses who do end up in jail or prison generally commit minor offenses, often related to survival strategies (Hiday & Burns, 2010). In response to the criminalization of those with mental illnesses, some are calling for stricter commitment criteria and an expanded role for mental institutions (Early, 2006). Rather than address the sources of violence in our society, we build more prisons and incarcerate more and more of those with mental health problems under the guise of their dangerousness to society (Parry, 2013). Sociologists point to the failure of the mental health system and the lack of community-based services as the source of the problem, not commitment criteria (Hiday & Burns, 2010). Seung-Hui Cho, the student who killed 32 people at Virginia Tech before committing suicide, was at that time under an involuntary outpatient commitment order. Other mass shootings have resulted in greater public pressures for more social control of those with mental illnesses who may become dangerous and harm others. Obviously, an important (and long-standing) institutional demand is the protection of society from harm as opposed to protecting the rights of the individual. Both Mental Health America (formerly, the Mental Health Association) and the Bazelon Center for Mental Health Law have policy statements opposing involuntary commitment unless the individual is in imminent likelihood of significant harm and when no least restrictive is available. Even in these cases, individuals need to be afforded full procedural protections and should be found either legally incompetent or provide informed consent for mental health treatment.

Adherents of recovery models are also critical of involuntary commitment given their emphasis on self-directed treatment and choice (Henwood, 2008). Wales and Hiday (2006) are critical of the leverage of outpatient commitment, arguing that we need to replace persuasion, leverage, or coercion (PLC) with tender loving care (TLC) – or improved patient centered treatment and assertive outreach. The dearth of community supports remains a central issue in renewed calls for expanded civil commitment criteria. Sederer and Sharfstein (2014) provide a very concise summary of exactly what kinds of community-based services individuals with serious mental illnesses need – the issue is how to provide the diverse array of needed services and supports in an era of cost containment and restricted public funding. In the wake of even more recent violent events (i.e., Sandy Hook), the conflict between calls for greater recovery efforts as well as stronger controls over those with mental health disabilities in the community will have a strong impact on both federal and state-level mental health policy. Yet the institutional logic of commodification, cost containment, and efficiency remains salient and it is obvious considerations of cost will have an important role in resolving policy debates.

A Framework for Understanding How Conflicting Institutional Demands Are Resolved

While institutional theory provides a useful model for understanding conflicting institutional demands, little attention has been paid to how such conflicts are resolved. This is in part due to institutional theory's early emphasis on organizational isomorphism – that is, organizations responding to similar demands were likely to exhibit similar changes in organizational structures and activities. In addition, institutional theory has paid less attention to how organizations deal with diverse institutional demands. Mental health organizations are expected to provide for continuity of care, fight stigma, protect the public from dangerous individuals, and also protect the civil rights of patients in their care. Both economic as well as social values shape care and treatment norms, and there continues to be a general lack of consensus about both the source of mental health problems as well as adequate treatment. Most clinicians adhere to a bio-psychosocial model which integrates biological mechanisms, psychological processes, and social influences; "treatment" focuses on the consequences (rather than the causes) of mental health problems (Scheid, 2004). Both medication and psychosocial rehabilitation are used, although criteria of medical necessity currently utilized for reimbursement limit the provision of psychosocial rehabilitation and social support services, including case management. The diversity of the mental health workforce (Morris & Lezak, 2010; Scheid, 2004) also contributes to ambiguity over treatment with 20 different disciplines providing mental health care, and different treatment orientations or ideologies exerting pressures within organizations which also creates conflict over organizational priorities. Conflict exists in both the external demands placed on mental health organizations, and from the internal demands of organizational participants.

There is also conflict between "ought" and the "is" goals–organizations often cannot do what they ideally would like to do because they lack the means to do so – and may experience goal incongruence as ideal goals are replaced by more realistic goals. In analysis of 29 outpatient mental health organizations, Scheid and Greenley (1997) found that levels of goal congruence were important to understanding evaluations of organizational effectiveness. In the current era of assessment and evaluation of both individual and organizational performance (an institutional demand made by the commodity model), goal incongruence is likely to be even greater than in the past. Abravanel (1983) referred to the difference between the "ought" and the "is" goals as conflict between fundamental goals (what should be done) and operative goals (what can be done). Ideally and fundamentally, community-based treatment and recovery call for client self-determination and community integration as well as improved quality of life (whether within or without the mental health system). Realistically and operatively some level of medication maintenance or short-term improvements may be all we can do with current funding constraints. This is especially likely given the lack of community supports or alternatives to traditional mental health care.

Abravanel (1983) has examined the role of mediatory myths in overcoming overt contradictions with an organization's ideology or belief system. In fact, he argues that faith in an organization myth is the only effective mechanism for reducing or bridging organizational contradictions and ambiguities (Abravanel, 1983, p. 273). Mediatory myths allow organizations to "get on" with their work by providing them with ideological justifications for their actions. For example, outpatient commitment can be seen as a mechanism to meet the contradictory purposes of enhanced social control over individuals with mental illnesses while also providing for a less restrictive alternative, thus protecting patient liberty. When originally implemented, the primary purpose of an outpatient commitment order to was to ensure patients went to their CMHC and received medication. The belief in the efficacy of psychiatric medication constituted the critical mediatory myth which allowed clinicians to mitigate (or mediate) the contradictory expectations of social control and least restrictive alternative (Scheid, 1993; Scheid-Cook, 1988). The belief in the efficacy of psychiatric medication is even stronger than it was 30 years ago (Frances, 2013; Smith, 2014; Whitaker, 2010) and managed care arrangements have reinforced medicalization

(Conrad, 2007). However, medication and medication compliance are weak substitutes for community-based care or recovery.

I speculate that the belief that the goals of community care and recovery can be met by adherence to EBPs is another mediatory myth which allows both providers and researchers to reconcile the contradictions posed by the community model and the commodity model. For example, Morris and Lezak (2010, p. 84) call for a transformed mental health system that is "consumer centered, grounded in the expectations of recovery, and built on a foundation of EBPs that generate measureable, quality outcomes." They see system fragmentation as the major barrier to this ideal (and system fragmentation is certainly a major problem), but they do not see the inherent contradiction between practices that enable recovery and which are at the same time evidence based. Just as researchers were not able to effectively quantify quality of life (Rapley, 2003), it is hard to imagine how any scale or measure can adequately capture the individual's experience of recovery. As Dobransky (2014) found, client level empowerment is ambiguous and difficult to define, while reduced use of services is much easier to measure and also meets standards for bureaucratic accountability.

Sociological theories of domain separation (Rundall, Alexander, & Shortell, 2004) and network embeddedness (Wholey, Christianson, Draper, Lesser, & Burns, 2004) can help understand how communities and organizations respond to competing institutional demands. Relevant stakeholders (health care providers, advocacy groups, for profit managed care organizations, local business interests, neighborhood associations) in a given community may have fairly high degrees of domain separation, or they may be more integrated – leading to either high or low degrees of network embeddedness. The resolution of conflict over competing institutional demands is in part a social process – who defined the problem to be addressed, who is sitting on what special commission to undertake an analysis of the problem, what groups are charged with implementing suggested reforms. As Binder (2007, p. 549) describes the process, "people go about squaring those (institutional) demands with their own local meaning systems, personal commitments, and professional obligations … and they do so in interaction with others." In North Carolina private business interests promoting privatization controlled the reform process while in Wisconsin reform was the result of an inclusive body of constituents who sought to maintain local community control over mental health care (Scheid, 2008). The different mental health policy outcomes in these two states are the result of different institutional actors who were able to advocate or their own institutional logics, and who were able to marshal legislative support for reforms that reflected these logics.

In terms of the future sociological work, much needs to be done to examine how the competing institutional demands I have described will be resolved. Negotiation is certainly central, and can often involve political battles (Thorton, Ocasio, & Lounsbury, 2012). Where there are high degrees of domain integration and network embeddedness, there is greater likelihood that conflicting demands will be recognized, and an increased emphasis on the resolution of conflicts to the benefit of all groups involved. Where there is a high degree of domain separation, and low levels of network embeddedness, those groups with the most power will have their demands met. Currently, under the commodity model, "power accrues to those having the tools with which to maximize efficiency outcomes" (Meyer, 1990, p. 211). That said, the logic of commodification will most likely continue to prevail beyond the era of post-deinstitutionalization.

CONCLUSION

The current state of public sector mental health is one of disarray, with very few of those with serious mental illness receiving appropriate care or treatment (Sederer & Sharfstein, 2014). That so many receive care in jails or prisons is "a situation which should embarrass all thoughtful citizens" (Mechanic, 2006, p. 80). Instead, we continue to focus on cost and hold mental health providers and clients accountable for meeting outcomes defined within the framework of cost containment. Yet cost containment itself is a constructed reality. For example, we do not actually access the true costs of inadequate mental health care, which are born by the wider community and the stress on other service systems (Mechanic, 1999). Instead, we focus on narrowly defined client outcomes and the implementation of EBPs without taking into account that system factors (financing and the organization of services) are more powerful predictors of patient outcomes (Carney, 2008).

Ultimately, we need to move beyond the individual level to more complex understandings of systems of care. Furthermore, we will have to confront the reality that the current system has been developed and is organized around the precept that health care is a commodity, and that profits and the accumulation of wealth are the primary goals motivating key stakeholders who control the "system." Rather than incremental reform, our health care nonsystem needs to be fundamentally reorganized around a different goal – not efficiency (i.e., cost), but effectiveness (access to and quality of care). The values of quality care, or greater access to care, are goals that health care providers and patients have control over, while corporate forces push for the priority of the accumulation of wealth as a primary goal. The contradiction between providing the full continuum of care needed by chronic care populations and a system designed to provide as little care as possible (or the minimal amount of care that one can afford) is becoming increasingly obvious. The 2000 and 2001 Institute of Medicine reports on quality care identify contradictory principles for quality care: effectiveness, efficiency, patient centered, safe, timely, and equitable (Timmermans & Berg, 2003). Each priority is also to subject to processes of subjective interpretation and redefinition, with notable variations in what counts for effective treatment.

Stylianos and Kehyayan (2012) see advocacy as a critical component to comprehensive mental health care. However, neither patients nor their providers are empowered to serve as effective advocates in the current environment. Community-based groups and advocates as well as researchers are forced to compete for funding to support research and services which do not lead to any kind of significant changes to the system of care. Consequently, community-based advocacy efforts need to move beyond market-based models of patient choice and consumerism to true democratic deliberation (Grob & Schlesinger, 2011). As noted by Tomes and Hoffman (2011, p. 13), patient empowerment takes place in an environment of "pervasive social and economic inequality. Differences of power, income, resources, and access to the media shape the ability of patient groups to affect policy." The consumer-survivor movement in mental health cannot counter the power of the pharmaceutical industry, the medical profession, or governmental agencies (Tomes, 2011). The major obstacles to patient empowerment described by Grob and Schlesinger (2011) target cultural and system level barriers to social change, which I would identify as overarching social inequalities, a medicalized and individualized approach to disease, and a concern with technocratic rationality which emphasizes clinical efficacy and cost effectiveness rather than system wide improvement.

Ultimately advocacy is about changing policy. It doesn't matter if these efforts are successful (Epstein, 2011); what matters is that people are working to change the rules by which the game is played and to enhance the sense of the public good and collective patient identity

(Grob & Schlesinger, 2011). However, advocacy has to be collective in order to improve the agency of individuals (Yanos, Knight, & Roe, 2007). Advocates, both consumers and providers, need to band together and become an effective countervailing power to those who benefit from the logic of commodification. A first step to changing mental health policy is to focus on public perception. Researchers and advocates in the United States need to follow the United Kingdom in seeing mental illness as a disability, which entails a shift from a medical model to a social model (Keith & Keith, 2013; Spandler, Anderson, & Sapey, 2015). Disability is not just a matter of individual health (or psychiatric symptoms); the roots of disability lie not in the individual – but in society. Disabilities are made worse by society's inability to either provide or create supportive environments (Keith & Keith, 2013).

Advocates can also learn from successful legal efforts. The 1990 Americans with Disabilities Act (ADA) sought to reduce discrimination in the workplace and improve the employment of those with mental impairments. While the ADA articulated a new set of legal and normative standards, the practical meaning and compliance of employers depended on how they interpreted the law (Scheid & Suchman, 2001). Not surprisingly, stigma played a major role in employer's responses to the ADA and their beliefs about mental disability were critical to the development of supportive work environments (Scheid, 2005). Hernandez and Uggen (2012) provide an institutional analysis of the factors which influenced the passage of state mental health parity laws. They found that mental health parity laws were less likely to pass in states with more conservative governmental ideology and in times of high unemployment. Advocacy was also important; those states with a stable National Alliance for Mental Illness Association were more likely to pass parity legislation.

At the federal level, there are currently two bills in Congress seeking to improve mental health. The "Helping Families in Mental Health Crisis Act" a bipartisan bill introduced by Timothy Murphy and it has been criticized by Mental Health America for reducing critical services and programs, for its expanded use of involuntary outpatient treatment, and for a number of measures which undermine the authority of SAMHSA and the Department of Health and Human Services (Mental Health America, 2014). The other bill, "Strengthening Mental Health in Our Communities" introduced by Ron Barber has been criticized for doing too little (Sederer & Sharfstein, 2014). Both laws ultimately seek to further reduce federal responsibility for mental health service delivery. Advocates must work to raise public awareness of the negative impact of these laws, despite their euphemistic titles. Further sociological work on the social factors influencing both advocacy and reform in mental health is needed.

In lieu of any major legal reforms, and in recognition of the fact that laws often follow social practices rather than create them, how else should advocacy work to effect change in mental health care? Carney (2008) argues that we need to emphasize the citizen rights of those with mental illness, rather than merely focusing on civil liberties. Advocates can fight for the individual's right to social supports and health services. We also need to focus on accountability measures which guarantee access to care and treatment and needed social supports. Another avenue is to fight for the inclusion of an ethical foundation by which we can evaluate policy reforms and service offerings. Just as we evaluate the merits of new drugs, we need to evaluate the merits of policy initiatives on the basis of higher moral standards (Russell, 2011). However, in the evaluation of services, "the language of social justice is largely absent" (Farmer, 2005, p. 177). The insistence on a moral, or ethical, foundation would be a direct counter to the logic of commodification and cost containment. Health policy has been the result of shifting preferences for access (the Affordable Care seeking to increase access), quality (as evidenced by current quality improvement efforts), and cost containment (Mendal & Scott, 2010). It is time to add a fourth pillar – an ethic of care or social justice.

Paul Farmer is well known for linking his own advocacy efforts to larger issues of social justice; he (2005, pp. 152–3) argues that "the commodification of medicine invariably punishes the vulnerable ... there is an enormous difference between seeing people as victims of innate shortcomings and seeing them as victims of structural violence." Structural violence accounts for the systematic exclusion of individuals with schizophrenia from society (Kelly, 2005). A focus on individual risk factors (or populations at risk) too often ends in blaming the victim (Farmer, 2005) and the reinforcing levels of cultural stigma which then serve as powerful obstacles to prevention and care. The social exclusion of those with severe mental illness is rooted in structural and socioeconomic conditions (Kelly, 2005). Rather than a rights-based framework for justice, Farmer (2005) advocates "preferential justice" – a system of care that sees the poor and disenfranchised as more, not less, deserving of care. As advocates and citizens we need to work to change the culture and social structures which surround the individual patient. As researchers we can contribute to understanding how different groups are able to mobilize resources and political support which will be critical to the future of public sector mental health.

NOTE

1. The correct referent for the individuals served in the public mental health sector varies considerably: Individuals with serious (or severe) and persistent (or chronic) mental illnesses (or disorders, or mental health problems). In this chapter, I will generally use the terms used by the authors when citing their work; otherwise I will use the term severe mental disability. Severe captures both the seriousness and the persistence of the mental health disability. The use of disability includes functional limitation, and also places emphasis on the social environment, whereas the use of illness or disorder focuses attention on the individual and their symptoms.

REFERENCES

Abravanel, H. (1983). Mediatory myths in the services of organization ideology. In L. Pondy, P. J. Frost, G. Morgan, & T. Dandridge (Eds.), *Organizational symbolism* (pp. 273–293). Greenwich, CT: JAI Press.

Anthony, W. A., & Ashcraft, L. (2010). The recovery movement. In B. Lubotsky Levin, K. D. Hennessy, & J. Petrila (Eds.), *Mental health services: A public health perspective* (3rd ed., pp. 465–480). New York, NY: Oxford University Press.

Binder, A. (2007). For love or monday: Organizations' creative responses to multiple environmental logics. *Theory and Society*, *36*, 547–571.

Blue Ribbon Commission of Mental Health Care. (1997). *The Blue Ribbon Commission on Mental Health: Final Report*. Submitted to Governor Tommy Thompson.

Bonnie, R. J., & Monahan, J. (2005). From coercion to contract: Reframing the debate on mandated community treatment for people with mental disorders. *Law and Human Behavior*, *29*, 485–503.

Campbell, S. M., Roland, M. O., & Buetow, S. A. (2000). Defining quality of care. *Social Science and Medicine*, *51*, 1611–1625.

Carney, T. (2008). The mental health service crises of neoliberalism – An antipodean perspective. *International Journal of Law and Psychiatry*, *31*, 101–115.

Conrad, P. (2007). *The medicalization of society: On the transformation of human conditions into treatable disorders*. Baltimore, MD: John Hopkins University Press.

Dobransky, K. M. (2014). *Managing madness in the community: The challenge of contemporary mental health care*. New Brunswick, NJ: Rutgers University Press.

Doub, T. W., Morrison, D. P., & Goodson, J. (2010). Community mental health centers. In B. Lubotsky Levin, K. D. Hennessy, & J. Petrila (Eds.), *Mental health services: A public health perspective* (3rd ed., pp.349–374). New York, NY: Oxford University Press.

Early, P. (2006). *Crazy: A father's search through American's mental health madness*. New York, NY: G.P. Putnam's Sons.

Epstein, S. (2011). Measuring success: Scientific, institutional, and cultural effects of patient advocacy. In B. Hoffman, N. Tomes, R. Grob, & Schlesinger (Eds.), *Patients as policy actors* (pp. 255–277). New Brunswick, NJ: Rutgers University Press.

Farmer, P. (2005). *Pathologies of power: Health, human rights, and the new war on the poor*. Berkely, CA: University of California Press.

Flood, A. B. (1994). The impact of organizational and managerial factors on the quality of care in health care organizations. *Medical Care Review*, *38*, 396–427.

Frances, A. (2013). *Saving normal: An insider's revolt against out-of-control psychiatric diagnosis, DSM-5, big pharma, and the medicalization of ordinary life*. New York, NY: Harper-Collins.

Grob, R., & Schlesinger, M. (2011). Principles for engaging patients in U.S. health care and policy. In B. Hoffman, N. Tomes, R. Grob, & M. Schlesinger (Eds.), *Patients as policy actors* (pp. 278–292). New Brunswick, NJ: Rutgers University Press.

Harcourt, B. E. (2011). An institutionalization effect: The impact of mental hospitalization and imprisonment on homicide in the United States. *The Journal of Legal Studies*, *40*, 39–83.

Hasenfeld, Y. (1992). *Human services as complex organizations*. Newbury Park, NJ: Sage.

Henwood, B. (2008). Involuntary inpatient commitment in the context of mental health recovery. *American Journal of Psychiatric Rehabilitation*, *11*(3), 253–266.

Hernandez, E. M., & Uggen, C. (2012). Institutions, politics, and mental health parity. *Society and Mental Health*, *2*, 154–171.

Hiday, V. A., & Burns, P. J. (2010). Mental illness and the criminal justice system. In T. L. Scheid & T. N. Brown (Eds.), *Handbook for the study of mental health* (2nd ed., pp. 478–498). New York, NY: Cambridge University Press.

Jacobson, N. (2004). *In recovery: The making of mental health policy*. Nashville, TN: Vanderbilt University Press.

Jacobson, N., & Greenley, D. (2001). What is recovery? A conceptual model and explication. *Psychiatric Services*, *52*(4), 482–485.

Karp, D. (2001). *The burden of sympathy: How families cope with mental illness*. New York, NY: Oxford University Press.

Keith, H. E., & Keith, K. D. (2013). *Intellectual disability: Ethics, dehumanization, and a new moral community*. Malden, MA: Whiley-Blackwell.

Kelly, B. (2005). Structural violence and schizophrenia. *Social Science and Medicine*, *61*, 721–730.

Markowitz, F. E. (2001). Modeling processes in recovery from mental illness: Relationships between symptoms, life satisfaction, and self concept. *Journal of Health and Social Behavior*, *42*, 64–79.

McLean, A. H. (2000). From ex-patient alternatives to consumer options: Consequences of consumerism for psychiatric consumers and the ex-patient movement. *International Journal of Health Services*, *30*, 821–847.

McSween, J. L. (2002). The role of group interest, identity, and stigma in determining mental health policy preferences. *Journal of Health Politics, Policy, and Law*, *27*, 773–800.

Mechanic, D. (1999). *Mental health and social policy: The emergence of managed care*. Boston, MA: Allyn and Bacon.

Mechanic, D. (2006). *The truth about health care: Why reform is not working in America*. New Brunswick, NJ: Rutgers University Press.

Mechanic, D., & Rochefort, D. (1990). Deinstitutionalization: An appraisal of reform. *Annual Review of Sociology*, *16*, 301–327.

Mechanic, D., Schlesinger, M., & McAlpine, D. D. (1995). Management of mental health and substance abuse services: State of the art and early results. *Milibank Quarterly*, *73*(1), 19–55.

Mendal, P., & Scott, W. R. (2010). Institutional change and the organization of health care: The dynamics of "Muddling Through". In C. E. Bird, P. Conrad, A. M. Fremont, & S. Timmermans (Eds.), *Handbook of medical sociology* (6th ed., pp. 249–260). Nashville, TN: Vanderbilt University Press.

Mental Health America. (2014). *Mental health America faults rep. Tim Murphy's legislation for jeopardizing role for consumers and their recovery.* Statement of D. Stern, Ph.D. President and CEO Mental Health America. Retrieved from www.mentalhealthamerica.net/mental-health-americ-faults-pre-tim-murphy. Accessed on May 3, 2014.

Meyer, J. W., & Scott, W. R. (1983). *Organizational environments: Ritual and rationality.* Beverly Hills, CA: Sage.

Meyer, M. W. (1990). The Weberian tradition in organizational research. In C. Calhoun, M. W. Meyer, & W. R. Scott (Eds.), *Structures of power and constraint* (pp. 191–215). New York, NY: Cambridge University Press.

Minkoff, K. (1997). Public sector managed care and community mental health ideology. In K. Minkoff & D. Pollack (Eds.), *Managed mental health in the public sector* (pp. 13–22). Amsterdam: Harwood Academic Publishers.

Morris, R., & Lezak, A. (2010). Workforce. In B. Lubotsky Levin, K. D. Hennessy, & J. Petrila (Eds.), *Mental health services: A public health perspective* (3rd ed., pp. 83–114). New York, NY: Oxford University Press.

National Institute of Mental Health. (2008). *The use of mental health services and treatment among adults.* Retrieved from www.nimh.nih.gov/health/statistics/prevalence/use-of-mental-health-services-and-treatment-among-adults.shtml. Accessed on July 6, 2015.

Neugeboren, J. (1999). *Transforming madness: New lives for people living with mental illness.* Berkeley, CA: University of California Press.

Parry, J. W. (2013). *Mental disability, violence, and future dangerousness.* Lanham, MD: Rowman & Littlefield.

Paulson, R. (1992). Advocacy and empowerment: Mental health care in the community. *Community Mental Health Journal, 28*, 70–71.

Rapley, M. (2003). *Quality of life research: A critical introduction.* London: Sage.

Rose, S. P., & Black, B. L. (1985). *Advocacy and empowerment: Mental health care in the community.* Boston, MA: Routledge and Kegan Paul.

Rundall, T., Alexander, J., & Shortell, S. (2004). A theory of physician-hospital integration. *Journal of Health and Social Behavior, 45*, (Special Issue), 102–117.

Russell, B. J. (2011). How research ethics' protections can contribute to public policy: The case of community treatment orders. *International Journal of Law and Psychiatry, 34*, 349–353.

Scheid, T. (1993). Controller and controlled: An analysis of participant constructions of outpatient commitment. *Sociology of Health and Illness, 15*, 179–193.

Scheid, T. L. (2003). Managed care and the rationalization of mental health services. *Journal of Health and Social Behavior, 44*(1), 142–161.

Scheid, T. L. (2004). *Tie a knot and hang on: Delivering mental healthcare in a turbulent environment.* Hawthorne, NY: Aldine De Gruyter Press.

Scheid, T. L. (2005). Stigma as a barrier to employment: Psychiatric disability and the impact of the American with disabilities act. *International Academy of Psychiatry and Law, 28*, 670–690.

Scheid, T. L. (2008). Competing institutional demands: A framework for understanding mental health policy. *Social Theory and Health, 6*, 291–308.

Scheid, T. L., & Greenley, J. R. (1997). Evaluations of organizational effectiveness in mental health programs. *Journal of Health and Social Behavior*, *38*, 403–426.

Scheid, T. L., & Suchman, M. C. (2001). Ritual conformity to the Americans with disabilities act: Coercive and normative isomorphism. *The Organizational Response to Social Problems*, *8*, 105–140.

Scheid-Cook, T. L. (1988). Mitigating organizational contradictions: The role of mediatory myths. *The Journal of Applied Behavior Science*, *24*, 161–171.

Schlesinger, M. J., & Gray, B. H. (1999). Institutional change and its consequences for the delivery of mental health services. In A. V. Horwitz & T. L. Scheid (Eds.), *A handbook for the study of mental health* (pp. 427–448). New York, NY: Cambridge University Press.

Schutt, R. K., & Goldfinger, S. M. (2011). *Homelessness, housing, and mental illness.* Cambridge, MA: Harvard University Press.

Sederer, L. I., & Sharfstein, S. S. (2014). Fixing the troubled mental health system. *JAMA*. doi:10:1001/jama.2014.10369

Smith, D. T. (2014). The diminished resistance to medicalization in psychiatry: Psychoanalysis meets the medical model of mental illness. *Society and Mental Health*, *4*, 75–91.

Spandler, H. (2014). Letting madness breathe? Critical challenges facing mental health social work today. In J. Weinstein (Ed.), *Mental health: Critical and radical debates in social work* (pp.26–38). Bristol: Policy Press.

Spandler, H., Anderson, J., & Sapey, B. (2015). *Distress and disability: Madness and the politics of disablement.* Bristol: Policy Press.

Spandler, H., & Stickley, T. (2011). No hope without compassion: The importance of compassion in recovery-focused mental health services. *Journal of Mental Health*, *20*, 555–566.

Stern, R., & Minkoff, K. (1979). Paradoxes in programming for chronic mental patients in a community clinic. *Hospital and Community Psychiatry*, *30*, 613–617.

Stylianos, S., & Kehyayan, V. (2012). Advocacy: A critical component in a comprehensive mental health system. *American Journal of Orthopsychiatry*, *81*, 115–120.

Substance Abuse Mental Health Services Administration. (2014). *State estimates of adult mental illness from the 2011 and 2012 National Surveys on Drug Use and Health.* The NSDUH Report. February 28, 2014. Retrieved on 7/6/15.

Sullivan, K. (2000). On the efficiency of managed care plans. *Health Affairs*, *19*, 139–148.

Swanson, J. W., Van Dorn, R. A., Monahan, J., & Swartz, M. (2006). Violence and leveraged community treatment for persons with mental disorders. *American Journal of Psychiatry*, *163*, 1404–1411.

Test, M., & West, S. G. (2010). Civil commitment in the United States. *Psychiatry*, *7*(10), 30–40.

Tew, J. (2012). Recovery capital: What enables a sustainable recovery from mental health difficulties? *European Journal of Social Work*, *16*, 360–374.

Thorton, P. H., Ocasio, W., & Lounsbury, M. (2012). *The institutional logics perspective: A new approach to culture, structure and process.* Oxford: Oxford University Press.

Timmermans, S., & Berg, M. (2003). *The gold standard: The challenge of evidence based medicine and standardization in health care.* Philadelphia, PA: Temple University Press.

Tomes, N. (2011). From outsiders to insiders: The consumer-survivor movement and its impact on U.S. mental health policy. In B. Hoffman, N. Tomes, R. Grob, & M. Schlesinger (Eds.), *Patients as policy actors* (pp. 113–131). New Brunswick, NJ: Rutgers University Press.

Tomes, N., & Hoffman, B. (2011). Patients as policy actors. In B. Hoffman, N. Tomes, R. Grob, & M. Schlesinger (Eds.), *Patients as policy actors* (pp. 1–16). New Brunswick, NJ: Rutgers University Press.

U.S. Department of Health and Human Services. (1999). *Mental health: Report of the surgeon general.* Washington, DC: US Governmental Printing Office.

US Department of Justice. (2006). *Bureau of justice statistics special report: Mental health problems of prison and jail inmates.* Office of Justice Programs. September 2006, NCJ 213600.

Wales, H., & Hiday, V. (2006). PLC or TLC: Is outpatient commitment the/an answer? *International Journal of Law and Psychiatry*, *29*(6), 451–468.

Whitaker, R. (2010). *Anatomy of an epidemic: Magic bullets, psychiatric drugs, and the astonishing rise of mental illness in America.* New York, NY: Broadway Paperback (a division of Random House).

Wholey, D., Christianson, J., Draper, D., Lesser, C., & Burns, L. (2004). Embedded responses of communities to national healthcare firms. *Journal of Health and Social Behavior*, *45*, (Extra Issue), 118–135.

Wolff, N. (2002). Risk, response, and mental health policy: Learning from the experience of the United Kingdom. *Journal of Health Politics, Policy and Law*, *27*, 801–832.

Yanos, P. T., Knight, E. L., & Roe, D. (2007). Recognizing a role for structure and agency: Integrating sociological perspectives into the study of recovery from severe mental illness. In W. R. Avison, J. D. McLeod, & B. A. Bescosolido (Eds.), *Mental health, social mirror* (pp. 407–433). New York, NY: Springer Science and Business Media, LLC.

Yates, I., Holmes, G., & Priest, H. (2012). Recovery, place and community mental health services. *Journal of Mental Health*, *21*, 104–113.

PART II
COMMUNITY REINTEGRATION AND THE SOCIAL ENVIRONMENT

SOCIAL ENVIRONMENT AND MENTAL ILLNESS: THE PROGRESS AND PARADOX OF DEINSTITUTIONALIZATION

Russell K. Schutt

ABSTRACT

Purpose – *Reexamination and reinterpretation of the process of deinstitutionalization of public mental hospital inpatients.*

Methodology/approach – *A comprehensive review of related research is presented and lessons learned for the sociology of mental health are identified.*

Findings – *The processes of both institutionalization and deinstitutionalization were motivated by belief in the influence of the social environment on the course of mental illness, but while in the early 19th century the social environment of the mental hospital was seen as therapeutic, later in the 20th century the now primarily custodial social environment of large state mental hospitals was seen as iatrogenic. Nonetheless, research in both periods indicated the benefit of socially supportive environments in the hospital, while research on programs for*

50 Years after Deinstitutionalization: Mental Illness in Contemporary Communities
Advances in Medical Sociology, Volume 17, 91–118

ISSN: 1057-6290/doi:10.1108/S1057-629020160000017004

deinstitutionalized patients and for homeless persons indicated the value of comparable features in community programs.

Research limitations/implications – *While the process of deinstitutionalization is largely concluded, research should focus on identifying features of the social environment that can maximize rehabilitation.*

Practical implications – *The debate over the merits of hospital-based and community-based mental health services is misplaced; policies should instead focus on the alternatives for providing socially supportive environments. Deinstitutionalization in the absence of socially supportive programs has been associated with increased rates of homelessness and incarceration among those most chronically ill.*

Originality/value – *A comprehensive analysis of deinstitutionalization that highlights flaws in prior sociological perspectives and charts a new direction for scholarship.*

Keywords: Deinstitutionalization; mental health; mental health services; social environment

On May 8, 1889, Vincent Van Gogh admitted himself to the mental asylum near Saint-Rémy-de-Provence. More a struggling artist at the time than the renowned French post-Impressionist he became posthumously, Van Gogh's efforts to develop an artists' community in southern France had failed – most dramatically after cutting off his own ear during an argument with roommate Paul Gauguin – and local townspeople, tired of his bizarre and unpredictable behavior, petitioned for his removal. Although Van Gogh had previously experienced periods of severe depression and apparent psychosis, at this low point he had decided the asylum walls would protect him as he looked forward to "a new life" (Mullins, 2015, p. 32). After nine months of "treatment" that included a controlled diet, regular doses of bromide, twice weekly baths, and many periods of calm punctuated by four more mental breakdowns – as well as 150 paintings, Van Gogh felt he had recovered and left the asylum, but then committed suicide two months later (Mullins, 2015).

The meaning of community, asylum, preferences, mental illness, each of the concepts required for understanding deinstitutionalization's sources, processes, and outcomes are represented in the Van Gogh story. Of course the story is distant in time and place and remarkable only because of the artistic legacy, but it is precisely for this reason that it is a useful starting point for developing a comprehensive understanding of deinstitutionalization. I will review the reasons for and process of development of state psychiatric hospitals, the evidence of this strategy's failure, and the process and results of the subsequent deinstitutionalization. I will focus particular attention on the social context in which these policies developed and the evidence of their impact. I will then suggest lessons learned and propose further steps for sociological research and theory about the delivery of mental health care.

THE DEVELOPMENT OF PUBLIC MENTAL HOSPITALS

Community-based responses to persons with serious mental illness were a cruel parody of the concept of "care" in the American colonies and the early United States. Although confinement in basements and backyard shacks, jails, workhouses, and almshouses may have been more humane than the alternative of community expulsion – not to mention the Middle Ages "ships of fools" that had once sailed between European ports, it is only by recognizing such practices as reflecting prevailing misconceptions of mental illness as possession by the devil, divine punishment, or becoming a beast that we can avoid seeing our forebears as other than morally depraved (Talbott, 1978, pp. 14–15). In the 1839 words of the Pennsylvania Legislature:

> It has been well said that were a system now to be devised, whose express object it should be to drive every victim of insanity beyond the limits of hope, it would scarcely be in the power of a perverse ingenuity to suggest one more infallible than that, which for so many years has been in practical operation among us. (p. 12)

Encouraged by Enlightenment ideals and reformist proselytizing, a new approach emerged early in the 19th century. Phillippe Pinel's celebrated removal (or support for the removal) of chains from mentally ill inmates in France and the success of the Quaker's York Retreat in England demonstrated the value of what came to be called "moral treatment" (simply meaning psychologically oriented treatment, in the original French) and the importance of the social environment for understanding both causes of and cures for mental illness (Grob, 1994, p. 27). In the United States, proponents of moral treatment believed that increasing geographic and social mobility, indulgent families, economic pressures, and prolonged schooling had created a stressful and disordered environment that caused insanity, and so reasoned that "a setting which eliminated the irritants could restore the insane to health" (Rothman, 1990, pp. 115–127, 129). New York State's Legislature adopted this approach in 1856:

> To diminish lunacy ... relief must be of a special nature .... Institutions ... which, by their order and quiet, may afford moral treatment, while intelligent medical direction should control their operation. (p. 16)

Asylums in tranquil rural settings would replace the "irritants" of prior family and community life with a calm, disciplined – but nonpunitive – and regular routine including daily physical labor, educational lectures and libraries, close interpersonal ties to staff, and a kindly, paternalistic relationship with the superintendent (Grob, 1973, pp. 176–180; Rothman, 1990, pp. 134–149). "Respect them," urged one superintendent, "and they will respect themselves" (Grob, 1973, p. 180). Even though the proponents of moral treatment viewed its primary goal as renewed conformity to social norms and the process of treatment as learning to internalize societal values (Grob, 1994, p. 27) – rather than patient empowerment as it is understood today – Van Gogh's decision to seek solace in such a calm and controlled environment is understandable.

Seeking to extend their influence and standardize their methods, hospital superintendents formed in 1844 a professional association – the Association of Medical Superintendents of American Institutions for the Insane – and supported the national campaign led by Dorothea Dix to make humane, hospital-based care the norm for both indigent and affluent persons with serious mental illness (Grob, 1994, p. 39; Osborn, 2009). As a result, 140 new asylums were constructed between 1840 and 1870 (Osborn, 2009), with public mental hospitals founded in 28 of the then 33 states by 1870, and the percentage of mentally ill persons receiving care in psychiatric hospitals rose from 15% in 1840 to 70% by 1890 (Grob, 1973, pp. 98–105; Segal & Aviram, 1978; Talbott, 1978, pp. 15–20). A newspaper article heralding the expansion of Worcester State Hospital in Massachusetts captured the supportive cultural milieu (Grob, 1973):

> We like the doctrine, that the State is the parent of the people. It is a genuine part of republicanism. (p. 111)

Hortatory calls for new mental hospitals often relied on easily impugned claims of 80–100% rates of cure, but an 1876 article by Pliny Earle, a contrarian asylum superintendent, largely discredited the empirical basis for these claims (Torrey & Miller, 2007, pp. 258–259). Nonetheless, one careful study with a long-term follow-up identified 58% of former inpatients in one hospital as permanently cured and another estimated that two-thirds of inpatients recovered in hospitals using moral treatment methods, while in decent custodial hospitals only one-third recovered spontaneously (Grob, 1973, pp. 181–182). A supportive social environment seemed to make a difference.

THE FAILURE OF PUBLIC MENTAL HOSPITALS

But the new hospital system was soon a victim of its own success. Rapid population growth in the United States and growing willingness of state governments to fund public hospitals for the indigent led to growth so rapid that the ability to provide even a semblance of moral treatment was eviscerated. The size of state mental hospitals and the heterogeneity and chronicity of those institutionalized rose rapidly in the second half of the 19th century. Patients arrived with illnesses ranging from dementia and syphilis to alcoholism and criminal psychopathy, from increasingly diverse and often foreign social backgrounds. Between 1850 and 1890, the population of the United States grew by a factor of 3.7, while the mental hospital population grew by a factor of 29 (Segal & Aviram, 1978). By 1870, state hospitals had an average census of 400–1,000 – far in excess of the 200–250 patients considered to be the upper limit for maintaining an environment conducive to moral treatment (Grob, 1973, pp. 181–182, 188–193, 322–323). By 1909, the doctor/patient ratio in state hospitals was 500:1 and the nurse/patient ratio was 1,320:1 (Osborn, 2009).

The asylum model developed by Superintendent Dr. Thomas Kirkbride at the Pennsylvania Hospital for the Insane (1841–1883) was widely adopted. It emphasized imposing architecture, beautiful grounds, and staff compassion – but also intensive security, physical regimentation, and manual labor (Chapin, 1898; Osborn, 2009, pp. 222–225). A decentralized model of care developed in Gheel, Belgium to enhance community integration was rejected by American superintendents as giving patients too much liberty (Grob, 1994, pp. 110–112). Bureaucratization seemed the only alternative for hospital management and custodial care became its primary service (Rothman, 1990, pp. 265–285). "At the least, the asylum would shield society from disorder and contamination" (Rothman, 1990, p. 286). While the community of Saint-Rémy-de-Provence may still have seen such a hospital as a desirable placement for a troubled member like Van Gogh, it is unlikely that anyone so troubled would have sought admission.

The status quo of custodial care prevailed and the inpatient count continued to increase until the second half of the 20th century (Torrey & Miller, 2007, p. 289). With its concentration of largely poor, often immigrant, and usually chronically ill patients, and an increasing fraction of elderly demented patients, the state hospital population was isolated from and of little interest to the larger community; a reflection of problems rather than a means for their solution (Grob, 1994, pp. 118–119). The profession of psychiatry shifted its attention away from what seemed the fruitless task of curing inpatients to focus on those with psychiatric disorders in the community (Grob, 1994, pp. 135–145). Leaders of the developing medical specialty of neurology impugned the efficacy of asylums and the integrity of their superintendents – those "shallow pretenders and ignorant indifferentists" (an 1878 speech quoted in Torrey & Miller, 2007, p. 263).

Hopes for asylum cures were largely abandoned as support for social Darwinism increased in the early decades of the 20th century, with 30 states adopting sterilization laws as a means to supposedly eliminate insanity from the gene pool (Dowdall, 1996, p. 40; Grob, 1994, pp. 159–162). Neither a consumer-led "mental hygiene movement" in the early part of the century nor an AMA-sponsored exposé of state hospitals in the 1930s generated enough concern to increase funding and alter policy (Grob, 1994, pp. 152–158; Johnson, 1990, p. 14, 18–19).

It took the major social disruptions of the Second World War to renew social concern with mental illness, interrupt the state hospital status quo, and create a turning point in the treatment of serious mental illness (Grob, 1991, pp. 5–23; Sareyan, 1994). The wartime draft highlighted the prevalence of mental illness when the Army rejected 17% of potential draftees for psychiatric reasons (similar to its experience in World War I), while subsequent military service made it apparent that even this percent was an underestimate: 1.1 million men were hospitalized during the war for neuropsychiatric conditions that often seemed to have antedated the war – in spite of the screening.

The extreme stress of warfare itself drew attention to the link between the social environment and mental illness (Grob, 1994, p. 191; Talbott, 1978, pp. 20–25). Even soldiers who entered service in good mental health could struggle with psychological reactions to traumatic combat experience. Military psychologists also learned that soldiers were more likely to recover, and to recover quickly, when they received immediate treatment for these traumatic stress reactions near their units, rather than in remote hospitals where they were isolated and disengaged. Engagement in a meaningful social community mattered.

The mobilization for World War II also had an indirect impact on mental health services policy that was even more important, albeit unanticipated. Three thousand Conscientious Objectors were assigned to state psychiatric hospitals for their alternative service during the war and as a result were exposed to conditions that they found appalling (Sareyan, 1994, p. 15). These religious, educated men did not keep their reactions to themselves; their experiences and the reports they compiled led to an exposé in *Life* magazine and many newspaper articles during the war; to a book, *Out of Sight, Out of Mind*, immediately after the war (Sareyan, 1994, pp. 15–20, 65–76); and to organized efforts to destigmatize mental illness and reform care of the mentally ill (Sareyan, 1994). The Mental Hygiene Program organized by the COs was expanded into the National Mental Health Foundation in 1946, which merged in 1950 into the new National Association for Mental Health (Sareyan, 1994, p. 147, 208). Publication of journalist Albert Deutsch's (1948) *The Shame of the States* and the 1946 release of Mary Jane Ward's *The Snake Pit* – one of that year's five most popular movies – sustained this renewed attention and strengthened popular support for institutional change (Grob, 1991, pp. 14–43, 70–92). The burgeoning subdiscipline of social psychiatry also renewed attention to social factors (Talbott, 1978, pp. 24–25).

These intense pressures for change generated calls for both reform and abolition of the state hospital system. Calls for reform led initially to some impressive efforts. The Veterans Administration expanded hospital facilities for psychiatric care (spending by 1960 $12 per patient per day in psychiatric wards, compared to $4 per patient in state and local psychiatric hospitals) (Grob, 1991, pp. 44–69). The American Psychiatric Association began a hospital standards program (Grob, 1991, pp. 80–81). Some hospitals developed "milieu therapies" and group therapy approaches, and some encouraged "open-door" relations with the surrounding community and close connections with community-based services (Grob, 1991, pp. 139–146, 157–180, 1994, pp. 227–228; Talbott, 1978, pp. 24–25). Research increased about the "treatment environment" on hospital wards (Moos, 1974). The Russell Sage Foundation funded an experiment at three Boston-area psychiatric hospitals to test the effect of developing close community relations and a supportive milieu, without seclusion or restraint and including what were considered to be appropriate medical treatments. The results included much higher rates of return to the community across diagnostic categories and so led to recommendations for improvements in the hospital environment (Greenblatt, 1955, p. 237, 424). It seemed possible that the compelling model of moral treatment could be improved considerably on a foundation of new research and with a less paternalistic, more empowering approach.

THE PROCESS OF DEINSTITUTIONALIZATION

But the possibility of and vision for reform was overwhelmed by growing calls for abolition (Ahmed & Plog, 1976; Okin, 1983). Sociologist Goffman's (1961) ethnography of a state mental hospital provided a compelling explanation of patient behavior as an unavoidable adaptation to the social expectations of this "total institution." The picture that Goffman painted from his vantage point within an asylum's walls was that of patients adapting as best they could to staff and routines that were meant to manage, but not to treat.

> Quiet, obedient behavior leads to the patient's promotion in the ward system; obstreperous, untidy behavior to demotion. (p. 361) A refraction of conduct thus occurs, the walls of the institution acting like a thick and faulted prism. (p. 360)

To many readers of *Asylums*, defending such a system would seem at best to disregard human potential; at worst, to violate the Hippocratic oath. More radical critiques questioned the concept of mental illness and thus the legitimacy of psychiatry itself (Grob, 1994, pp. 271–273).

Any nascent interest in hospital reform that remained was swept aside by a budget-breaking 226% rise in state mental health expenditures from 1939 to 1949 (compared to an increase in the CPI of 71%) and growing interest in community-based approaches (Johnson, 1990, p. 90). The National Mental Health Act of 1946 founded the National Institute of Mental Health with an interdisciplinary research mission including the behavioral and social sciences and goals of preventing mental illness and encouraging mental health, not treatment of chronic mental illness (Grob, 1991, pp. 44–69). Increasing support in the American Psychiatric Association for a psychodynamic orientation and growing concern with social issues led its president in 1953 to call for reexamining the functioning of state hospitals and then, in 1958, to declare that state hospitals were "rapidly becoming obsolete" (Grob, 1994, p. 232). Congress established in 1955 a Joint Commission on Mental Illness and Health that, in its 1961 report, *Action for Mental Health*, reported 80% of state hospitals offered only custodial care and then recommended severe limits on the size and proliferation of hospitals in addition to a focus on active treatment (Grob,

1994, pp. 241–261). President Kennedy's subsequent 1963 Presidential Address on Mental Illness and Mental Retardation led to the Community Mental Health Centers Act of 1963 and a goal of reducing the long-term hospital population by 50% within 10–20 years (Grob, 1991, pp. 181–208; Kramer, 1977, p. 2; Mechanic & Rochefort, 1990, p. 302; Talbott, 1978, pp. 28–29). The civil rights movement in the 1960s and 1970s stimulated a patient rights movement that challenged the legitimacy of involuntary treatment, emphasized the right to adequate treatment, and urged more respect for patient preferences (Grob, 1994, pp. 274–275; Mollica, 1983; Robitscher, 1976, p. 143; Talbott, 1978, pp. 33–34).

Discovery of new psychotropic medications added another critical incentive to deinstitutionalize. Chlorpromazine (1954) and reserpine (1953) relieved the psychotic symptoms of some patients and resulted in more sedated behavior on hospital wards, while antidepressants (1956) reduced the distress of many with affective disorders. While the immediate effect of these medications was to facilitate inpatient management, they also made evident a much greater potential for patient success after discharge (Grob, 1991, pp. 146–156). The other pressures for deinstitutionalization in the United States during this period ensured that these drugs would be touted as justification for opening the asylum doors, even while some European countries maintained high rates of institutional treatment in spite of widespread use of psychotropic medication (Mechanic & Rochefort, 1990, pp. 314–315).

These cultural, medical, fiscal, and policy pressures explain why the state hospital census began to decline in 1955, but it was not until new programs allowed states to shift much of the financial burden of care to the federal government that the inpatient count dropped rapidly (Mechanic & Rochefort, 1990, pp. 310–11). Begun in 1965, Medicaid allowed states to transfer elderly state hospital patients (about one-third of the total) to nursing homes with federal funding; then in 1974, the implementation of Social Security Income (SSI) for indigent disabled persons facilitated further decline in the state hospital population (Johnson, 1990, pp. 94–99). While from 1955 to 1965 the public hospital population declined only by 1.75% per year, the annual rate accelerated to 8.6% between 1965 and 1975, with a total 80% decline from the 1955 peak (Mechanic & Rochefort, 1990, pp. 302–305). Although the rate of decline slowed after 1980, it continued through 2010 (Torrey, Fuller, Geller, Jacobs, & Ragosta, 2012, p. 24).

The change is clearer when standardized for population size. The rate of 339 per 100,000 hospitalized in state mental institutions in 1955 dropped

91% by the early 1990s to 31 per 100,000 (Bachrach, 1999) and by 2010 to just 14.0 (Torrey et al., 2012) (Fig. 1). The rate of admissions to state and county hospitals per 100,000 civilian population dropped from 139 in 1986 to 80 in 2002, although it then increased slightly to 89 in 2004 (National Center for Health Statistics [NCHS], 2009, Table 97). Even by 1994, Torrey (1997) projected that 92% of the people who would have been living in public psychiatric hospitals on any given day in that year were not doing so after deinstitutionalization; this rate declines to 84% if those in psychiatric beds in general hospitals and community mental health centers are included as hospitalized, but even with this adjustment the 1963 Community Mental Health Center Act's goal of a 50% reduction seems almost laughably conservative. Deinstitutionalization became the new reality.

Although the downward trend decelerated, other changes indicated an accelerating crisis of insufficient alternative placements for persons suffering from chronic mental illness. From 1956 to 1965 – the first phase of the deinstitutionalization process – it was primarily the less impaired long-term residents and some of those newly admitted who were transferred to alternative settings, but between 1966 and 1975 there were relatively

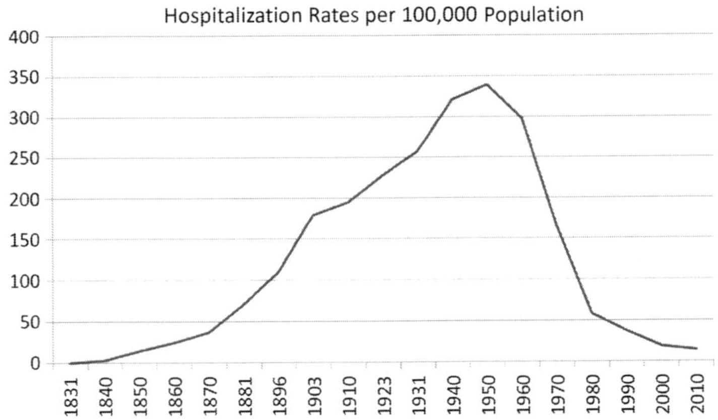

Fig. 1. Public Mental Hospital Patients, 1831–2010. *Sources*: Torrey et al. (2012). Data for 1831–1980 taken from Stroup and Manderscheid (1988). Data was obtained from the National Association of State Mental Health Program Directors (NASMHPD) Research Institute in Alexandria, Virginia. Collected in early 2012, data included the number of patients on January 1, 2010. 2010 census numbers were used to develop bed population rates per population.

indiscriminate massive diversions and patient discharges. Inpatient episodes did not begin to decline until 1965, but then fell 44% by 1983. The median length of stay declined by 43% (41–23 days) from 1970 to 1980 and the number of inpatient beds per 100,000 population dropped by 72% (1970–1984). It was not until after 1986 that the number of state and county mental hospitals themselves began to decline, but state hospital budgets then decreased dramatically and 18% of state hospitals were closed or in the process of closing (McGrew, Wright, & Pescosolido, 1999; Mechanic & Rochefort, 1990, pp. 307–309; Witkin, Atay, & Manderscheid, 1996). The destination of those discharged also changed as the proportion that were chronically ill increased: in two studies in New York, 66% of those discharged in the mid-1960s returned to their families, but in 1975 only 23% did so (Johnson, 1990, pp. 73–75).

The declining role of state hospitals was also reflected in increasing use of community-based services. The percentage of all psychiatric treatment episodes provided in state hospitals dropped from 49% in 1955 to just 9% in 1977. In 1977, community mental health centers already accounted for 32% of all treatment episodes; by 1993, expenditures for community mental health services exceeded those for state mental hospital inpatient services (McGrew et al., 1999; Mollica, 1983).

In spite of this resource shift, the demand created by the rapidly increasing number of chronically mentally ill patients discharged from state hospitals – or not being admitted in the first place – was not matched by a corresponding increase in the supply of alternative placements. There were four problems: (1) Not enough of the community mental health centers envisioned by the CMHC Act of 1963 were built. By 1989, 786 CMHCs had been opened, but 2,400 would have been needed to meet the expectations of the 1963 CMHC Act (Grob, 1991, pp. 293–272; Mechanic & Rochefort, 1990, pp. 304–305). (2) Most CMHCs, like the 1963 Act itself, did not focus on services for the seriously and chronically mentally ill population (Grob, 1991, pp. 293–272; 1994, pp. 279–280). Many CMHCs offered psychotherapy for diverse mental health problems to the "worried well" and abjured treating former hospital patients (Grob, 1994, pp. 213, 263–264). Later, younger, impoverished minorities and community members with substance abuse problems who would not have been sent to state hospitals in previous years became their primary concern (Grob, 1991, pp. 293–272; Mechanic & Rochefort, 1990, p. 313). (3) Affordable residential opportunities were vanishing in many cities as urban renewal progressed through the 1970s. Boston lost more than 90% of its single room occupancy (SRO) lodgings and similar declines occurred nationally, even as welfare benefits were reduced dramatically for impoverished able-bodied men (Burt, 1992, p. 33; Jencks, 1994, pp. 61–74; Rossi, 1989, p. 192; Schutt, 2011a, p. 50). (4) Clinicians found that younger persons suffering from severe mental illness – "young adult chronics" – often resisted diagnosis as mentally ill, abused alcohol and drugs, and were uncooperative with treatment (Grob, 1995; Mechanic & Rochefort, 1990, p. 316). Vincent Van Gogh's willingness to seek treatment, whatever the foundation, seemed increasingly anachronistic.

OUTCOMES OF DEINSTITUTIONALIZATION

Research on the fate of discharged patients indicated both the potential for deinstitutionalization and the challenges it created. A 1982 transitions program that emphasized training in social skills and connections to local CMHCs succeeded in reducing hospital use by about three-quarters and achieved an acceptable quality of life for patients after discharge (Sullivan, 1999). A study of patients after closing a large state hospital in Indiana found generally improved patient functioning, quality of life, and cost savings for those placed in the community (McGrew et al., 1999). Another study after closure of a Massachusetts hospital found that 90% of patients liked their new community placements better than the hospital (Greenblatt & Glazier, 1976, p. 129). Former inpatients discharged after further hospital closings in Massachusetts, and their family members, reported generally positive results (Upshur et al., 1997).

By contrast, many studies focusing specifically on residential outcomes and community functioning reached less favorable conclusions (McGrew et al., 1999). In a seven year study of 55 former patients from Boston State Hospital, Scheper-Hughes found that all continued to function entirely within the confines of the mental health system, including occasional hospitalizations, and that there had not been "a single staff-supported graduation into independent community living" (Mollica, 1983, p. 370). In a four-year follow-up study, three-quarters of 46 inpatients discharged from Vermont State Hospital to community mental health services after 1989 were still in structured community housing at the time of the follow-up, compared to just one expatient who had remained in independent housing for more than one year; moreover, 87% had been rehospitalized at some point and their social contacts were primarily case managers and other staff. "Isolation, separation, stigma-related loneliness, and pervasive hard times were the dominant themes" and few expressed "even a remote interest in work" (Dewees, Pulice, & McCormick, 1996, pp. 1091–1092). Estroff (1981, pp. 188–189) found that living in a community residence did not mean integration in the community for most clients in Wisconsin's post-hospital support program. Elderly patients experienced 2–3 times more deaths and considerable deterioration after relocation from one hospital (Marlowe, 1976), although in another study there had been no increase in mortality (Markson & Cumming, 1976).

This evidence of negative outcomes soon after the shift to community living can now be balanced with more positive outcomes after a longer-term follow-up period and more attention to services delivered in the community. The multidisciplinary service teams of the highly regarded Program for Assertive Community Treatment (PACT) succeeded in keeping 80–85% of traditional patients out of the state mental hospital, although more intensive services up to and including hospitalization were required for the rest (Monroe-DeVita, & Mohatt, 1999, p. 93). One 20–25 year follow-up of 269 persons who had been severely ill at the time of their release from Vermont's state hospital found that 55% (of the two-thirds who were still alive) evinced slight to no impairment in overall function and three-quarters led a "moderate to very full life" (Harding, Brooks, Ashikaga, Strauss, & Breier, 1987, p. 723). These positive outcomes improved considerably on an earlier 5–10 year outcome study of the same deinstitutionalized patients, when the researchers had concluded that successful outcomes required intensive service provision and substantial contact with rehabilitation workers (Harding et al., 1987, p. 720). In Saskatchewan, research on the effects of closing a psychiatric hospital indicated that care could be shifted completely to the community if the hospital census was reduced gradually through declining admissions and accompanied by an extensive preparatory rehabilitation program for inpatients, as well as careful planning for assimilation into home communities (LaFave, Grunberg, Woodhouse, & Barrington, 1976, p. 190). In Australia, a two-year study of deinstitutionalized patients in a well-staffed and carefully designed program found improved psychiatric symptoms and life satisfaction as former patients were able to function more independently from staff, self-confidence and relations with community members also increased (Newton, Rosen, Tennant, & Hobbs, 2001, p. 160). A cross-sectional study of deinstitutionalized clubhouse members in New Jersey found that vocational services and use of an empowerment approach were associated with more life satisfaction (Rosenfield, 1992, pp. 310–311).

Patient outcomes after deinstitutionalization thus could be largely positive when support in the community was intensive, when the setting provided a supportive cultural tradition and a more comprehensive care system, and when stabilization efforts had decades to have an effect. It is clear that the mixed research outcomes reflect in part the differing needs of different patients; those with less chronic psychiatric problems or who responded more readily to currently available drug treatment fared much better after deinstitutionalization. It is also clear that some patients with severe and chronic mental illness recover over the course of decades and that the quality of services and community supports can alter the likelihood of recovery (Green et al., 2013; Harding et al., 1987). Many persons who formerly were institutionalized or would have been institutionalized in the past are more satisfied with their lives as a result of deinstitutionalization and some are productively employed and live independently (Bachrach, 1999, p. 96).

LONG-TERM CONSEQUENCES OF DEINSTITUTIONALIZATION

Although decentralized delivery of community-based mental health services clearly was feasible, its success was contingent on being able to engage potentially high cost patients with effective interventions that could maintain their health and improve their quality of life (Taube & Goldman, 1989, p. 155). Inadequate community-based care arrangements combined with the loss of much low-cost housing in the inner city instead resulted in the failure of many of those who formerly would have been institutionalized to find stable community living arrangements (Schutt, 2011a, p. 50). Homelessness and incarceration were too often the result (Bassuk & Lamb, 1986; Lamb, 1984; Schutt, 2011a, pp. 51–52).

By the mid-1990s, the lifetime risk of homelessness among persons hospitalized with a psychotic disorder for the first time was five times that for the general population (Herman, Susser, Jandorf, Lavelle, & Bromet, 1998). Almost one in five state hospital patients in the New York City area had been homeless in the preceding three months and more than one-quarter had been homeless at some prior time (Susser, Lin, & Conover, 1991). Among 10,340 adult public mental health patients who had received treatment at least once for schizophrenia, bipolar disorder or major depression in fiscal year 1999–2000, 15% had been homeless within the preceding year (Folsom et al., 2005, p. 372). Surveys of the adult homeless population indicated that between one-quarter and more than half had significant psychiatric symptoms (Kahn, Hannah, Hinkin, & Montgomery, 1987; Mechanic & Rochefort, 1990, p. 317). Homeless persons surveyed in Los Angeles had been homeless nearly twice as long if they had previously been hospitalized for psychiatric problems (Gelberg, Linn, & Leake, 1988).

The first estimates of serious mental illness among inmates of jails and prisons ranged from 6% to 15% after deinstitutionalization began in earnest, with methods ranging from diagnostic interviews to surveys of jail directors (Guy, Platt, Zwerling, & Bullock, 1985; James, Gregory, Jones, & Rundell, 1980; Jemelka, Trupin, & Chiles, 1989; Steadman, Fabisiak, Dvoskin, & Holohean, 1987; Teplin, 1990; Whitmer, 1980). A Los Angeles study of homeless persons with a history of psychiatric hospitalization found that three-quarters had been arrested at some time (Gelberg et al., 1988). Among former mental hospital patients with a diagnosis of schizophrenia, bipolar illness, or major depressive disorder who were discharged from a state hospital in Ohio in 1985, one-third were arrested and jailed within six months (Belcher, 1988). A recent Bureau of Justice Statistics report (James & Glaze, 2006) identified more than half of inmates in federal and state prisons and local jails as having symptoms of mental illness within the past year, using DSM-IV criteria or recent clinical diagnosis or treatment. A review of studies across 12 western countries involving 23,000 inmates indicated rates of psychotic disorders and major depression of 2–4 times that of the general population, and a rate of antisocial personality disorder that is 10 times higher among inmates than in the general population (Fazel & Danesh, 2002). Current estimates still vary widely due to differences in measurement (affecting particularly cross-national estimates of antisocial personality disorder), timing in relation to incarceration, participation rate, and also the ability of most studies to distinguish mental disorders that preceded imprisonment from those emerging as a result of it (Andersen, 2004).

Research indicates a link between deinstitutionalization and the prevalence of mental illness among prisoners and inmates. In a sample of 81 U.S. cities with a population greater than 50,000, public psychiatric hospital capacity was associated inversely with rates of crime and arrest (Markowitz, 2006). Torrey and Miller's (2007) review of multiple studies supports a conclusion that the proportion of inmates in jails and prisons increased as a result of deinstitutionalization and that it has been common in some jurisdictions to jail seriously mentally ill persons because of noncriminal aberrant public behavior related to their illness or simply as a means to provide shelter and food. Yet upon release, former inmates with mental illness or addiction are less socially integrated, have less secure housing and achieve lower employment levels than others (Western, Braga, Davis, & Sirois, 2015).

For seriously mentally ill persons who receive housing after hospital discharge or homelessness, social integration is a key factor in achieving greater residential stability and quality of life. Graduates of an experimental program in independent living had much larger social networks and reciprocal relationships, as well as more contact with voluntary social groups and less use of mental health services than a comparison group; they also worked more and were hospitalized less (Pilisuk, 2001). Residents in housing providing more informal staff-resident interaction and more social skills training were more integrated in their communities (Kruzich, 1985). Mutually beneficial peer relationships reduced the likelihood of becoming passive service recipients (Weinberg & Marlowe, 1983).

The most compelling evidence for the importance of social engagement comes from the only randomized trial of group homes compared to independent apartments for homeless persons with serious mental illness, funded by the National Institute of Mental Health and conducted by Goldfinger, Schutt, Seidman, and others at the Massachusetts Mental Health Center. The risk of housing loss was higher during the project for participants who were randomized to independent living with case management support and access to other mental health services (35%) rather than group homes with equivalent case management support and service access (20%) (Fig. 2). In a 20-year follow-up after their initial housing placement, the cumulative rate of housing loss rose to almost 60% of those originally assigned to independent apartments (for the three-quarters of project participants having long-term housing records), compared to 33% of those initially assigned to the group homes, in spite of the continuing use of case managers for all (Schutt, 2011a, p. 247).

Qualitative data from case managers indicated that residents who retained their housing during the project tended to have supportive social ties with others, while those who lost housing did not (Schutt, 2011a, p. 246). Analysis of quantitative data indicated a difference in the individual-level predictors of housing loss for those assigned to group and independent housing. For participants randomized to independent housing, being African-American (the only minority group represented in the project) was strongly associated with likelihood of housing loss, as was a lifetime diagnosis of substance abuse (Table 1). Among those randomized to group housing, however, strength of preference to live independently was the only

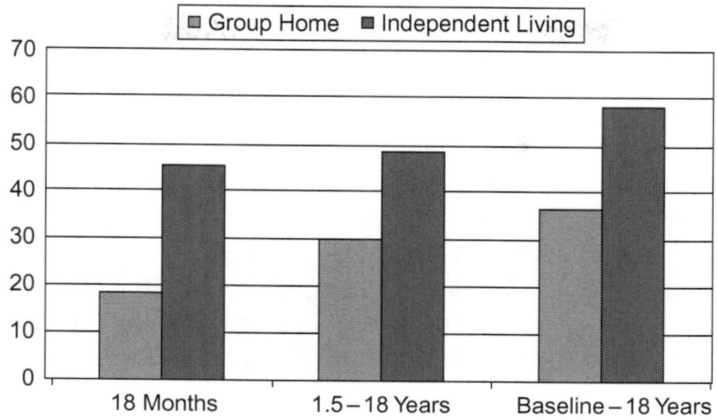

Fig. 2. Any Homelessness by Housing Type and Follow-Up. *Source*: Based on Schutt (2011a, p. 247) (only data for 75 project participants who appeared in Department of Mental Health housing records). *Notes*: 18 months: From baseline to end of randomized trial of housing types; 1.5–18 years: From project end at 18 months to end of housing records; Baseline–18 years: From baseline to end of housing records.

Table 1. Regression Analysis of Logged Days Homeless, in McKinney Project.[a]

Variable	Total[b]	Group	Independent
Independent apartment	.22*	–	–
Minority	.21*	.01	.48***
Age	.04	−.00	.12
Female	.14	.12	.14
Education	.13	.06	.19
Schizophrenia or SchizAff	.04	.03	−.03
Lifetime substance abuse	.29**	.26	.44**
Prefers independent living	.19*	.34**	−.00
Clinician recommends group	.34***	.33*	.45**
R^b	.31	.30	.44
N	107	59	48

Source: Schutt (2011a, p. 247).
[a]Eighteen-month period.
[b]Beta coefficients.
*$p < .05$; **$p < .01$; ***$p < .001$.

other individual-level predictor of housing loss. In other words, living in a staffed group home reduced the overall risk of housing loss as well as the additional risk due to being a member of a minority group or a substance abuser, but it increased the risk of housing loss for those who had been most eager to live independently at the time they were placed in housing. Overall, living in a group home reduced the variance explained in housing loss by individuals' characteristics by one-third compared to the variance explained by individuals' characteristics for those living in an independent apartment (from .44 to .30). Nonetheless, those participants who clinicians had rated at baseline as most in need of a staffed, group home subsequently proved to be more at risk of housing loss no matter which type of housing they received.

Group living also was associated with cognitive gains in executive functioning, while living independently was associated with cognitive losses (Fig. 3). These differences were maintained 18 months after the project ended, but they did not occur for those diagnosed with a lifetime history of substance abuse. Thus, this risk factor that increased housing loss among

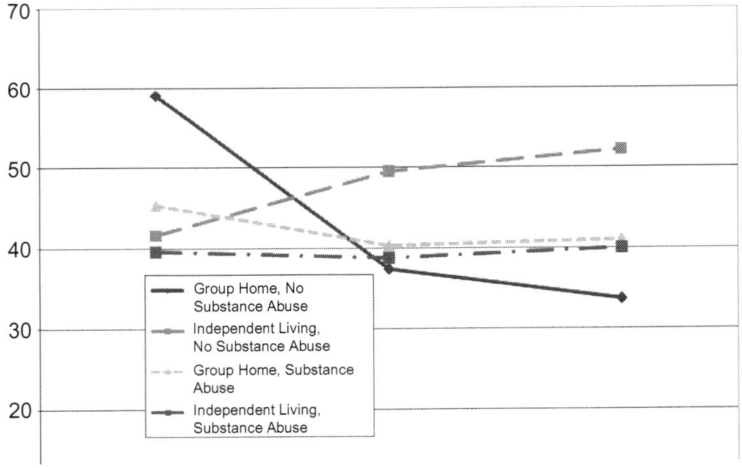

Fig. 3. Executive Functioning (total perseverations, Wisconsin Card Sort (higher scores indicate more impairment)) by Housing Type, Substance Abuse, and Follow-Up. *Source*: Based on Caplan, Schutt, Turner, Goldfinger, and Seidman (2006, p. 82). *Notes*: Neuropsychological Functioning Assessment Points: Time 1: Project baseline. Time 2: Project end at 18 months after baseline. Time 3: 36 months after baseline.

those living independently also interfered with cognitive benefit from group living.

The apparent benefits of living in group housing would be compelling evidence for mental health policies favoring such placements were it not for a widespread preference for independent living. Between 50% and 90% of mental health service consumers say that they prefer independent living (Holley et al., 1998; Keck, 1990; Neubauer, 1993; Schutt, 2011b; Tanzman, 1993; Yeich & Mowbray, 1994). The drive to normalize residential arrangements through independent living placements in response to consumer preferences can thus undermine the development of social group support among persons with serious mental illness (Mandiberg, 1999). As a result, rates of housing loss among formerly homeless persons diagnosed with severe mental illness are likely to be as high as 40–50% within 5–20 years after placement in independent apartments without supportive social ties or very intensive services (Lipton, Siegel, Hannigen, Samuels, & Baker, 2000; Wong et al., 2006, pp. 39–40).

Even for those at the furthest remove from hospital care, the paradox apparent through the deinstitutionalization process appeared. The most effective programs that enhanced the social environment were more difficult to implement, in part due to disinterest in services or social contact by the intended beneficiaries.

DISCUSSION

With mixed research findings and a perennial gap between resources and needs, controversy has erupted repeatedly about the propriety of the deinstitutionalization process and the feasibility of the goal itself (Mendel, 1976; Rachlin, 1976). Governor Reagan's 1973 plan to close all mental hospitals in California was terminated after public and legislative opposition (Greenblatt, 1976, pp. 19–20). A decade later, Goldman, Taube, Regier, and Witkin (1983, p. 296) concluded that "we have learned that simply closing the state mental hospital will neither replace its function nor change the social and historical forces that have preserved it." At the start of the next decade, medical sociologist David Mechanic declared that "deinstitutionalization remains an unfulfilled promise" that some considered to be "one of the era's most stunning public policy failures" (Mechanic & Rochefort, 1990, p. 302, 324), while at its conclusion sociologist Bachrach (1999, pp. 15–17) asked whether it is "time to reinstate our state mental hospitals as the central loci in our system of care" because they "may well be the only facilities that provide even the most minimal care and asylum to persons in grave need of assistance."

Even the most ardent proponents of a community-based mental health system that "will totally obviate any need for the state hospital" recognized that a solution must first be found "for patients who are too debilitated medically or psychiatrically or too violent to be allowed into the decentralized system" (Mollica, 1983, p. 368); those who "do not take their medicine, they do not seek help, they do not show up for appointments, they are lost in the anonymity of the community" (Robitscher, 1976, p. 164). Yet no such solution was in place by the time deinstitutionalization began in earnest.

Deinstitutionalization is thus a policy that succeeded in its proximate objective but failed in its ultimate goal. Although the process required much more time and encountered many more difficulties than initially anticipated, deinstitutionalization succeeded in reducing dramatically the use of public mental hospitals for persons diagnosed with chronic mental illness. In this achievement, deinstitutionalization can rightfully be considered as one of the most important and successful intentional public policy changes in United States history. Both the numbers affected and the practices changed are, in retrospect, remarkable. But in terms of what can arguably be considered its ultimate goal – creating a more humane and effective mental health system for those reliant on public resources – this success has been overshadowed by unintended effects that worsened conditions for many of those most in need.

In spite of this conflicted history and these disparate results, the American experience with institutionalization and deinstitutionalization over more than two centuries can yield compelling lessons about the treatment of mental illness and the perspectives of social science. After reviewing these lessons, I will suggest the most productive directions they suggest for sociological theory and research.

Early public and professional enthusiasm for psychiatric institutions as well as later decisions to seek their demise reflected certainty in the power of the social environment to shape mental health and functioning. In the first half of the 19th century, it was widely felt that a controlled social environment was needed to ameliorate the psychic effects of an increasingly inchoate community environment. In the second half of the 20th century, it was this controlled social environment – in a shockingly diminished form – that was felt to threaten mental health, while the social environment in the larger community was seen to have curative potential. Both perspectives, no matter how inapposite on their face, were supported by empirical evidence available at the time: Hospitals offering a "moral treatment" environment seemed beneficial for patients, while their much expanded progeny offering only custodial care in a demeaning social environment seemed quite harmful.

This fundamental lesson from the historical record about the importance of the social environment was reinforced by the findings of more recent empirical research. The hospital environment could again become ameliorative if it was redesigned to reflect the principles of a therapeutic community, while the benefit of community programs was enhanced when they provided a socially supportive environment. Support programs could smooth the transition from the hospital to the community environment if they focused on developing social supports before and after the move. When hospital discharge was instead treated as simply a change of address, deterioration, readmission, as well as homelessness or incarceration were much more likely.

But this lesson must be balanced with another that is equally important even though it may be harder to accept. In one form or another, this lesson emerged repeatedly as social scientists, historians, and clinicians reviewed the experience of deinstitutionalization at different times and from different vantage points. The dominant vision that generated the policy of deinstitutionalization was fundamentally flawed.

> Eligibility criteria and funding levels for community-based rehabilitation were designed to reduce support services as soon as a patient is stabilized, with no attention to development of new adaptive skills or gradual improvement of functioning over time. Funding levels were clearly insufficient to provide rehabilitation over a time period necessary for a meaningful benefit to any but the least disabled recipients. (Sullivan, 1999, p. 51)

Deinstitutionalization policy, that is, has been based on "neglect and a failure to appreciate the scope, severity, and degree of dysfunction and suffering associated with mental disorder" (Mechanic & Rochefort, 1990, p. 324). Proponents of deinstitutionalization "sometimes failed to understand the human and social needs of the very persons they wanted to help" (Grob, 1991, p. 304). Even Goffman (1961, p. 384) averred that his emphasis on the limitations of total institutions did not allow him "to claim that I can suggest some better way of handling persons called mental patients."

Of course if mental illness means no more than a label attached by observers to behavior arbitrarily considered aberrant, the lesson has no value except for those seeking a basis with which to reproach others for their insensitivity. It is only if mental illness is conceptualized as in some way involving dysfunction of the human organism that consideration of appropriate treatment becomes as necessary as in the war against cancer and the effort to cure heart disease. To diminish any action to prevent the human suffering that mental illness can produce as only an effort to "satisfy their [the relatives' and authorities'] needs" (Goffman, 1961, p. 334) is to demean the value of human life and to discredit the personally experienced psychic maladies that diminish human potential – potential that Van Gogh seemed desperate to restore when he voluntarily became an inpatient.

CONCLUSIONS

While the primary causes of the inpatient census decline beginning in 1955 and its precipitous drop after 1965 were, respectively, the introduction of psychotropic drugs and the start of Medicaid and Medicare (and then SSI), changes in politics, fiscal pressures, and psychiatrists' orientations also helped to sustain the rapid decline in inpatients through the 1980s, at which time it could be said that only the most chronic and severe cases and, in many states, only those at risk of harming themselves or others, remained on the hospital wards. Continued reductions in the hospital census caused in many states further decline in even this fraction of the inpatient population.

But in spite of the fact that this broad perspective on both the causes and consequences of deinstitutionalization makes evident how essential understanding of the phenomenon is to further advances in the sociology of medicine, it also diverts attention from the central issue. The debate over the superiority of hospital-based or community-based care "neglects the complex nature and variety of mental disorders and the full spectrum of service programs required" (Mechanic & Rochefort, 1990, p. 324). The central issue is how to improve the social environment experienced so that it diminishes insofar as possible the likelihood of onset of severe mental illness and maximizes the prospects for rehabilitation and even recovery of those who become severely mentally ill. This issue is of equal importance whether the setting is a hospital, a health center, or a community residence.

Although 19th century neurologists had little scientific knowledge of the human brain on which to base their efforts to expose the flawed reasoning and compromised standards of that era's mental hospital superintendents, neuroscience research in the 21st century has begun to identify the specific neural structures and processes that are associated with mental illness and that can alter perceptions, feelings, and actions. Such research has helped to explain the failure of reductionist models of genetic determination and of inflated expectations for neuroleptic medication, but most noteworthy in relation to the history of deinstitutionalization is how much the environments of the past and the experiences of the present shape neural processes in ways that in turn influence future behavior. And it has become clear that in this ongoing process of interaction between the human brain and its environment, it is social relations that connect the two.

Human action in the social world is shaped by evolved neural structures in the human brain that support social interaction, while human reactions to the social world are embodied through neuroplastic response and epigenetic adaptation (Schutt, Seidman, & Keshavan, 2015). Although the policy debate over deinstitutionalization is largely over, a new agenda for advancing scholarship reflecting the importance of the social environment for the effective design of mental health services is only now emerging. Investigation of the many ways in which the social environment can be enhanced in order to maximize the expression of human sociality and identify the multiple traits and experiences that diminish individuals' abilities to benefit from the social environment are the key to further progress in mental health services. More effective mental health services will result from improved social organization, not from changes in physical location.

ACKNOWLEDGMENT

I am grateful for the comments of the two anonymous expert reviewers.

REFERENCES

Ahmed, P. I., & Plog, S. C. (Eds.). (1976). *State mental hospitals: What happens when they close*. New York, NY: Plenum.

Andersen, H. S. (2004). Mental health in prison populations: A review – With special emphasis on a study of Danish prisoners on remand. *Acta Psychiatrica Scandinavica, 110*(Suppl. 424), 5–59.

Bachrach, L. L. (1999). The state of the state mental hospital at the turn of the century. *New Directions for Mental Health Services, 84*, 7–24.

Bassuk, E. L., & Lamb, H. R. (1986). Homelessness and the implementation of deinstitutionalization. *New Directions for Mental Health Services, 30*, 7–14.

Belcher, J. R. (1988). Are jails replacing the mental health system for the homeless mentally ill? *Community Mental Health Journal, 24*, 185–195.

Burt, M. (1992). *Over the edge: The growth of homelessness in the 1980s*. New York, NY: Russell Sage.

Caplan, B., Schutt, R. K., Turner, W. M., Goldfinger, S. M., & Seidman, L. J. (2006). Change in neurocognition by housing type and substance abuse among formerly homeless seriously mentally ill individuals. *Schizophrenia Research, 83*, 77–86.

Chapin, J. B. (1898). Dr. Thomas story Kirkbride: An address on the presentation of his portrait to the college of physicians, Philadelphia, January 5, 1989. *American Journal of Insanity, 55*, 119–127.

Deutsch, A. (1948). *The shame of the states*. New York, NY: Harcourt, Brace.

Dewees, M., Pulice, R. T., & McCormick, L. L. (1996). Community integration of former state hospital patients: Outcomes of a policy shift in Vermont. *Psychiatric Services, 47*, 1088–1092.

Dowdall, G. W. (1996). *The eclipse of the state mental hospital: Policy, stigma, and organization*. Albany, NY: SUNY Press.

Estroff, S. E. (1981). *Making it crazy*. Berkeley, CA: University of California Press.

Fazel, S., & Danesh, J. (2002). Serious mental disorder in 23,000 prisoners: A systematic review of 62 surveys. *Lancet, 359*, 545–550.

Folsom, D. P., Hawthorne, W., Lindamer, L., Gilmer, T., Bailey, A., Golshan, S., … Jeste, D. P. (2005). Prevalence and risk factors for homelessness and utilization of mental health services among 10,340 patients with serious mental illness in a large public mental health system. *American Journal of Psychiatry, 162*, 370–376.

Gelberg, L., Linn, L. S., & Leake, B. D. (1988). Mental health, alcohol and drug use, and criminal history among homeless adults. *American Journal of Psychiatry, 145*, 191–196.

Goffman, E. (1961). *Asylums: Essays on the social situation of mental patients and other inmates*. New York, NY: Doubleday.

Goldman, H. H., Taube, C. A., Regier, D. A., & Witkin, M. (1983). The multiple functions of the state mental hospital. *American Journal of Psychiatry, 140*, 296–300.

Green, C. A., Perrin, N. A., Leo, M. C., Janoff, S. L., Yarborough, B. J. H., & Paulson, R. I. (2013). Recovery from serious mental illness: Trajectories, characteristics, and the role of mental health care. *Psychiatric Services, 64*, 1203–1210.

Greenblatt, M. (1955). *From custodial to therapeutic care*. New York, NY: Russell Sage Foundation.

Greenblatt, M. (1976). Historical factors affecting the closing of state hospitals. In P. I. Ahmed & S. C. Plog (Eds.), *State mental hospitals: What happens when they close* (pp. 9–20). New York, NY: Plenum.

Greenblatt, M., & Glazier, E. (1976). Some major issues in the closing of the hospitals. In P. I. Ahmed & S. C. Plog (Eds.), *State mental hospitals: What happens when they clos* (pp. 127–139). New York, NY: Plenum.

Grob, G. N. (1973). *Mental institutions in America: Social policy to 1875*. New York, NY: The Free Press.

Grob, G. N. (1991). *From asylum to community: Mental health policy in modern America*. Princeton, NJ: Princeton University Press.

Grob, G. N. (1994). *The mad among us: A history of the care of America's mentally ill*. New York, NY: The Free Press.

Grob, G. N. (1995). The paradox of deinstitutionalization. *Society* [Special issue], (July–August), 51–59.

Guy, E., Platt, J. J., Zwerling, I., & Bullock, S. (1985). Mental health status of prisoners in an urban jail. *Criminal Justice and Behavior, 12*, 29–53.

Harding, C. M., Brooks, G. W., Ashikaga, T., Strauss, J. S., & Breier, A. (1987). The Vermont longitudinal study of persons with severe mental illness, I: Methodology, study sample, and overall status 32 years later. *American Journal of Psychiatry, 144*, 718–726.

Herman, D. B., Susser, E. S., Jandorf, L., Lavelle, J., & Bromet, E. J. (1998). Homeless among individuals with psychotic disorders hospitalized for the first time: Findings from the Suffolk county mental health project. *American Journal of Psychiatry, 155*, 109–113.

Holley, H. L., Hodges, P., & Jeffers, B. (1998). Moving psychiatric patients from hospital to community: Views of patients, providers, and families. *Psychiatric Services, 49*, 513–517.

James, D. J., & Glaze, L. E. (2006). *Mental health problems of prison and jail inmates.* Washington, DC: Bureau of Justice Statistics. NCJ 213600.

James, J. F., Gregory, D., Jones, R. K., & Rundell, O. H. (1980). Psychiatric morbidity in prisons. *Hospital & Community Psychiatry, 11*, 674–677.

Jemelka, R., Trupin, E., & Chiles, J. A. (1989). The mentally ill in prisons: A review. *Hospital & Community Psychiatry, 40*, 481–485.

Jencks, C. (1994). *The homeless.* Cambridge, MA: Harvard University Press.

Johnson, A. B. (1990). *Out of bedlam: The truth about deinstitutionalization.* New York, NY: Basic Books.

Kahn, M. W., Hannah, M., Hinkin, C., Montgomery, C., & Pitz, D. (1987). Psychopathology on the streets: Psychological assessment of the homeless. *Professional Psychology: Research & Practice, 18*, 580–586.

Keck, J. (1990). Responding to consumer housing preferences: The Toledo experience. *Psychosocial Rehabilitation Review, 13*, 51–58.

Kramer, M. (1977). *Psychiatric services and the changing institutional scene, 1950–1985* (pp. 77–433). DHEW Publication No. (ADM). Washington, DC: National Institute of Mental Health.

Kruzich, J. M. (1985). Community integration of the mentally ill in residential facilities. *American Journal of Community Psychology, 13*, 553–564.

LaFave, H. G., Grunberg, F., Woodhouse, R. W., & Barrington, L. (1976). Is the community ready? In P. I. Ahmed & S. C. Plog (Eds.), *State mental hospitals: What happens when they close* (pp. 177–203). New York, NY: Plenum.

Lamb, H. R. (1984). Deinstitutionalization and the homeless mentally ill. *Hospital & Community Psychiatry, 35*, 899–907.

Lipton, F. R., Siegel, C., Hannigen, A., Samuels, J., & Baker, S. (2000). Tenure in supportive housing for homeless persons with severe mental illness. *Psychiatric Services, 51*, 479–486.

Mandiberg, J. M. (1999). The sword of reform has two sharp edges: Normalcy, normalization, and the destruction of the social group. *New Directions for Mental Health Services, 83*, 31–44.

Markowitz, F. E. (2006). Psychiatric hospital capacity, homelessness, and crime and arrest rates. *Criminology, 44*, 45–72.

Markson, E. W., & Cumming, J. H. (1976). The posttransfer fate of relocated patients. In P. I. Ahmed & S. C. Plog (Eds.), *State mental hospitals: What happens when they close* (pp. 97–109). New York, NY: Plenum.

Marlowe, R. A. (1976). When they closed the doors at Modesto. In P. I. Ahmed & S. C. Plog (Eds.), *State mental hospitals: What happens when they close* (pp. 83–95). New York, NY: Plenum.

McGrew, J. H., Wright, E. R., & Pescosolido, B. A. (1999). Closing of a state hospital: An overview and framework for a case study. *The Journal of Behavioral Health Services & Research*, *26*, 236–245.

Mechanic, D., & Rochefort, D. A. (1990). Deinstitutionalization: An appraisal of reform. *Annual Review of Sociology*, *16*, 301–327.

Mendel, W. M. (1976). The case for closing of the hospitals. In P. I. Ahmed & S. C. Plog (Eds.), *State mental hospitals: What happens when they close* (pp. 21–44). New York, NY: Plenum.

Mollica, R. F. (1983). From asylum to community: The threatened disintegration of public psychiatry. *The New England Journal of Medicine*, *308*, 367–373.

Monroe-DeVita, M. B., & Mohatt, D. F. (1999). The state hospital and the community: An essential continuum for persons with severe and persistent mental illness. *New Directions for Mental Health Services*, *84*, 85–97.

Moos, R. H. (1974). *Evaluating treatment environments: A social ecological approach.* New York, NY: Wiley.

Mullins, E. (2015). *Van Gogh: The asylum year*. London: Unicorn Press.

National Center for Health Statistics [NCHS]. (2009). *Health, United States, 2009, with special feature on medical technology*. Hyattsville, MD: NCHS.

Neubauer, R. (1993). Housing preferences of homeless men and women in ashelter population. *Hospital and Community Psychiatry*, *44*, 492–494.

New York State Legislature. (1856). Report and memorial of the county superintendents of the poor of New York State on lunacy and its relation to pauperism, and for relief of insane poor. Albany: New York State Legislature, Senate Document No. 17, January 23. Reprinted In G. N. Grob (Ed.), 1973. The origins of the state mental hospital in America. New York, NY: Arno Press.

Newton, L., Rosen, A., Tennant, C., & Hobbs, D. (2001). Moving out and moving on: Some ethnographic observations of deinstitutionalization in an Australian community. *Psychiatric Rehabilitation Journal*, *25*, 152–162.

Okin, R. L. (1983). The future of state hospitals: Should there be one? *American Journal of Psychiatry*, *140*, 577–581.

Osborn, L. A. (2009). From beauty to despair: The rise and fall of the American state mental hospital. *Psychiatric Quarterly*, *80*, 219–231.

Pennsylvania Legislature. (1839). Report in relation to an asylum for the insane poor, March 11. Harrisburg: Pennsylvania Legislature. Reprinted. In G. N. Grob (Ed.), 1973. The origins of the state mental hospital in America. New York, NY: Arno Press.

Pilisuk, M. (2001). A job and a home: Social networks and the integration of the mentally disabled in the community. *American Journal of Orthopsychiatry*, *71*, 49–60.

Rachlin, S. (1976). The case against closing of state hospitals. In P. I. Ahmed & S. C. Plog (Eds.), *State mental hospitals: What happens when they close* (pp. 31–44). New York, NY: Plenum.

Robitscher, J. (1976). Moving patients out of hospitals – In whose interest? In P. I. Ahmed & S. C. Plog (Eds.), *State mental hospitals: What happens when they close* (pp. 141–175). New York, NY: Plenum.

Rosenfield, S. (1992). Factors contributing to the subjective quality of life of the chronic mentally ill. *Journal of Health and Social Behavior*, *33*, 299–315.

Rossi, P. H. (1989). *Down and out in America: The origins of homelessness*. Chicago, IL: University of Chicago Press.

Rothman, D. J. (1990). *The discovery of the asylum: Social order and disorder in the new republic, revised edition*. Boston, MA: Little, Brown.

Sareyan, A. (1994). *The turning point: How men of conscience brought about major change in the care of America's mentally ill*. Washington, DC: American Psychiatric Press.

Schutt, R. K. (2011a). *Homelessness, housing, and mental illness*. Cambridge, MA: Harvard University Press.

Schutt, R. K. (2011b). Maximizing the benefit of housing: Consumer preferences, clinician recommendations, social processes and outcomes. Keynote address for VISN 1 VA Clinical Staff Conference. Ending a National Shame: Addressing Homelessness among Veterans. Hanscom Air Force Base, Bedford, MA, May 6.

Schutt, R. K., Seidman, L. J., & Keshavan, M. S. (Eds.). (2015). *Social neuroscience: Brain, mind, and society*. Cambridge, MA: Harvard University Press.

Segal, S. P., & Aviram, U. (1978). *The mentally ill in community-based sheltered care: A study of community care and social integration*. New York, NY: Wiley.

Steadman, H. J., Fabisiak, S., Dvoskin, J., & Holohean, E. J. (1987). A survey of mental disability among state prison inmates. *Hospital & Community Psychiatry*, *38*, 1086–1090.

Stroup, A. L., & Manderscheid, R. W. (1988). The development of the state mental hospital system in the United States: 1840–1890. *Journal of the Washington Academy of the Sciences*, *78*, 59–68.

Sullivan, M. (1999). The unique roles of state hospital programs: Keeping what works in an evolving system. *New Directions for Mental Health Services*, *84*, 47–55.

Susser, E. S., Lin, S. P., & Conover, S. A. (1991). Risk factors for homelessness among patients admitted to a state mental hospital. *American Journal of Psychiatry*, *148*, 1659–1664.

Talbott, J. A. (1978). *The death of the asylum: A critical study of state hospital management, services, and care*. New York, NY: Grune & Stratton.

Tanzman, B. (1993). An overview of surveys of mental health consumers' preferences for housing and support services. *Hospital and Community Psychiatry*, *44*, 450–455.

Taube, C. A., & Goldman, H. A. (1989). State strategies to restructure psychiatric hospitals: A selective review. *Inquiry*, *26*, 146–156.

Teplin, L. A. (1990). The prevalence of severe mental disorder among male urban jail detainees: Comparison with epidemiologic catchment area program. *American Journal of Public Health*, *80*, 663–669.

Torrey, E. F., Fuller, D. A., Geller, J., Jacobs, C., & Ragosta, K. (2012). *No Room at the inn: Trends and consequences of closing public psychiatric hospitals, 2005–2010*. Arlington, VA: Treatment Advocacy Center.

Torrey, E. F., & Miller, J. (2007). *The invisible plague: The rise of mental illness from 1750 to the present*. New Brunswick, NJ: Rutgers University Press.

Torrey, E. F., Stieber, J., Ezekiel, J., Wolfe, S. M., Sharfstein, J., Noble, J. H., & Flynn, L. M. (1992). *Criminalizing the seriously mentally ill*. Washington, DC: National Alliance for the Mentally Ill and Public Citizen Health Research Group.

Upshur, C. C., Benson, P. R., Clemens, E., Fisher, W. H., Leff, H. S., & Schutt, R. K. (1997). Closing state mental hospitals in Massachusetts: Policy, process, and impact. *International Journal of Law & Psychiatry*, *20*, 199–217.

Ward, M. J. (1946). *The snake pit*. Toronto: Random House of Canada.

Weinberg, R. B., & Marlowe, H. (1983). Recognizing the social in psychosocial competence: the importance of social network interventions. *Psychosocial Rehabilitation Journal*, *6*(4), 25–34.
Western, B., Braga, A. A., Davis, J., & Sirois, C. (2015). Stress and hardship after prison. *American Journal of Sociology*, *120*, 1512–1547.
Whitmer, G. E. (1980). From hospitals to jails: The fate of California's deinstitutionalized mentally ill. *American Journal of Orthopsychiatry*, *50*, 65–75.
Witkin, M. J., Atay, J., & Manderscheid, R. W. (1996). Trends in state and county mental hospitals in the U.S. from 1970 to 1992. *Psychiatric Services*, *47*, 1079–1081.
Wong, Y. I., Hadley, T. R., Culhane, D. P., Poulin, S. R., Davis, M. R., Cirksey, B. A., & Brown, J. L. (2006). *Predicting staying in or leaving permanent supportive housing that serves homeless people with serious mental illness*. Final Report prepared for U.S. Department of Housing and Urban Development, Office of Policy Development and Research. Center for Mental Health Policy and Services Research, University of Pennsylvania, Philadelphia.
Yeich, S., & Mowbray, C. T. (1994). The case for a 'supported housing' approach: A study of consumer housing and support preferences. *Psychosocial Rehabilitation Journal*, *18*, 75–86.

THE REVOLVING DOOR: PATIENT NEEDS AND NETWORK TURNOVER DURING MENTAL HEALTH TREATMENT

Will R. McConnell and Brea L. Perry

ABSTRACT

Purpose – *While much research examines the consequences of deinstitutionalization for caregivers, few studies address support mobilization strategies used by patients themselves. We examine the relationship between mental health patients' needs, their activation of network ties for health discussion, and network dynamics during the course of treatment. We hypothesize that patients strategically activate their network ties for support that matches their needs. Linking activation to network dynamics, we also propose that patients with greater needs exhaust their supportive relationships and experience more network turnover.*

Methodology/approach – *We draw on a dataset of new mental health patients (*N=*173) and their associated network members (*N=*4,144) observed over three years. Random-intercept regression models test the relationship between patients' needs and (1) network tie activation for health discussion and (2) network turnover.*

50 Years after Deinstitutionalization: Mental Illness in Contemporary Communities
Advances in Medical Sociology, Volume 17, 119–145

ISSN: 1057-6290/doi:10.1108/S1057-629020160000017005

Findings – *Although the overall level of need does not predict network tie activation, mental health patients are more likely to activate network ties who provide support that matches their expressed needs for discussion, emotional, and financial support (although not instrumental or informational support). In addition, patients with elevated needs experience increased network turnover. Strategic activation and its unintended consequence together suggest a revolving door of support for patients in crisis.*

Practical implications – *In the post-deinstitutionalization era, patients' informal social safety nets must compensate for needs that are left unmet by deficits in the formal treatment system. We find that patients seek out network members who are well-equipped to help them cope with the onset of illness. At the same time, network activation may lead to instability as high-need patients churn through supportive relationships. Future research should examine the consequences of tie activation and support needs for network dynamics in different treatment contexts.*

Keywords: Network turnover; mental illness; social support; egocentric social networks; deinstitutionalization

INTRODUCTION

Beginning with Goffman's (1961) seminal work on institutionalized mental healthcare, scholars have recognized that illness experiences are shaped through dynamic interactions with healthcare providers and the treatment system (Pavalko, Harding, & Pescosolido, 2007). The mental health system in the United States has undergone substantial changes during deinstitutionalization, particularly with respect to treatment methods, the organization of inpatient care, and the role of professionals in care delivery (Mechanic & Rochefort, 1990). In recent years, ideas about mental illness recovery have shifted from emphasizing the elimination of symptoms toward promoting successful illness management, reintegration into social roles, and maintaining a positive quality of life (Markowitz, 2001). Although deinstitutionalized mental health treatment necessarily involves increased responsibility for patients and their community caregivers, few studies have examined the consequences of deinstitutionalization for informal networks of support (Carpentier & Ducharme, 2003). In this chapter we ask two research questions. First, how do mental health patients post-deinstitutionalization draw on their informal networks to supplement or replace professional resources? Second, what are the consequences of elevated needs and informal support seeking for social network dynamics?

Mounting evidence suggests that patients organize their social networks deliberately in order to cultivate a wide range of resources that can address health needs as they arise (House, Landis, & Umberson, 1988; Perry & Pescosolido, 2010; Smith & Christakis, 2008; Wellman & Wortley, 1990). Yet the value of network resources depends upon strategic "activation" of network ties to access needed support (Lin, 1999; Perry & Pescosolido, 2015). Researchers know relatively little about patients' goal-directed network activation strategies and how those strategies may drive network dynamics during crises (Carpentier & Ducharme, 2003; Perry & Pescosolido, 2012). In particular, recent research has noted that core networks display a surprising amount of churn beneath overall structural stability (Sasovova, Mehra, Borgatti, & Schippers, 2010; Small, Pamphile, & McMahan, 2015). We address this research gap through an examination of the relationship between network tie activation for health discussion and network instability over time. We propose that network activation has an unintended consequence – patients with elevated needs exhaust their supportive relationships and consequently experience more network turnover. The Network Episode Model provides a framework for developing hypotheses (Pescosolido, 1991, 1992; Pescosolido, Gardner, & Lubell, 1998). We test hypotheses using a detailed dataset of new mental health patients (N = 173) and their associated network members (N = 4,144). Results from random-intercept longitudinal regression models provide evidence that patients strategically activate network members to address needs, although only in certain domains. We also demonstrate a dynamic consequence of activation: patients with elevated needs experience increased network turnover.

BACKGROUND

Activating Network Ties during Mental Health Crises

Our theoretical starting point is the Network Episode Model (NEM) first formulated by Pescosolido (1991, 1992, 2006). In contrast to individualistic models for understanding healthcare decision-making, the NEM locates healthcare experiences within informal (i.e., lay or personal) and formal (i.e., professional) social networks. As a basic premise, the NEM argues that individuals strategically leverage their network members to address problems that exceed their individual capacity for coping (Bury, 1982; Wellman, 2000). When confronted with health problems, individuals cope through interactions with lay and professional network members who may discuss or dismiss their symptoms, recommend or provide services, and influence health behaviors and treatment compliance. Through these embedded interactions, social networks influence individuals' health decision-making, shape the course of treatment, and impact health outcomes (Pescosolido et al., 1998; Thoits, 2011).

Relationships with mental health professionals act as both "safety nets" and "brokers" during treatment, in that they provide critical professional care and connect patients to other supportive resources (Carpentier & Ducharme, 2003; Gage-Bouchard, LaValley, Panagakis, & Shelton, 2015; Perry & Pescosolido, 2012). Given the growing reliance on deinstitutionalized mental health services and chronic illness management, however, informal support networks hold perhaps equally as much potential to impact the treatment process. While the NEM emphasizes that others' concerns or perceptions of increased need can motivate their involvement during treatment, it acknowledges that individuals purposefully reach out to others during the crisis and uncertainty that may accompany illness.

Following the "functional specificity hypothesis" (Cutrona & Russell, 1990; Penning, 1990), the NEM proposes that informal resources are sometimes accessed deliberately through targeted "activation" of network ties (Perry & Pescosolido, 2015, 2010). When faced with disruptive life events like the onset of illness, the decision of whom to approach for support represents a crucial step in recovery (Perry & Pescosolido, 2010). One might interpret network ties as "boutiques" where individuals "shop" for needed goods and services (Wellman & Wortley, 1990). While much prior work emphasizes the social and institutional constraints that confront persons with mental illness, the idea of network activation acknowledges the agency of those individuals to leverage network ties and make decisions that affect the course of their treatment and recovery (Pescosolido et al., 1998).

The functional specificity hypothesis emphasizes that network tie activation attempts to match perceived needs with the complementary skills, resources, and information available in the network (Cutrona & Russell, 1990; Karp, 2000; Perry, 2011; Perry & Pescosolido, 2012). Consistent with this expectation, Perry and Pescosolido (2015) found that new mental health patients activate ties for health discussion who are best suited to help with the problem at hand. Specifically, patients draw on their most intimate relationships – ties who trust doctors and those who had experience with a similar mental health problem. Strategic network activation appears in other cases of illness as well. Gage-Bouchard et al. (2015) found that new cancer patients sought logistical support from existing ties with friends and family members. For informational and emotional support, however, they established new ties with other families and health professionals who had dealt with similar circumstances. In effect, these patients sought "experiential homophily" that enriched the value of the support (Thoits, 2011). When patients activate ties strategically they show improved health outcomes. In contrast, mental health patients who activate ties injudiciously report poorer functioning, difficulty performing social roles, and worse social satisfaction and quality of life (Perry & Pescosolido, 2015).

Although network tie activation has demonstrable effects on the course of treatment, relatively little is known about why patients choose to activate particular ties (Gage-Bouchard et al., 2015; Perry & Pescosolido, 2015). Recent work has examined how patients deploy targeted discussions regarding health services, compliance, behaviors, and beliefs in order to inform their decision-making (Abbott, Bettger, Hanlon, & Hirschman, 2012; Cornwell & Waite, 2012; Perry & Pescosolido, 2010; Schafer, 2013). Building on this line of work, we examine how patients' needs inform their decision to activate different network members for health discussion. Mental health patients encounter a wide variety of social, emotional, and financial challenges; we test whether patients activate network ties who provide support for specific needs in multiple life domains. In addition, we note that the consequences of network tie activation have only been studied with reference to health outcomes. In the following section, we propose that network tie activation during crises can have unintended consequences for the architecture of networks themselves.

Network Dynamics during Treatment

A second basic premise of the NEM is that illness episodes impact social network dynamics, influencing the structure, function, and content of individuals' relationships (Pescosolido, 1991, 1992). Serious illness creates a "network crisis" that has the capacity to disrupt everyday life and individuals' most basic identities (Abbott et al., 2012; Bury, 1982; Lipton, Cohen, Fischer, & Katz, 1981). Studying persons with arthritis, Bury (1982) describes serious illness as "the kind of experience where the structures of everyday life and the forms of knowledge which underpin them are disrupted" (p. 169). When a person faces a health crisis of this kind, empirical evidence suggests that their social network responds in both positive and negative ways. Patients entering treatment enjoy larger and more functional networks relative to members of the general population (Gage-Bouchard et al., 2015; Perry & Pescosolido, 2012). In some ways disruption can be seen as an opportunity to form new relationships or strengthen existing ones. First responders in patients' networks provide critical support, advice, and advocacy to address the immediate problems that motivated help-seeking (Carpentier, Lesage, & White, 1999; Muhlbauer, 2002). At this early stage of the treatment process, network members may be called upon to provide atypical services like treatment advice, financial support, or a place to stay (Pescosolido et al., 1998).

Although network activation in response to illness can be beneficial, heightened reliance on network members can also bring about negative consequences for patients. The role of reciprocity in relationships can elicit feelings of dependence, a perceived obligation to repay social debts, or promote relationship dissatisfaction (Fehr, Fischbacher, & Gächter, 2002). In addition, discussion of a stigmatized health problem like mental illness could provoke negative reactions from network members, especially those on the periphery of the network (Perry, 2011; Wahl, 2012). In keeping with these expectations, new mental health patients' networks significantly decrease in size during treatment relative to the general population, a shift which has been linked to worse health outcomes among older adults (Cornwell, Laumann, & Schumm, 2008; Perry & Pescosolido, 2012). In addition, Perry and Pescosolido (2012) found evidence that networks of patients with severe mental disorders become increasingly unstable as treatment progresses. In particular, extended kin tend to provide elevated levels of support during the initial stages of illness, but their level of involvement tapers off as mental health conditions become chronic.

In sum, prior research suggests that initially robust support in mental health patients' networks eventually gives way to instability and attrition, although functionality stays relatively constant (Perry & Pescosolido, 2012). Perry and Pescosolido (2012) describe several possible explanations for this pattern (see also Carpentier & Ducharme, 2003). First, dynamic network changes may reflect the replacement of informal relationships with professional support (Carpentier et al., 1999; Karp, 2000; Muhlbauer,

2002). After contacting formal services, family members and other initial supporters may withdraw support that is no longer necessary. That said, about two-thirds of persons with mental health problems exit professional care within several months (Kessler et al., 2005), which suggests that formal support is short-lived. Second, network attrition may result from increased stigmatization following formal labeling with a mental illness. This would be the case if judgmental ties withdraw their support or if patients limit contact with acquaintances in order to avoid stigmatization (Link, Cullen, Struening, Shrout, & Dohrenwend, 1989; Perry, 2011). Third, elevated levels of support may not be as critical later in the illness career after patients have experienced and subsequently managed the fall-out from the initial crisis period of acute mental illness.

These explanations no doubt play some role in patients' network dynamics, but they leave some patterns unexplained. First, prior explanations account for network attrition, but do not address the surprising instability of patients' relationships. Rather than just losing ties, patients tend to churn through them, cycling in new members to replace others (Perry & Pescosolido, 2012). Second, these explanations do not consider the actions and goals of patients themselves, and how those actions might contribute to network dynamics.

The Revolving Door

We propose a link between tie activation and network instability during treatment. In forging this link we rely on a NEM framework and previous research. The onset of serious illness can be understood as a "biographical disruption" that reverberates through an individual's life and social relationships (Perry & Pescosolido, 2012; Pescosolido, 1991, 1992). As is the case with other disruptive life events, individuals must adapt to unfamiliar challenges, needs, and obligations that arise from illness. At this juncture, social networks become vital sources of advice and support (Abbott et al., 2012). Patients recruit or compel network members to provide resources that address their needs (Pescosolido, 1992; Wellman, 2000). One important way in which mental health patients activate their networks in response to illness is in seeking out health discussion partners (Perry & Pescosolido, 2015). Following this logic, our first hypothesis is that new mental health patients with elevated needs will be more likely to activate network ties for health discussion.

Hypothesis 1. Greater support needs are associated with increased probability of a network member entering (or remaining in) the health discussion network.

Expanding on this hypothesis, mental health patients derive the greatest benefit when network resources address specific challenges that they face (Cutrona & Russell, 1990; Horowitz et al., 2001). For example, Horowitz et al. (2001) describe experimental evidence that individuals respond more positively to social support that addresses an implied problem. Depending on a patient's life circumstances or their stage in the treatment process, they may have a greater need for certain kinds of support (e.g., financial rather than emotional). In fact, individuals seem to curate networks in exactly this way, retaining certain ties to provide specific services (Wellman & Wortley, 1990). This suggests a more refined activation hypothesis.

Hypothesis 2. Network members who provide support functions that compliment patients' expressed needs are more likely to enter (or remain in) the health discussion network than those who do not.

Although much attention has been paid to stable cores of highly functional network members, our literature review suggests that network activation is not constant over time. Instead, when selecting whom to leverage for support, patients respond to new circumstances during treatment and dynamic changes in relationships. Rather than relying on a firm core of intimate confidants, patients may draw on the best available ties to meet the challenges at hand. This idea is consistent with recent suggestions that researchers' emphasis on stable cores ignores more subtle network dynamics (Sasovova et al., 2010; Small et al., 2015). Although overall network characteristics like size and density tend to remain stable, the individuals who constitute networks change with great frequency (Morgan, Neal, & Carder, 1997; Wellman, Wong, Tindall, & Nazer, 1997). Small et al. (2015) argue that the surprising instability of core discussion networks is a result of individuals entering new social contexts, which brings about concomitant changes in obligations and routine behaviors (Feld, 1981). Rather than being dominated by stable cores, this research suggests that informal networks are "highly contextual" or composed of fleeting attachments made to meet functional goals in different institutional contexts (Small, 2013; Small et al., 2015).

Mental health treatment is plainly a new institutional context in this sense, with numerous changes to one's life and social relationships

(Pescosolido, 1991, 1992). Research shows that network instability in the general population is common, with perhaps only one-third or one-fourth of individuals' network members persisting over a decade (Suitor & Keeton, 1997; Wellman et al., 1997). In the demanding context of serious illness we anticipate that network instability is even more pronounced. Prior research suggests that strong initial support for mental health patients eventually gives way to instability although functionality remains stable (Carpentier & Ducharme, 2003; Perry & Pescosolido, 2012). Rather than attributing this pattern to formal replacement of informal support or the influence of stigma, we look to strategic network activation for an explanation. We argue that opportunistic leveraging of social ties by mental health patients can exhaust supportive relationships, leading to network instability.

Hypothesis 3. Greater support needs are associated with increased turnover in the health discussion network.

This hypothesis suggests a "revolving door" in patients' informal support networks. Patients may seek out relationships to cope with the onset of illness, cycling in new ties when old ties depart, become unsupportive, or are no longer needed. The revolving door metaphor is consistent with evidence from prior work, although it has not yet been proposed in the context of mental health treatment. For example, in his ethnography of the urban poor, Desmond (2012) found that people in poverty relied on "disposable ties" to address essential needs like housing and companionship. These relationships are best described as high intensity but ultimately fragile ties that are quickly formed and discarded. People dealing with serious illness can exhibit similar actions, as when mental health patients recruit previously peripheral ties like extended kin to help in the early stages of treatment but later separate from them again (Gage-Bouchard et al. 2015; Karp, 2000; Perry & Pescosolido, 2012). Some ties could be cast off by patients when they no longer provide useful support, whereas others may simply become exhausted and withdraw. Caregivers for persons with a mental illness face social, emotional, and economic burdens that tend to make those relationships imbalanced and fragile (Carpentier & Ducharme, 2003; Pavalko & Woodbury, 2000; Perlick, Hohenstein, Clarkin, Kaczynski, & Rosenheck, 2005). Thus, involvement during treatment is sure to fluctuate along with caregivers' own needs and feelings of obligation (Carpentier & Ducharme, 2003; Muhlbauer, 2002). Following this logic we expect that patients' needs and corresponding network activation may be an unexplored source of network instability during treatment.

DATA AND METHODS

Sample

The Indianapolis Network Mental Health Study (INMHS) took place from 1990 to 1997 at two large hospitals, one public and one private.[1] Researchers contacted all individuals who had a mental health history of no more than two years and who were making their first major contact with mental health services.[2] Of all clients beginning treatment during the study period, 66.4% consented to an initial interview. Participants were administered the Structured Clinical Interview for DSM-III-R (Spitzer, Williams, Gibbon, & First, 1992). Those who received a research diagnosis of any major Axis I disorder (schizophrenia, bipolar disorder, or major depression) were recruited to the study. Baseline in-depth interviews were generally conducted within 1 month of contact with the hospital, and two follow-up interviews occurred between 10 and 24 months later. A total of 173 individuals participated in the study, providing information about a total of 4,144 network ties over three waves of interviews. The INMHS remains one of the largest and most detailed studies of its kind, providing near comprehensive information about patients' social networks. Although observation begins following the initial decision to seek treatment and ends after 24 months, the INMHS captures a sizeable portion of new mental health patients' early "illness careers" (Aneshensel, 2013).[3]

Demographic characteristics of the baseline sample indicate that over half the respondents are female (64%), and three quarters are white (73%). The mean age is 31, with a range from 16 to 72 and an average of 11.6 years of schooling (63% had a high school diploma or equivalent). Half of the patients were diagnosed with major depression (53%), 6% with bipolar disorder, 13% with schizophrenia, and 27% with a different mild disorder. Two respondents had missing data on variables used in analyses, leaving an effective sample size of 171 at the patient level at baseline. The 171 patients could be observed up to three times, for a potential 513 total observations. Only 376 patient-level observations were obtained, with 140 (27%) lost due to respondent attrition. Prior analysis of this data suggests that bias from the missing cases is not severe (Perry & Pescosolido, 2012). In addition, we will employ multilevel models that allow for analysis of the unbalanced sample (see below).

Measures

Researchers collected information about network members through a wide variety of name generators, which solicit information from patients about their relationships. The name generators in the INMHS ask about family, household, romantic, work, and school relationships, as well as friends, acquaintances, people with common mental health problems, and treatment providers. Respondents could list any number of individuals in response to each name generator, and network members could be listed in multiple groups. The outcome of this detailed approach is a near census of respondents' personal networks (Wellman, 2005). Here we examine one type of network in particular – the core health discussion network. This is a variant of the "important matters" name generator from the General Social Survey (Marsden, 1987). The health discussion network name generator asks participants to list individuals who they talk to about health matters, who approach them to talk about health matters "whether you want them to or not," and who talk to the participant about their own health problems. In general, these network members are the persons with whom the respondent engages in discussions about health on at least a somewhat regular basis. Previous research suggests that the health discussion network is a stronger predictor of health and treatment outcomes than the more general "important matters" network (Perry & Pescosolido, 2010). Examining this network also fits our theoretical interest in identifying how patients leverage some ties for health discussion, and what the consequences of that leveraging may be.

Dependent Variables

Our first dependent variable is health core activation. This is a binary variable where 1 indicates that a network tie was a member of the health discussion network, 0 otherwise. Our second dependent variable is health discussion network turnover. This continuous variable is calculated using two waves of data. Network turnover equals the percentage of health discussion network members who are added or dropped between one wave and the next. To calculate this variable we determined the total number of health discussion network members across two consecutive waves, tallied the number of members who appear in only one of the two waves (i.e., ties added or dropped), and divided the second number by the first to obtain the percentage of unstable ties. Because this variable uses two consecutive waves of data, the maximum number of observations for each respondent is two. In effect, analyses of turnover are based on a subsample of 108 respondents who were observed in two or more waves (62% of the original sample).[4]

Independent Variables

Network members can provide new mental health patients with a variety of support functions that may or may not address their needs. Support functions are measured by five binary variables, including discussion partner ("listening to you"), emotional support ("telling you they care"), information and advice ("making practical suggestions"), instrumental support ("helping with things like chores or transportation"), and financial support ("giving/loaning you money"). Respondents were asked if each network member contributed that type of support; these variables are coded 1 if yes and 0 otherwise. Descriptive statistics for these and other variables described in this section are available in Table 1.

To measure patients' needs we calculated two sets of binary variables and a scale variable. First, we identified variables in the dataset that corresponded to each of the five support domains. For example, for emotional support, respondents could report that they had a "Very" or "Sorta" stressful social life or family life. If a respondent reported stress in either of those areas, they were coded as needing emotional support. Similar procedures were followed for each of the five support domains, resulting in five indicators of patient need (or lack there of), based on 10 underlying survey items in all. Second, the five needs variables were then used to calculate a set of five binary variables at the network tie level. We created five "function-need matching" variables where 1 indicates that a network tie provides a support function that a patient expressed as a need, 0 otherwise. For example, a network member who provides financial support to a patient who expressed a need for financial support is coded as 1 on the financial support match variable. Finally, in addition to the five function-need matching binaries we also calculated a needs scale. This scale is the patient-level average of the 10 survey items used to indicate the five categories of patient needs. The scale is calculated using the items' original four-point response values (patient needs help 1 "Never" to 4 "Daily"), thus the resultant needs scale can range from 1 to 4, with higher values indicating greater overall need.[5]

Table 1 presents descriptive statistics for all variables. First, our models include controls for characteristics of patients that could influence the dependent variables. These are patient's sex (1 if female, 0 if male), age (10 years), race (1 if white, 0 if black), education (years), and psychiatric

Table 1. Descriptive Statistics for Dependent and Independent Variables.

Variable	*N*	Mean (%)	SD	Min	Max
Network tie variables[a]					
Dependent variables					
Health core activation	3,547	(27.4)		0	1
Independent variables					
Support functions					
Discussion partner	3,547	(71.2)		0	1
Emotional support	3,547	(62.8)		0	1
Information and advice	3,547	(55.6)		0	1
Instrumental support	3,547	(30.4)		0	1
Financial support	3,547	(32.4)		0	1
Function-need matching					
Discussion partner	3,547	(29.8)		0	1
Emotional support	3,547	(50.9)		0	1
Information and advice	3,547	(21.7)		0	1
Instrumental support	3,547	(10.2)		0	1
Financial support	3,547	(26.2)		0	1
Is female	3,547	(56.5)		0	1
Age (10 years)	3,547	3.13	1.00	1.6	7.2
Shares mental health problem	3,547	(6.2)		0	1
Relationship type					
Friend	3,547	(24.3)		0	1
Parent/spouse	3,547	(13.8)		0	1
Medical professional	3,547	(7.3)		0	1
Other relationship	3,547	(54.6)		0	1
Patient and network variables[b]					
Dependent variables					
Percent health discussion network turnover (10s)[c]	173	5.87	2.76	0	10.0
Patient variables					
Needs scale	160	1.40	0.46	1	3.5
Is female	171	(63.7)		0	1
Is white	171	(73.1)		0	1
Education (years)	171	11.59	2.00	6	16
Age (10 years)	171	3.06	1.02	1.6	7.2
Diagnosis					
Mild disorder	171	(27.3)		0	1
Major depression	171	(53.2)		0	1
Bipolar disorder	171	(6.4)		0	1
Schizophrenia	171	(12.9)		0	1
Network variables					
Health network size	171	3.82	2.31	0.0	11.0
Total network size	171	15.50	6.19	5.0	37.0
Average frequency of contact[d]	171	2.28	0.30	1.5	3.0
Percent female (10s)[d]	171	4.18	1.47	0.6	7.5
Percent kin (10s)[d]	171	4.57	1.74	0	10.0

[a]Level 1 statistics include pooled observations from all three waves.
[b]Level 2 statistics include sample of patients at baseline.
[c]Calculated for subsample interviewed in multiple waves ($N = 108$); includes 173 observations over waves 2–3.
[d]Calculated for total network.

diagnosis. The latter variable is coded as four dummy variables: 1 if mild disorder (e.g., adjustment disorder), major depression, bipolar disorder, or schizophrenia. The characteristics of network members may also influence their participation in treatment and provision of support (Gage-Bouchard et al., 2015; Marsden, 1987; Thoits, 2011). Consequently, we introduce multiple controls at the network tie level as well. Those members who share a common emotional or mental health problem with patients are coded 1, otherwise 0. Other variables include tie sex (1 if female, 0 if male), age (10 years), and relationship type. We collapsed an initial nine-category relationship type variable into four different mutually exclusive categories. Network members can be friends, parents/spouses/romantic partners, mental health/medical professionals, or other type. The "other" category includes respondents attached to any other name generators including roommates, coworkers, neighbors, acquaintances, etc.

Finally, several aggregate network-level variables are calculated using all of a patient's network members. These variables include number of persons in the health discussion network ("health network size"), number of persons in the total network based on all name generators ("total network size"), percent total network members who are female, percent total network members who are kin (by marriage or blood), and average tie frequency of contact in the total network. Frequency of contact was measured by the question "How often do you see or talk to the person?" with a three-point response scale ranging from "Very often/Often" to "Not very often/Hardly ever." This variable is coded such that higher values correspond to higher average frequency in the network.

Analytic Strategy

Because network members are associated with patients and observations were made longitudinally, normal independence assumptions for regression analysis do not hold. To address this problem we treat network members as nested within patients over time. Specifically, we employ random-intercept regression models that are appropriate for nested data in a longitudinal design (Raudenbush & Bryk, 2002). In these models, random intercepts at the network member and patient levels allow the over-time observations to freely vary with respect to the dependent variable. In other words, these are "mixed" models that include randomly varying intercepts as well as independent effects that are fixed to be the same across the higher level units. Because of our unbalanced sample, this modeling strategy is preferable to alternatives such as clustered standard errors (Raudenbush & Bryk, 2002). Our research design is consistent with prior multilevel analyses of egocentric networks (e.g., de Miguel Luken & Tranmer, 2010; Perry & Pescosolido, 2015). The chief advantage of this design is that it avoids the loss of information that results from aggregating data up to higher levels. Rather, it embraces complete egocentric networks without reduction to individuals or dyads.

We employ two sets of regression models. To control for variation in time between interview dates each model includes a variable equal to the number of years since the patients' baseline interview. This variable is coded as .08 (1/12) at baseline for all respondents because most interviews occurred within one month of entering treatment. To test Hypotheses 1 and 2 in the first set of models, we predict the odds that a network member enters or remains in a patient's health discussion network in any wave ("health core activation"). We model this outcome using three-level random-intercept logistic regression with network members nested in patients observed over time. To facilitate interpretation we also calculate predicted probabilities of health core activation based on the fixed effect estimates. Because our outcome of interest for Hypothesis 3 is health discussion network turnover, for the second set of models we collapse observations up to the patient level. We model turnover using two-level random-intercept regression with patients observed over time. We estimate all models using the Stata 13/SE statistical software.

RESULTS

Patient Needs and Network Activation

We first examine the relationship between patients' needs and activation of network members for health discussion. Table 2 contains results from three-level random-intercept logistic regression, with network members nested in patients over time. The non-significant effect for the needs scale variable in Panel 1 contradicts Hypothesis 1. Patients' overall support needs are not associated with increased odds of activating network ties for health discussion. In order to examine activation in more detail, we introduce five binary variables for different types of support in Panel 2. Here, the findings support the idea that patients activate ties strategically.

Table 2. Three-Level Random-Intercept Logistic Regression of Health Core Activation on Patient Needs.

	(1)		(2)		(3)	
	OR	SE	OR	SE	OR	SE
Patient variables (level 3)						
Is female	1.114	(0.13)	0.981	(0.20)	0.925	(0.19)
Is white	0.835	(0.21)	1.094	(0.23)	0.964	(0.21)
Education (years)	1.050	(0.16)	1.047	(0.05)	1.054	(0.05)
Age (10 years)	1.312**	(0.05)	1.375***	(0.13)	1.408***	(0.13)
Diagnosis[a]						
Major depression	1.137	(0.22)	1.143	(0.23)	1.460	(0.31)
Bipolar disorder	1.475	(0.55)	0.950	(0.38)	1.671	(0.68)
Schizophrenia	1.649	(0.51)	1.301	(0.41)	1.923	(0.64)
Total network size (log)	0.563**	(0.11)	0.633*	(0.13)	0.564**	(0.12)
Needs scale	0.903	(0.17)				
Network tie variables (level 2)						
Support functions						
Discussion partner			3.001***	(0.60)		
Emotional support			1.972***	(0.33)		
Information and advice			2.039***	(0.31)		
Instrumental support			1.800***	(0.28)		
Financial support			2.458***	(0.41)		
Function-need matching						
Discussion partner					2.513***	(0.41)
Emotional support					2.493***	(0.37)
Information and advice					1.244	(0.22)
Instrumental support					1.186	(0.27)
Financial support					3.267***	(0.55)

Is female	1.784***	(0.25)	1.550**	(0.21)	1.697***	(0.24)
Age (10 years)[b]	1.147**	(0.06)	1.133*	(0.06)	1.127*	(0.06)
Shares mental health problem	6.900***	(1.85)	4.135***	(1.02)	5.032***	(1.31)
Relationship type[c]						
Parent/spouse	14.420***	(3.90)	9.334***	(2.35)	11.600***	(3.06)
Medical professional	3.537***	(0.96)	5.873***	(1.57)	5.913***	(1.64)
Other relationship	0.667*	(0.11)	0.920	(0.15)	0.798	(0.13)
Time (years)	1.408***	(0.17)	1.319**	(0.12)	1.516***	(0.15)
Constant	0.081	(0.07)	0.005	(0.00)	0.013	(0.01)
Wald X^2	190.0***		246.4***		218.5***	
Observations	3547		3547		3547	

Note: Random effects not shown.
[a]Reference is "mild disorder."
[b]Centered at grand mean.
[c]Reference is "friend."
*$p < .05$; **$p < .01$; ***$p < .001$ (two-tailed test).

Patients have significantly greater odds of including a tie in the health discussion network if that tie listens to them (Odds Ratio = 3.0, $p < .001$, two-tailed test), or provides emotional (OR = 2.0, $p < .001$), informational (OR = 2.0, $p < .001$), instrumental (OR = 1.8, $p < .001$), or financial support (OR = 2.5, $p < .001$).

In Hypothesis 2 we propose that network members who provide support functions that compliment patients' expressed needs will be more likely to be activated than their peers. To test this possibility we introduce function-need matching variables in Panel 3 of Table 2. Patients have greater odds of activating ties who match their expressed needs in three of the five domains: discussion (OR = 2.5, $p < .001$), emotional support (OR = 2.5, $p < .001$), and financial support (OR = 3.3, $p < .001$). Although Panel 2 shows that patients activate ties who provide informational and instrumental support, results in Panel 3 suggest that those areas of activation are not necessarily driven by patients' needs. To aid interpretation we calculated predicted probability of health core activation using the fixed effects from the third model and holding other variables at their sample means. Network members who discuss problems with patients who need discussion have a 0.28 probability to enter or remain in the health discussion network, compared to a 0.17 probability for ties who are not a match (both significantly different from pr(Y) = 0, $p < .001$). The 0.11 difference in predicted probabilities is a statistically significant 65% increase (test of difference $p < .001$). Similarly, network members who provide needed emotional support have a 0.10 increase in probability of activation over non-matches; this is an increase of 62% (test of difference $p < .001$). For network members who provide needed financial support, the change in probabilities relative to non-matching network members is 0.15; this is an 86% increase (test of difference $p < .001$).

Overall, these results provide support for Hypothesis 2, that patients are more likely to activate network members who meet their expressed needs, although not in all five support domains. Lending credence to these results, each of the models includes controls for characteristics of both patients and network members. Looking to Panel 3, older patients have greater odds to activate network members for health discussion (OR = 1.3, $p < .001$) and patients with larger networks have decreased odds to activate any one particular tie (OR = 0.5, $p < .01$). A patient's gender, race, education, and diagnosis are not significant predictors. Looking to characteristics of network members, females (OR = 1.7, $p < .001$), older ties (OR = 1.1, $p < .05$), and those that share a mental health problem with the patient (OR = 5.0, $p < .001$) all have greater odds to be activated for health discussion. In addition, parents/spouses and medical professionals hold greater odds to be activated than friends (OR = 11.6 and 5.9, respectively, both $p < .001$). Finally, the linear effect for time spent in the treatment career indicates that the odds of a tie being activated increase by a factor of 1.5 for each year a patient is in treatment (OR = 1.5, $p < .001$).[6]

Health Discussion Network Turnover

We now examine the influence of patients' needs on health discussion network turnover. In this section we analyze the subsample of respondents who were interviewed in multiple waves. Among those 108 patients, health discussion network turnover is common. For 173 observations in waves 2–3, the average turnover from the previous wave is 58.7%. Table 3 presents results from two-level random-intercept regression of percent network

Table 3. Two-Level Random-Intercept Linear Regression of Percent Health Discussion Network Turnover (10s) on Patient Needs.

	(1)		(2)		(3)	
	β	SE	β	SE	β	SE
Patient variables (level 2)						
Needs scale	1.620**	(0.56)	1.442**	(0.53)	1.420*	(0.56)
Is female			0.029	(0.50)	−0.231	(0.54)
Is white			−0.523	(0.53)	−0.649	(0.58)
Education (years)			0.111	(0.13)	0.141	(0.13)
Age (10 years)			−0.004	(0.23)	0.054	(0.25)
Diagnosis[a]						
Major depression			0.666	(0.56)	0.886	(0.56)
Bipolar disorder			−0.138	(0.92)	0.001	(0.98)
Schizophrenia			0.900	(0.75)	1.186	(0.77)
Network variables (level 2)						
Health network size (log)					−0.743*	(0.33)
Average frequency of contact					−0.283	(0.72)
Percent female (10s)					0.323	(0.19)
Percent kin (10s)					−0.145	(0.12)
Time (years)	0.312	(0.32)	0.338	(0.32)	0.208	(0.33)
Constant	3.456	(0.90)	2.259	(2.29)	2.904	(3.13)
Wald X^2	8.77*		19.8*		36.7***	
Observations	173		173		173	

Notes: Robust standard errors; random effect not shown.
[a]Reference is "mild disorder."
*$p < .05$; **$p < .01$; ***$p < .001$ (two-tailed test).

turnover (10s) on patient needs. Controlling only for time, patients with higher support needs experience significantly increased network turnover relative to those with lower needs (β = 1.6, $p < .01$). This effect persists after introducing controls for characteristics of both patients and their networks in Panels 2 and 3, respectively. Using the fixed effects estimate from Panel 2, the average marginal effect of a one standard deviation increase on the patient needs scale is an additional 6.6% network turnover ($p <$ .01). This finding supports Hypothesis 3, that elevated needs predict increased network turnover.

Turning to the control variables in Table 3, Panels 2 and 3, few other variables are significant predictors of network turnover. The exception is health discussion network size: patients with larger core networks experience significantly less turnover than their peers (β = −0.7, $p < .05$). The random effects (not shown in Table 3) indicate that a substantial amount of variation in the outcome remain unexplained in these models, although alternative specifications did not improve model fit. As such, these results must be taken with caution. Nevertheless, level of need is an important building block for future work examining network dynamics and health.

DISCUSSION

Goffman (1961) examined how institutional settings transform individuals' lives. Half a century later, deinstitutionalization, the consumer movement, and the epidemiological shift to chronic illness have brought health and healing outside of the medical institution and into the community. Deinstitutionalized mental health treatment involves a complex set of professional and community organizations as well as relationships in patients' day-to-day lives (Mechanic & Rochefort, 1990). Consequently, deinstitutionalization raises important questions about the supportive resources available to patients and how they leverage those resources to cope with health problems. Whereas healthcare organizations and professionals once provided the majority of mental health support, the bulk of responsibility for managing health now falls to patients and their informal communities of support. In this chapter we examined how mental health patients post-deinstitutionalization seek resources from their network members during the transition into professional care. Building on the NEM and the functional specificity hypothesis (Cutrona & Russell, 1990; Pescosolido, 1991, 1992), we anticipated that patients activate network members in response to their needs in specific life domains, and that needs-based activation promotes network instability.

Contradicting Hypothesis 1, we find no evidence that elevated needs *in general* predict increased network activation for health discussion. All else equal, patients with greater needs do not seek additional help from network members. However, patients disproportionately recruit functional ties into their core health networks, preferring to draw on ties who provide any of the five forms of support. Investigating this further, results show that patients draw in network members whose supportive contributions match their expressed needs. In support of Hypothesis 2, patients activate ties who meet their needs for discussion as well as needs for emotional and financial support. The results for Hypotheses 1 and 2 suggests that patients leverage their network members carefully. Rather than activation being driven by overall level of need, activation is targeted to functional ties and in response to patients' specific needs. In contrast, when we examine network dynamics we find that elevated level of need corresponds to significantly increased instability. Patients who express greater overall need tend to churn through their supportive relationships, with supporters cycling in and out of the health discussion network. This provides strong evidence for Hypothesis 3, the *revolving door*. The revolving door phenomenon provides a compelling reminder that networks are more than the sum of their parts. Undue attention to overall level of functionality or stable cores of supportive ties overlooks surprising instability beneath the surface (Perry & Pescosolido, 2012; Sasovova et al., 2010; Small et al., 2015).

Taking a network perspective necessitates recognizing both the agency of individual patients and also the constraints imposed by their network members and life circumstances (Carpentier & Grenier, 2012; Pescosolido et al., 1998). As such, we suggest two complimentary interpretations of the revolving door phenomenon. First, patients may strategically seek out new sources of informal support when previously supportive ties are no longer useful or resources run out. Activating new relationships could avoid feelings of guilt, dependence, humiliation, or stigmatization that patients may experience when calling on the same ties again and again (Fehr et al., 2002; Perry, 2011). Second, the revolving door may arise from the actions and interests of network members. Caregivers may choose to withdraw support when faced with the social, emotional, and economic burdens that tend to accompany mental healthcare (Carpentier & Ducharme, 2003; Pavalko & Woodbury, 2000; Pavalko, Harding, & Pescosolido, 2005). Whatever the cause in any particular case, these patient- and network-focused interpretations can jointly explain the emergence of a revolving door of support for new mental health patients.

Limitations

The INMHS data contain neither information about social networks prior to the onset of illness nor information about comparison groups outside the population of new mental health patients entering care. The social networks of these individuals could differ in meaningful ways from people who do not have mental illnesses or who do not seek treatment. Consequently, the results presented here may only be applicable to mental health patients and possibly only those who have recently initiated their treatment careers. In addition, the INMHS sample is relatively small, particularly for the purposes of longitudinal analyses. In the second set of analyses, findings are restricted to patients who participated in the study through multiple waves and there is some evidence that this subsample is unique (see note 4). These limitations suggest that results must be taken with caution until corroborating studies are carried out. Limitations notwithstanding, the early stage of the treatment career captured by the INMHS data has the potential to be one of its most profoundly disruptive, considering the many changes that confront an individual and his or her social network (Pescosolido et al., 1998). Researchers can build on these findings to examine other circumstances in which network activation, patient needs, and network dynamics intertwine.

Implications and Directions for Future Work

Our findings have several implications for theory and practice. For research on networks and health, this study provides additional evidence for network activation and its consequences as mechanisms that drive network change (Perry & Pescosolido, 2015, 2010). Further, our results underscore the need for scholars to look beneath structural network indices (e.g., density, size) when studying network dynamics. To understand the relationship between health trajectories and network change, scholars should build on recent work that recognizes the surprising instability and situational flexibility of core networks (Small, 2013). For mental health professionals, the instability that follows from network involvement during treatment suggests a need to engage directly with caregivers, for example, in the form of training or resource provision. Deinstitutionalization and other societal shifts indicate that communities are more involved in mental healthcare than ever before. Whereas professional healthcare organizations are well-equipped to address patients' needs over a lengthy period of chronic illness, informal networks evidently suffer from the added burden. Social disruption in informal networks holds important implications for treatment outcomes; although disruption can facilitate the flow of new resources and opportunities, patients in unstable networks may lack support when it is needed most (Perry, 2006). As such, professionals should pursue initiatives promoting community-based care and caregiver outreach.

We note several promising directions for future work. First, our data does not allow us to examine domain-specific network activation at different stages of the treatment career (Aneshensel, 2013). We found that new mental health patients pursue ties that match their emotional, instrumental, and discussion needs. Future work might examine how patients leverage support in different domains at various stages of treatment, for example, at illness onset or during recovery. Further, additional research is needed to understand how these informal resources may supplement or replace professional support. Second, we have linked network activation to network instability, but the relationship between network dynamics and patient experiences during chronic illness requires further study. Dynamic changes in network properties such as size, density, functionality, and composition hold great potential to inform understanding of health trajectories (Abbott et al., 2012; Perry & Pescosolido, 2012). Third, this work was partly inspired by research in other contexts about network dynamics during crises (e.g., urban poverty in Desmond, 2012). Future work should examine network activation in response to different types of biographical disruption.

NOTES

1. Additional information at http://www.indiana.edu/~icmhsr/inmhs.html
2. Both inclusion criteria were assessed by self-report.
3. The INMHS data is a "treated" sample – only individuals who sought professional care for their mental health problems appear in the study. An important segment of the population of interest, those who did not seek care, are overlooked in this dataset; future research should examine this important population. For discussion of the decision to seek mental health treatment, see Pescosolido et al. (1998).
4. Sensitivity analyses indicate that this subsample does not significantly differ from the subsample of respondent contacted in only one wave, with one exception. Network members observed in only one wave have about one year less education,

on average. Consequently, results from the second set of analyses may not be generalizable to mental health patients with lower levels of education.

5. Additional notes on scale construction are omitted due to space limitations. An appendix that lists each needs item and details on scale construction are available on request.

6. Alternative non-linear specifications for time did not improve model fit.

ACKNOWLEDGMENTS

We gratefully acknowledge Bernice Pescosolido and the Indiana Consortium for Mental Health Services Research (ICMHSR) for providing access to the INMHS dataset. Financial support for INMHS was provided by the National Institute of Mental Health (grants K01MH00849, R29MH44780, and R24MH51669).

REFERENCES

Abbott, K. M., Bettger, J. P., Hanlon, A., & Hirschman, K. B. (2012). Factors associated with health discussion network size and composition among elderly recipients of long-term services and supports. *Health Communication*, *27*(8), 784–793.

Aneshensel, C. S. (2013). Mental illness as a career: Sociological perspectives. In *Handbook of the sociology of mental health* (pp. 603–620). Rotterdam: Springer.

Bury, M. (1982). Chronic illness as biographical disruption. *Sociology of Health and Illness*, *4*(2), 167–182.

Carpentier, N., & Ducharme, F. (2003). Care-giver network transformations: The need for an integrated perspective. *Ageing and Society*, *23*(04), 507–525.

Carpentier, N., & Grenier, A. (2012). Successful linkage between formal and informal care systems: The mobilization of outside help by caregivers of persons with Alzheimer's disease. *Qualitative Health Research*, *22*, 1330–1344.

Carpentier, N., Lesage, A., & White, D. (1999). Family influence on the first stages of the trajectory of patients diagnosed with severe psychiatric disorders. *Family Relations*, *48*, 397–403.

Cornwell, E. Y., & Waite, L. J. (2012). Social network resources and management of hypertension. *Journal of Health and Social Behavior*, *53*(2), 215–231.

Cutrona, C. E., & Russell, D. (1990). Type of social support and specific stress: Toward a theory of optimal matching. In I. Sarason, B. Sarason, & G. Pierce (Eds.), *Social support: An interactional view*. New York, NY: Wiley.

Cornwell, B., Laumann, E. O., & Schumm, L. P. (2008). The social connectedness of older adults: A national profile. *American Sociological Review*, *73*(2), 185–203.

de Miguel Luken, V., & Tranmer, M. (2010). Personal support networks of immigrants to Spain: A multilevel analysis. *Social Networks*, *32*(4), 253–262.

Desmond, M. (2012). Disposable ties and the urban poor. *American Journal of Sociology*, *117*(5), 1295–1335.

Fehr, E., Fischbacher, U., & Gächter, S. (2002). Strong reciprocity, human cooperation, and the enforcement of social norms. *Human Nature*, *13*(1), 1–25.

Feld, S. L. (1981). The focused organization of social ties. *American Journal of Sociology*, *86*, 1015–1035.

Gage-Bouchard, E. A., LaValley, S., Panagakis, C., & Shelton, R. C. (2015). The architecture of support: The activation of preexisting ties and formation of new ties for tailored support. *Social Science and Medicine*, *134*, 59–65.

Goffman, E. (1961). *Asylums: Essays on the social situation of mental patients and other inmates*. New York, NY: Anchor Books.

Horowitz, L. M., Krasnoperova, E. N., Tatar, D. G., Hansen, M. B., Person, E. A., Galvin, K. L., & Nelson, K. L. (2001). The way to console may depend on the goal: Experimental studies of social support. *Journal of Experimental Social Psychology*, *37*(1), 49–61.

House, J. S., Landis, K. R., & Umberson, D. (1988). Social relationships and health. *Science*, *241*(4865), 540–545.

Karp, D. A. (2000). *The burden of sympathy: How families cope with mental illness*. Oxford: Oxford University Press.

Kessler, R. C., Demler, O., Frank, R. G., Olfson, M., Pincus, H. A., Walters, E. E., & Zaslavsky, A. M. (2005). Prevalence and treatment of mental disorders, 1990 to 2003. *New England Journal of Medicine*, *352*(24), 2515–2523.

Lin, N. (1999). Building a network theory of social capital. *Connections*, *22*(1), 28–51.

Link, B. G., Cullen, F. T., Struening, E., Shrout, P. E., & Dohrenwend, B. P. (1989). A modified labeling theory approach to mental disorders: An empirical assessment. *American Sociological Review*, *54*(3), 400–423.

Lipton, F. R., Cohen, C. I., Fischer, E., & Katz, S. E. (1981). Schizophrenia: A network crisis. *Schizophrenia Bulletin*, *7*(1), 144–151.

Markowitz, F. E. (2001). Modeling processes in recovery from mental illness: Relationships between symptoms, life satisfaction, and self-concept. *Journal of Health and Social Behavior*, *42*(1), 64–79.

Marsden, P. V. (1987). Core discussion networks of Americans. *American Sociological Review*, *52*, 122–131.

Mechanic, D., & Rochefort, D. A. (1990). Deinstitutionalization: An appraisal of reform. *Annual Review of Sociology*, *16*, 301–327.

Morgan, D. L., Neal, M. B., & Carder, P. (1997). The stability of core and peripheral networks over time. *Social Networks*, *19*(1), 9–25.

Muhlbauer, S. A. (2002). Navigating the storm of mental illness: Phases in the family's journey. *Qualitative Health Research*, *12*(8), 1076–1092.

Pavalko, E. K., Harding, C. M., & Pescosolido, B. A. (2007). Mental illness careers in an era of change. *Social Problems*, *54*(4), 504–522.

Pavalko, E. K., & Woodbury, S. (2000). Social roles as process: Caregiving careers and women's health. *Journal of Health and Social Behavior*, *41*(1), 91–105.

Penning, M. J. (1990). Receipt of assistance by elderly people: Hierarchical selection and task specificity. *The Gerontologist*, *30*(2), 220–227.

Perlick, D. A., Hohenstein, J. M., Clarkin, J. F., Kaczynski, R., & Rosenheck, R. A. (2005). Use of mental health and primary care services by caregivers of patients with bipolar disorder: A preliminary study. *Bipolar Disorders*, *7*(2), 126–135.

Perry, B. L. (2006). Understanding social network disruption: The case of youth in foster care. *Social Problems*, *53*(3), 371.

Perry, B. L. (2011). The labeling paradox stigma, the sick role, and social networks in mental illness. *Journal of Health and Social Behavior*, *52*(4), 460–477.

Perry, B. L., & Pescosolido, B. A. (2010). Functional specificity in discussion networks: The influence of general and problem-specific networks on health outcomes. *Social Networks*, *32*(4), 345–357.

Perry, B. L., & Pescosolido, B. A. (2012). Social network dynamics and biographical disruption: The case of "first-timers" with mental illness1. *American Journal of Sociology*, *118*(1), 134–175.

Perry, B. L., & Pescosolido, B. A. (2015). Social network activation: The role of health discussion partners in recovery from mental illness. *Social Science and Medicine*, *125*, 116–128.

Pescosolido, B. A. (1991). Illness careers and network ties: A conceptual model of utilization and compliance. *Advances in Medical Sociology*, *2*(16), 164–181.

Pescosolido, B. A. (1992). Beyond rational choice: The social dynamics of how people seek help. *American Journal of Sociology*, *97*(4)1096–1138.

Pescosolido, B. A. (2006). Of pride and prejudice: The role of sociology and social networks in integrating the health sciences. *Journal of Health and Social Behavior*, *47*(3), 189–208.

Pescosolido, B. A., Gardner, C. B., & Lubell, K. M. (1998). How people get into mental health services: Stories of choice, coercion and "muddling through" from "first-timers." *Social Science and Medicine*, *46*(2), 275–286.

Raudenbush, S. W., & Bryk, A. S. (2002). *Hierarchical linear models: Applications and data analysis methods* (Vol. 1), Thousand Oaks, CA: Sage.

Sasovova, Z., Mehra, A., Borgatti, S. P., & Schippers, M. C. (2010). Network churn: The effects of self-monitoring personality on brokerage dynamics. *Administrative Science Quarterly*, *55*(4), 639–670.

Schafer, M. H. (2013). Discussion networks, physician visits, and non-conventional medicine: Probing the relational correlates of health care utilization. *Social Science and Medicine*, *87*, 176–184.

Small, M. L. (2013). Weak ties and the core discussion network: Why people regularly discuss important matters with unimportant alters. *Social Networks*, *35*(3), 470–483.

Small, M. L., Pamphile, V. D., & McMahan, P. (2015). How stable is the core discussion network? *Social Networks*, *40*, 90–102.

Smith, K. P., & Christakis, N. A. (2008). Social networks and health. *Annual Review of Sociology*, *34*, 405–429.

Spitzer, R. L., Williams, J. B., Gibbon, M., & First, M. B. (1992). The structured clinical interview for DSM-III-R (SCID): I: History, rationale, and description. *Archives of General Psychiatry*, *49*(8), 624–629.

Suitor, J., & Keeton, S. (1997). Once a friend, always a friend? Effects of homophily on women's support networks across a decade. *Social Networks*, *19*(1), 51–62.

Thoits, P. A. (2011). Mechanisms linking social ties and support to physical and mental health. *Journal of Health and Social Behavior*, *52*(2), 145–161.

Wahl, O. F. (2012). Stigma as a barrier to recovery from mental illness. *Trends in Cognitive Sciences*, *16*(1), 9–10.

Wellman, B. (2000). Partners in illness: Who helps when you are sick? *Complementary and Alternative Medicine: Challenge and Change*, *1*, 143–162.

Wellman, B. (2005). Community: From neighborhood to network. *Communications of the ACM*, *48*(10), 53–55.

Wellman, B., Wong, R. Y. L., Tindall, D., & Nazer, N. (1997). A decade of network change: Turnover, persistence and stability in personal communities. *Social Networks*, *19*(1), 27–50.

Wellman, B., & Wortley, S. (1990). Different strokes from different folks: Community ties and social support. *American Journal of Sociology*, *96*(3), 558–588.

UNDERSTANDINGS OF COMMUNITY AMONG PEOPLE USING PUBLICLY FUNDED COMMUNITY MENTAL HEALTH SERVICES

Alisa K. Lincoln and Wallis E. Adams

ABSTRACT

Purpose – *To understand how people using community public mental health services conceptualize community and their place within it within the post-deinstitutionalization era.*

Methodology/approach – *Two hundred ninety-four service users completed structured interviews in two urban, outpatient, public, and community mental health facilities in the Northeast. Quantitative and qualitative responses to the MacArthur Scale of Subjective Social Status, Community Ladder version, were analyzed to understand perspectives on community.*

Findings – *Mean subjective community status ladder score among participants was five (SD = 2.56). Participants identified four broad*

50 Years after Deinstitutionalization: Mental Illness in Contemporary Communities
Advances in Medical Sociology, Volume 17, 147–174

ISSN: 1057-6290/doi:10.1108/S1057-629020160000017006

categories of definitions of community: geographic community; community related to social definitions; contributing to society; and mental health service-user communities. Explanations for the location of their placement on the ladder (subjective community status) include comparisons to self and others, contributions to community, and social relationships. There was also a set of explanations that spoke to the intersection of multiple marginalizations and structural constraints. Finally, we explore relationships among understandings of community and perceptions of place within community.

Originality/value – *Community integration is a critical concept for community public mental health services, but little research has explored how mental health service users conceptualize their communities and their roles within them. Understandings of community are crucial to appropriately support peoples' needs within their communities. Furthermore, participants identify mechanisms that facilitate their personal community standing, and these are areas for potential intervention.*

Keywords: Community; mental health services; MacArthur ladder; community integration; serious mental illness

INTRODUCTION

The past decade has seen an increase in attention to how best to actualize calls for "a life in the community for all" for people with serious mental illness, as exemplified by the Substance Abuse and Mental Health Services Administration (SAMHSA) report "From Exclusion to Belonging: Transforming Mental Health Care in America" (Substance Abuse and Mental Health Service Administration [SAMHSA], 2006). Such efforts have been driven by policy makers, health care providers, researchers, advocacy groups, and mental health service users themselves. While these efforts have furthered exploration and dialogue on recovery and community integration, many important gaps in our knowledge remain. Despite increased attention to community integration many people with serious mental illness (SMI), particularly those using publicly funded services, remain marginalized and excluded from communities due to multiple factors including stigma, housing instability, poverty, and unemployment (Cook, 2006; Draine, Salzer, Culhane, & Hadley, 2002; Pescosolido, 2013; Rowe & Pelletier, 2012). Additionally, this lack of full community integration has been shown to impact mental health status as well as access to opportunity, leading to efforts to increase community integration as a critical component of mental health recovery (Bond, Salyers, Rollins, Rapp, & Zipple, 2004; Pahwa et al., 2014).

Despite calls for expanded community mental health services and focus on improved community integration, little is known about how community community mental health service users think about their communities and their place within them. Here we discuss the meaning of community in the lives of people with SMI as well as their place within these communities. We explore the ways in which understandings of community may relate to people's subjective social status (SSS) or perceived social position within their communities. Finally, we discuss implications of understanding community and the relationships among community and SSS for people with SMI.

We focus on the conceptualizations of community shared among people using public, urban, mental health services. The question of community is particularly relevant here, as mental health policy post-deinstitutionalization aimed to develop and expand community mental health services and supports and thus necessitated focus and attention on the meaning and processes of community inclusion and recovery for people with SMI. These efforts were driven by complex social, economic, and political forces well described elsewhere (Lamb & Bachrach, 2001; Paulson, 2012) and explicitly drew upon sociological conceptualizations of community as a framework for the design and structuring of community mental health centers and systems of care. However, others have argued that this was in fact a post-hoc application of sociological thinking (Hunter & Riger, 1986).

Sociological Understandings of Community

Exploration and understanding of community has been a central focus of sociological work for many years. Concepts of community are operationalized and engaged across multiple sociological sub-disciplines, informed by multiple theoretical perspectives, and vary in part by the function or role of community being examined. Most sociological understandings of community draw upon three components, albeit in varying ways: (1) shared geography or physical place; (2) people engaging in social interaction; and (3) shared ties or bonds (Goe & Noonan, 2007; Hillery, 1955).

The last few decades have seen a great increase in the amount and quality of scholarship related to place and health. In their work on "place effects," Macintyre, Ellaway, and Cummins (2002) brought to light the ways in which both material infrastructure and collective social functioning are important and interrelated explanations for health inequalities. While noting that place differences in health effects differ according to area, population and health outcomes, they also presented a framework for healthy neighborhood that includes both material opportunity structures and collective social functioning (Macintyre et al., 2002). Gesler's concept of a "therapeutic landscape" noted that the "social and the spatial are intimately intertwined" (1992, p. 774). The "therapeutic landscape," in which landscapes are associated with treatment and healing, is now a central tenant in many social scientific studies of place and health (Gesler, 1992; Williams, 2007).

Others have written about the social construction of community noting, "Community is not a received truth, something out there to which individuals simply relate; rather, a community is what people define it to be" (Hunter & Riger, 1986, p. 64). Furthermore, various levels of community exist, and people can identify with several communities simultaneously (Hunter & Riger, 1986). Multiple and coexisting meanings of community were present in ancient societies (Delanty, 2010), and the idea of community continues to be constructed and reconstructed today. Some have argued that the concept of community is particularly relevant for the contemporary era, due to an increased sense of insecurity and fragmentation of society (Delanty, 2010). Mulligan (2015) extends Delanty's work on community by proposing a differentiation between "grounded," or place-based, communities, and "projected" communities. In her 2009 ASA Presidential Address, Patricia Hill Collins highlighted the multiple ways of understanding and categorizing community, while proposing that community be reframed as a political construct. "The construct of community constitutes both a principle of actual social organization and an idea that people use to make sense of and shape their everyday lived realities, and it may be central to the workings of intersecting power relations in heretofore unrecognized ways" (Collins, 2010, p. 8). Further work on community attachment in rural communities has shown that individual experience, rather than aspects of the community itself, significantly impacts levels of community attachment (Flaherty & Brown, 2010).

Understandings of Community among Mental Health Service Users

While there is a long-standing sociological tradition of studying the broad meaning of community, few studies have explored how mental health service users understand community and whether people with SMI have a unique experience of community. Post-deinstitutionalization, the experience of long-term physical exclusion from community in psychiatric facilities is a far less frequent occurrence among people with SMI. However, new forms of both geographic and social exclusion have emerged and these have had a powerful impact on public mental health service users experience of community. Public mental health service users provide an important opportunity to examine understandings of community and people's perception of their place within community among a group that faces multiple sources of social marginalization, including stigma, high rates of poverty and unemployment, lack of access to stable housing, and high rates of trauma exposure. Given the demonstrated importance of social cohesion and social capital on the well-being of all community members, as well as the noted clinical importance of community integration for people with serious mental illness, attention to understandings of community and social position within communities is well needed for people using public mental health services. As Ware, Hopper, Tugenberg, Dickey, and Fisher (2007) noted, "Despite decades of deinstitutionalization and the best efforts of community mental health services, individuals with psychiatric disabilities living outside the hospital may be described as in the community but not of it" (p. 469).

Thus, recent qualitative work has focused on understanding how people with SMI think about community. These studies have found that, like people living without disabilities, most people with SMI define community in terms of places and people. However, other concepts have arisen in this work as well. Wong, Sands, and Solomon (2010) explored the concept of community through seven focus groups with mental health consumers, grouped by ethnicity and sexuality/gender identity. Consumers identified four types of communities: communities based on cultural identity, treatment communities, faith communities, and neighborhoods. Two conceptual domains were present in discussions of all of the types of communities: togetherness and community acceptance (Wong et al., 2010). The authors note that identities other than that of mental health service user, such as ethnic or gender identities, are central to understandings of community among people with psychiatric disabilities and that experiences of community exclusion are based on the intersection of multiple stigmatized identities (Wong et al., 2010).

More recently, Bromley et al. (2013) and Townley (2015) have emphasized the importance of sub-communities, particularly mental health communities, among people with serious mental illness. Both studies drew upon semi-structured interviews with participants receiving services at public mental health clinics and reported that the majority of participants identified both people and places as community, but each also highlighted the role of the mental health communities. Bromley et al. (2013) described four types of experiences that participants saw as critical to how they understand community: receiving help, minimizing risk, avoiding stigma, and giving back. Townley (2015) emphasized that the majority of participants provided definitions of community very much in keeping with the Miriam-Webster definition, "the people with common interests living in a particular area" (p. 117) but noted that participants also identified five types of sub-communities and belonged on average to three sub-communities. These included sub-communities related to: mental health, residential place, spiritual, leisure/recreational, and substance abuse. Two of the 30 participants identified as belonging to no sub-communities.

This literature suggests that people using mental health services think about and define their communities in multiple ways, some similar to people without SMI and others perhaps shaped by their unique lived experience (Bromley et al., 2013; Wong et al., 2010; Townley, 2015). Some mental health service users specifically identify the salience of mental health communities. Mandiberg (2010) has argued that enclave communities might provide the most social inclusion for people with psychiatric disabilities. In a recent study (Pahwa et al., 2014), ethnically diverse people with severe mental illness ($n = 33$) were interviewed for a study assessing community integration within both the mental health community and the non-mental health community. Among this sample people with severe mental illness most frequently rate themselves as primarily integrated into the mental health community. However, their social support networks and social capital are predominantly based within non-mental health communities. While these results vary by intensity of service use, this inconsistency between social integration and social capital (Pahwa et al., 2014) needs to be considered when thinking about the relationships between community definition and ones perceived status or role within community.

Subjective Social Status (SSS): Mental Health Service Users' Understandings of Their Place within Community

Just as people define communities in various ways, people also identify their role and status within those communities in complex ways. Subjective social status has originally been defined as "a person's belief about his location in a status order" (Davis, 1956). This is often operationalized as community status and questions asking about subjective social status may include asking participants to define their community, as well as their place within it. It has been demonstrated that a person's subjective social status is strongly influenced by their conceptualization of their reference group. In a study of subjective social status and referent group sensitivity, Wolff, Subramanian, Acevedo-Garcia, Weber, and Kawachi (2010) found that there is a stronger relationship between self-rated health and subjective social status when people are asked to compare themselves to distal referent groups, such as American society, than closer referent groups, such as ones neighbors or parents. Additionally, groups with certain stigmatized statuses report lower subjective social status than others. For example, formerly incarcerated persons and those who have spent time in a psychiatric hospital report lower subjective social status than the general population (Schnittker & Bacak, 2013).

Peoples' perceptions of their own social status are a strong indicator of multiple poor physical health measures, such as diabetes and respiratory illness, as well as depressive symptomology (Singh-Manoux, Adler, & Marmot, 2003). The relationships among subjective social status and poor mental health have also been found in United States immigrant populations (Nicklett & Burgard, 2009). Studies of subjective social status draw upon multiple methods but often utilize what has come to be known as the MacArthur Ladder, an instrument designed to measure perceptions of social or community status (Adler, Stewart, & Psychosocial Working Group, 2007). There are two versions of the MacArthur Ladder, one linked to traditional SES indicators (known as the society ladder) and a second linked to standing in one's community.

The relationships among subjective social status, as measured with the MacArthur ladder, and mental health and well-being has been examined among several populations. The Whitehall II study, a prospective cohort study of London-based civil service employees, demonstrated a significant relationship between GHQ depression and low subjective status (Singh-Manoux et al., 2003). Subjective social status has been found to be inversely associated with chronic stress, subjective stress, negative effect, and pessimism among women (Adler, Epel, Castellazzo, & Ickovics, 2000). In fact, there is some evidence that subjective social or community status may be an even more powerful predictor of mental health status than objective measures of social position. McLaughlin, Costello, Leblanc, Sampson, and Kessler (2012) demonstrated that subjective social status (as assessed with the community status ladder) was more consistently related to mental disorders among adolescents than either absolute or relative measures of SES.

In another study with adolescents, the community ladder rankings were more strongly associated with depressive symptoms than were the society ladder rankings (Goodman et al., 2001) demonstrating that understandings and experiences of local community may be particularly salient for adolescent mental health. The relationship between subjective social status and mental health has also been demonstrated among both American and British adults, with Adler et al. (2008) finding that lower social status is associated with depressive symptomology among male and female participants in both the Whitehall-II and CARDIA studies.

Each of the studies utilizing the MacArthur ladder to assess community social status drew upon quantitative analyses of the marked social position provided by participants. However, the MacArthur Ladder instrument also includes open-ended questions that allow participants to define their communities and explain how they decided their position on the ladder. Few studies have reported on these data. One of the exceptions is a recent British study exploring subjective social status among individuals living with chronic illness. This study utilized the MacArthur society ladder through a mixed methods approach (Daker-White et al., 2014; Vassilev et al., 2014). With their analyses of both the quantitative ladder rankings and qualitative responses, the authors suggest that social participation outside of the labor market might allow individuals to rebuild their subjective social status (Vassilev et al., 2014). Further qualitative analysis explored the narratives of low socioeconomic status respondents in this study who ranked themselves either high or low in terms of subjective social status (Daker-White et al., 2014). The community ladder and the associated qualitative questions were also examined among a subsample of black and white participants in the Coronary Artery Risk Development in Young Adults ($N = 60$) study (Adler, Stewart, & Psychosocial Working Group, 2007). Here participants most frequently defined community as their neighborhood and noted that their community status most commonly depended on everyday ways in which they did or did not give to others, such as volunteering and being good neighbors.

In this chapter we examine two important questions. First, how do people using urban, public mental health services think about, and define community? And, secondly, how do they understand their place within their communities (SSS)? Finally, we explore the potential relationships among understandings of community and SSS. To do this, we examine data collected as part of a larger inter-disciplinary NIMH funded study designed to examine the meaning and impact of limited literacy in the lives of people with serious mental illness and the ways in which limited literacies serve as barriers to recovery and social integration. Here the MacArthur Community Status Ladder was used to assess perceptions of subjective social status within self-defined community, how participants defined their community, and explanation as to why they placed themselves where they did on the ladder.

METHODS

Sample

Structured interviews (n = 294) were completed at two urban public mental health outpatient clinics in a Northeastern City in the United States as part of a study aimed at understanding the meaning and impact of limited literacy in the lives of people with serious mental illness. Individuals aged 18 and older who received services at one of the two clinics were not under guardianship, and were capable of communicating with their mental health providers in English were eligible to participate in the study. Participants were randomly recruited by study staff, although due to clinic specific factors this was done differently at the two sites. At one clinic every fifth patient presenting for care was eligible, and at the other clinic recruitment was randomized by day of the week. A rigorous consent process was utilized with an awareness of the challenges of limited literacy and the study was fully approved by multiple Institutional Review Boards.

The interview not only assessed multiple types of literacy (reading, numeracy and aural) but also collected information about each participant that could help us understand the relationships, and explore mechanisms, among psychiatric disorders, limited literacy and mental health service utilization. This included questions about participants' gender, race, ethnicity, immigration history, language, socioeconomic status, and education. Multiple tests of neurocognitive impairment were administered, as were measures of health care utilization, stigma, discrimination and understandings of recovery.

Assessment of social status was part of the demographic battery and included the MacArthur Scale of Subjective Social Status (the "MacArthur ladder") to assess participants' perception of their standing in the community (Kilpatrick & Cantril, 1960; Nicklett & Burgard, 2007). Respondents were shown a picture of a ladder with 10 rungs. They were instructed to mark an "X" on the rung that best represented where they stand in the community. The first rung (bottom rung) indicated the lowest standing in the community whereas the 10th rung (top rung) indicated the highest standing. If respondents put an "X" between two rungs, the interviewer would ask the respondent to choose the lower or higher rung. A few participants opted out of participating in the MacArthur ladder, leaving the sample size for this chapter at 276 individuals. After marking the ladder, three qualitative follow-up questions were asked to learn more about the participants' responses. These included: "Can you tell me briefly how you thought about community when you drew the 'X' on the ladder?"; "Can you tell me briefly why you put yourself where you did?"; and "How do you feel about being positioned where you feel you are?"

In this chapter, we utilize data gathered from the assessments of Social Status including the quantitative data derived from the participant's placement of the "X" on the ladder and their responses to the first two qualitative questions. Qualitative responses were read and analyzed by both authors and a coding scheme for responses was developed through an iterative process. Ultimately eight codes were created as a way to organize participants' understandings of community and those eight codes were grouped into four emerging themes (Table 2). Explanation for where people placed themselves on the ladder also fell into four categories as described below.

RESULTS

Demographics

The mean age of the participants was 45, ranging from 19 to 77 years of age. The sample was 57% female. Participants reflected the racial diversity of service users at both sites with an overall sample of 39% African American, 38% White, and 9% Hispanic ethnicity. Reflective of public mental health services users, individual yearly income was quite low, with over two thirds of participants earning less than ten thousand dollars per year. There was a range of income, however, with one participant earning over $100,000 per year and two participants between $40,000 and $49,999 per year. Educational attainment also varied, with over a quarter of participants not completing High School and eight participants obtaining a post-graduate degree. Demographic characteristics are presented in Table 1.

Quantitative Ladder Results

Participants rated their subjective community status by indicating where they believed they stood on the community status ladder. Participants

Table 1. Demographics and Ladder Scores.

	N	Valid Percentage	Mean Ladder Score	Standard Deviation
Sample	276		5.00	2.558
Site				
Medical Center	189	68.5	5.08	2.568
Public Mental Health Center	87	31.5	4.84	2.542
Age				
18–49	155	56.4	4.68*	2.512
>50 years	120	43.6	5.40	2.565
Gender				
Male	116	42.3	4.65*	2.595
Female	158	57.7	5.27	2.458
Ethnicity				
Latino/Hispanic	24	8.8	5.04	2.971
Non-Latino/Hispanic	150	91.2	5.01	2.505
Race				
White	104	37.7	4.65	2.421
Black	110	39.9	5.31	2.587
2+ Races	34	12.3	5.24	2.618
Other	28	10.1	4.82	2.816
Country of birth				
Born Outside the United States	31	11.2	5.13	2.419
US born	245	88.8	4.99	2.579
Incarceration				
Ex-inmates	135	49.3	4.60*	2.604
Not previously incarcerated	139	50.7	5.33	2.427
Yearly income (individual)				
<$10,000	181	67.8	4.80	2.480
$10–19,999	60	22.5	5.15	2.748
>$20,000	26	9.7	6.04	2.425
Educational attainment				
Did not complete high school	73	26.4	5.25	2.727
High school diploma/GED	93	33.7	4.91	2.408
Some college/vocational	84	30.4	4.75	2.620
Bachelor's degree and above	26	9.4	5.46	2.404
Housing status				
Lives alone	92	34.6	5.52**	2.522
Group/supported housing	32	12	4.16	2.371
No stable housing/shelter	62	23.3	4.26	2.605
Family/spouse	80	30.1	5.48	2.460

$^{*}p < .05$; $^{**}p < .01$.

identified themselves at the bottom of the ladder (ladder score = 0), at the top of the ladder (ladder score = 10), and at every ladder rung between those two extremes. Of the participants who completed the ladder task ($n = 276$), the mean ladder score is 5.00. The median ladder score is 5.00, while the mode is 6. The standard deviation for the sample is 2.56.

Differences in mean ladder scores were tested across subgroups using independent sample t-tests and one-way analysis of variance. Statistically significant differences in mean ladder scores were observed between those over and under 50 years of age, with those 50 years and older reporting higher subjective community status. Other significant mean differences were observed according to gender, as well as history of incarceration. Men and those participants indicating a history of incarceration reported lower ladder scores than women and participants not previously incarcerated, respectively. Ladder means according to housing status was also statistically significant, with those living alone and with family reporting higher ladder scores than those living in group homes, supported housing, shelters, or without stable housing. Both significant and non-significant mean ladder score differences are also reported in Table 1.

Qualitative Results: Meaning of Community

Our participants defined community in many ways, and individual participants often had multiple definitions. Participant understandings of community draw upon four aspects of community: place/geographic location; social relationships; community as people who "contribute"; and peer or recovery communities.

Neighborhood and Place

More than three-quarters of our participants defined community as a physical place, primarily a neighborhood or city. This was often described as the "neighborhood where I live" or by specific neighborhood names. Others defined their community by a specific building or housing structure, "I was thinking about my building, cause there's, like I said there is over 50 people in it … that's what I was referring, mostly to the building because it is a community within itself" (RID 011). Residential programs and clubhouses, as physical places, were also frequently mentioned in definitions of community.

> Community is, I guess it's around where you live and stuff, and my community revolves around the Clubhouse because I go there three days a week and go out to dinner once a month, and they got me a job. (RID 097)

Several described Public Housing as their community. "So I live in a public housing development that I've lived for almost 8 years. And we're a tightknit community" (RID 219). Often neighborhood definitions included discussion of the people within the neighborhoods, "the people around me," and institutions within neighborhoods which contributed in positive ways to their sense of community. Definitions of community included places such as libraries, churches, pools, schools, police and community centers as well as "getting together with other people and, volunteering, or, visiting the community centers, or any other facilities in the community like the pool or something like that" (RID 077). Discussions of neighborhood also included many discussions of fear of crime and violence and challenging neighborhood conditions. As described by one participant, "I don't care for my community. It's like dangerous" (RID 160). Another noted:

> RID 263: The community where I am living at there is a lot of problems...there is always a lot of gang fights out in the areas, and shootings and stuff like that.
>
> Interviewer: And what does the word community mean to you?
>
> RID 263: Um community I thought of as violent

Challenges to place-based definitions of community were found among people with no permanent home. As 23% of our sample reported having no permanent home this represents a significant portion of our population and reflects the high rates of housing instability among public mental health service users. Many homeless participants described feeling that the neighborhood community did not include them. As one noted, "I don't believe this community feels that I'm a viable part at all … well because of my present situation. Homeless, not working, Black, um, male, kind of large, I feel that sometimes people are kind of intimidated because of those things" (RID 131). Participants with no permanent home sometimes described shelters as their community but more often spoke of the lack of community because they were homeless. One defined community as "the environment that I live in, just, I'm homeless" (RID 125). Finally a handful of participants defined community in a more expansive way, as the "whole world" or the "whole United States."

Social Explanations of Community

The second most common type of community definition included friends and family, and "people they can be around" or "associate with on a daily basis." These understandings of community rested heavily on spending time with people in recreational activities as well as descriptions of people within participants' social network on whom they could rely for various types of social support (instrumental, emotional). Often people described what community meant to them, but then followed with the ways that it actually played out in their lives. "A bunch of people getting along … getting together, hanging out. But then again, I've only met one person [in my neighborhood] who I've talked to" (RID 211).

Social definitions of community extending beyond family and friends most often included descriptions of "people who care and want to help" (RID 087), "people working together and saying they can … looking out for one another" (RID 110), "community is just like helping people" (RID 276), and other examples of working together to make something better or improve conditions. Some were more general describing community as all of the people they interact with.

People Who Contribute to Society

Community was often defined as made up of those people "contributing" to society. "Community. I thought about it as people that are, you know, that own homes and businesses" (RID 197). Many people defined community as "people having employment" (RID 047), or jobs, or without a criminal record. "I mean the citizens who don't have, who don't share the same criminal record" (RID 051). When asked how they thought about community another noted, "I just thought about people that are educated and smart and work and you know, live, have houses and families" (RID 169). Another said, "I just think about like all the normal people with good jobs that don't do drugs, and haven't been to jail, and always done the right thing" (RID 296). While some participants spoke of being a part of community by contributing to the community, by "giving back," "being able to help somebody" (RID 055), or helping others often through volunteering or work and employment, most saw their lack of employment and social instability as excluding them from "community." Their descriptions of other community members looked very different from their own lives. Several participants responded that they had no community, were not a part of a community or were alone. "I just see all the people around me and I just feel all alone and like I have no one and that it's going to be like that forever. In essence I don't have a community" (RID 118).

Mental Health Communities

Finally, our participants described the importance of specific service-user communities, specifically disability communities, mental health communities, communities focused on sobriety and "staying clean," and recovery. Some people described having a strong mental health community or recovery community, but not being part of a larger community. "I mean the only real ties that I have are the mental health community. Ya know some clients like myself, and then the staff too like this whole sort of circle" (RID 094). Others described their community as AA, NA or other self-help communities. One noted, "a community where my peers, my neighbors, or my community in my methadone clinic" (RID 137). Or, "yeah, people in recovery that I hang out with, and don't use" (RID 145). There was also discussion of being separated from communities of people using drugs and alcohol by their choices to try to get or stay clean.

Qualitative Results: Explanations for Ladder Locations

In addition to asking participants to discuss how they defined their community, interviewers prompted participants to discuss the reasons why they placed themselves on the ladder at the level they chose. Responses to this question included a variety of explanations and explorations of the mechanisms that facilitated their ladder placement or their SSS within their community. Qualitative analysis of these responses revealed four different types of explanations: comparative explanations; contribution-based explanations; relationship focused explanations; and a set of explanations related to experiences of marginalization. Participants frequently drew upon two or more types of explanations in their discussions.

Comparative Explanations

The community mental health service users that we spoke with often engaged in comparitive appraisals when discussing the reasons for their placement on the ladder. Service users located themselves on the ladder in relation to the perceived location of others. Their comparisons were both negative and positive, in that they identified lower or higher on the ladder than their chosen comparison group. One participant explained their centralized location on the ladder: "Because I'm not any worse .... There are people that are doing worse than I am and people that are doing better than I am. So kind of equal centered, not so high centered, but more down in the center" (RID 130). In this case, she located her status within the community in contrast to a generalized other. However, other participants compared themselves to specific people with whom they have interaction. "Cause I see my other neighbors, I mean, you know they involved in things like the crime watch and they got houses and cars and stuff and doing something with their life" (RID 174). In contrast to his neighbors, this participant notes that he is neither fully engaged in community activities nor in possession of the material status symbols.

One of the most frequently evoked explanations centered on the participants' own histories. Participants frequently described their current community standing in contrast to how they conceptualize their past experiences, behaviors, and social standing. One participant explained their new, lower position:

> Um well I had it rough the past 2 years I've been out of homeless shelters and like I've been um a van ... which is really like tough place and um, So I'm dealing, I'm getting SSI which is not like the best income you could have. I used to have two jobs, so it's like...right now it's like I'm not really at my best. Like I'm not really like 10% of what I used to be so it's really bad (RID 068).

This participant located himself on the second rung of the ladder at this point in his life. Several participants presented a personal narrative of "falling" down the ladder due to both health-related and economic circumstances, which made current difficulties harder to bear when compared to previous successes. A present but less common personal narrative reflected an improvement in circumstance over time, as demonstrated by this man who located himself on the eighth rung of the ladder: "I was down there at the bottom of the ladder and I built up people's trust and stuff and the past six years I've been volunteering, cooking and everything" (RID 073). Personal changes in housing stability and status impact perceived standing, with one reflecting, "I would have put myself at the bottom of the ladder when I was homeless but I have my place now" (RID 211). In contrast, another noted, "like I backtracked now I'm homeless again" (RID 212).

Comparative explanations juxtapose not only one's current perceived standing with one's past, but also with one's goals and idealized future selves. Service users report disappointment when they perceive themselves as failing to achieve what they believe to be possible for them. Multiple participants repeat this sentiment: "I feel like I'm not living up to my potential" (RID 077); "I'm not fulfilling my goals" (RID 231); "I could do more with my life" (RID 249); "I'm not where I want to be" (RID 225); "I should be farther along in my life" (RID 296). In these cases, subjective standing within the community does not reflect a comparison with others or even with one's own past standing. Rather, ladder placement reflects perceived personal failures and unreached life goals.

Community Contribution Explanations
Contribution to community plays an important role in locating a person's status within that community. A person who located himself on the ninth rung explained that his high location on the ladder is, "because I do a lot for my community. And I participate a lot in the community that I live in. That's why I put myself there. And I help my community a lot" (RID 180). Service users describe a wide variety of ways in which people can contribute to society that range from broad to the specific, and economic to social.

Specific activities that service users report when explaining their location includes: volunteering in various capacities with multiple organizations, participating in tenant associations and neighborhood task forces, employment, and paying taxes. "[I teach] English and shopping, and I work in food pantries to help out" (RID 122). The contributions to society did not have to be through formal means or organizations. Several participants reflected on assisting older adults in their neighborhood or apartment complex with daily tasks. "The older people on my street, they made me feel responsible because they are asking me to do things" (RID 297). Relationships with neighbors and other community members are central to community standing.

Participants reflected upon contribution to community both when they believed they did contribute, and when they did not. After marking the second rung, one explained: "I do not have anything good that I can contribute to society right now, you know, as far as what is going on my life right now, that's why I put myself so low on the, on the ladder, you know?" (RID 185). Location on the ladder was explained by both the provision and the absence of contribution. Furthermore, several participants despaired that they were using community or governmental resources, rather than contributing. A participant explained why he located himself on the first (lowest) rung of the community ladder, "Because I'm getting help from the community and not giving it" (RID 138) while another person described "depending on the state for my livelihood … I am depending on them to feed me, house me" (RID 023). This is in stark contrast to the prideful discourse surrounding employment and community contribution.

Relationship-Based Explanations
Relationships with others, or lack of relationships, determined ladder location for a great number of the people that spoke with us. These

relationships were based on community participation and contribution, as discussed above, but also invoked narratives of reputation and standing, as well as intimacy with friends and family. For a number of people, experiences of isolation, or lack of interpersonal relationships, were used to explain subjective community standing. For others, religion, or relationships with God, played a central role in their understandings of ladder locations.

Reputation and standing within the general community or neighborhood factors into a person's community standing score. Some participants are well known within their communities, while others are not. Several people discussed the importance of being respected within their community. One man explained the reasoning behind his score of nine on the community status ladder, "I get along with most everybody, uh, landlord is good, you know, I'm, I'm pretty respected and honest, I've gotten some breaks because of that. My word is generally regarded as good. I'm still living where I'm living at because my word is generally regarded as good. Yeah, I enjoy a good reputation with the people that I'm around" (RID 011). He does not explicitly identify the people that he is "around" other than his landlord, instead indicating that he has positive relationships with a group of people that make up his community. Other participants identify relationship with specific people, frequently friends or family members, as critical elements in determining where they place themselves on the ladder.

For a subset of the participants, explanations of subjective community standing centered on their relationships with God and religion. Many of these people identify their religiosity as a factor associated with higher standing. One participant explains marking rung 7 on the community ladder by noting that she is "work[ing] at becoming Christ-like which makes me become more righteous as I get older. Which is a good thing. Righteousness is a good thing for society" (RID 144). Others explicitly place God at the top of the ladder, and determine their ladder locations based on their relationships with God. Another man explained that the top rung (score of 10) is God, and that he is located on the eighth rung (RID 108). Those "individuals in the world that understand God" are also located on the upper part of the ladder, while "the rest of the world are on the lower rungs."

While many participants discussed positive relationships with their community, people within their lives, and God, there were a large number of people who discussed experiences of social isolation. Lack of relationships with others is a common explanation for community standing among our participants. One participant placed herself on the second rung because "in the community where I live, most people don't know me, you know I just live there and I feel like I don't even exist, I feel like people don't know that I'm there. Maybe people don't know that I'm there. I feel invisible" (RID 287). Other participants talked in depth about the lack of ties that they have to their neighborhoods, lack of social engagement, and feelings of segregation. In general, participants discussing their experiences of isolation placed themselves on the bottom few rungs of the community status ladder, "At the bottom, its like the very, it not, its not part of it, its not participating, its going in a closed area, like solitary confinement" (RID 020). These service users are indicating a distinct lack of community integration.

Explanations of Stigmatized Status and Structural Constraints

The final type of explanations that participants utilized in discussing their subjective community status speaks to experiences of marginalization. This set of explanations includes the intersection of multiple stigmatized statuses, alongside lower socioeconomic positions and other structural constraints. A few of the participants discussed the stigma of experiences of mental illness, mental health services utilization, and medication management, but a far greater number of participants discussed other types of stigmas and obstacles.

Participants disclosed marginalization and stigma related to history of incarceration, history of and current drug use, challenges with medication management and mental health, disability, educational attainment, race, immigration status, housing status, and gender identity. Having a criminal background was cited as reasons for having a low community standing, but it was also used to explain how their standing has improved over time. Most commonly, participants discussed multiple stigmatized statuses when discussing experiences of marginalization. As one woman explained, she feels, "less than, because I don't have a job and I'm on disability and people judge you and I look like a certain way. They look at me like I'm an addict, and I am a previous addict. It's just um, how you feel as you go on and how people look at you" (RID 300). Participants described how they are treated and responded to due to multiple stigmatized statuses. Two participants who placed themselves on the second rung of the ladder cited multiple stigmatized identities, with the first citing lack of education and being transgender, and the latter indicating that her low community status is due to her race and being in a wheelchair (RID 65 and RID 214).

Finally, poverty was a pervasive topic, with participants discussing lack of housing and material possessions as primary explanations for their ladder locations. Socioeconomic standing and employment are vitally important factors in determining community standing. A woman explains her location on the second rung of the ladder: "Because right now I'm homeless, I've lost my job, I'm having problems with my mental illness, and um I don't feel I'm in good standing with my community. Even though I'm an honest person. Plus I'm poor" (RID 260). Others echoes these concerns, "I'm very poor. I'm very poor and mentally ill, and I'm don't have a job. I'm close to being homeless" (RID 074). The challenges of poverty were often exacerbated by episodic illness as described by this woman:

> I get admitted into the hospital, come out and my gas is off. So now all I have is my electricity. Everything is shut off. My insurance is canceled on my car. The registry wants my license plates; they don't even want me to drive. I need my car to go to work. I don't have my disability; I only got a little part time job to support me and my sixteen-year-old son. And... uh now I can't even take a shower. My refrigerator is on the fritz; my microwave is about to go. Everything is just like crap in my life right now. I have nothing, nothing. (RID 232)

Exploring the Relationships among Definitions of Community and SSS

Finally, we examine how community definitions relate to perceptions of place within community (SSS). As seen in Table 2, ladder score differed

Table 2. Exploring the Relationships among Definitions of Community and SSS.

Definitions of Community Themes and Codes	Description	*N*	Ladder Mean
Theme 1: Neighborhood/place			
Neighborhood	Neighborhood definitions	113	5.32
Macro place	Place-based definitions on a broad scale, including country and society	34	4.28
Housing and facilities	Buildings, housing units, programs, and facilities	32	5.90
Theme 2: Social explanations of community			
Friends, family, and daily relationships	Community is ones friends, family, neighbors, and other individuals with whom one has a daily relationship	62	5.37
Lack of community	Individuals state that they do not belong to any community	19	2.94
Theme 3: People who contribute to society			
Volunteering and giving back	Contribution through "giving back," including volunteering	33	5.55
Employment and ownership	Individuals who are employed and/ or have home/ car ownership	22	4.29
Theme 4: Mental health communities	Peer communities, NA, AA and other recovery communities	11	4.90
Entire sample		276	5.0

substantially by definition of community. In these preliminary analyses we examined the global association of mean ladder score across the eight community definition variables in a regression model with a partial F-statistic (8 numerator df). Analyses demonstrated that there are overall statistically significant differences in the mean ladder scores across the groups (p = 0.0014). Thus, as suggested by others (Wolff et al., 2010), SSS in part depends on the reference group, the defined community. People using public mental health services have multiple comparative explanatory frames for their own position within community. Further work is needed to disentangle these findings and to understand the relationships among community definitions and other factors related to SSS such as experiences of discrimination or stigma, poverty, and other markers of social exclusion.

DISCUSSION

This sample of public mental health service users report SSS (mean ladder score of 5.00) that is lower than previously found in both national population samples and those of others who use mental health services. This is in keeping with previous literature that shows that people with mental illness experience high levels of stigma and discrimination. Schnittker and Bacak (2013) report that the mean community ladder score for male participants in a nationally representative sample with a psychiatric disorder over their lifetime is 6.19, while the mean community ladder score for those participants who have previously been in a psychiatric hospital is even lower, at 5.78. However, these mean scores are still higher than those found in the current study of public sector outpatient mental health service users. The mean ladder score among men in our study was lower than that of women, at 4.65 in comparison to 5.27.

While experiences of stigma and discrimination are important factors in understanding SSS, our qualitative analyses provide insight into other factors that might be contributing to these lower reported scores through understanding how our participants think about community and their place within it. Our participants first and foremost define community through the use of place. They see community as their multi-residence buildings, public housing or residential programs. Yet, they also see community as their neighborhood and city. Institutions and programs, such as libraries, community and recreation centers, schools, and health care facilities are important components of community. Other participants chose to define community in more social terms, the people they interact with, their families and friends. Often these definitions focused on people who helped and supported them, or less frequently, people they were able to support and help. These understandings resonate with prior sociological work on community.

However two important aspects of understanding community stand out for our participants. First, as seen in prior work, our participants described the importance of mental health communities. These were described in multiple ways including people using services at the same clinics they did, participation in support groups such as AA or NA, or just more generally as a community of people with shared experiences of health and stigma. Secondly, participants spoke of community as people helping each other, supporting each other and working toward a common goal of making things better. As in Bromley's work (Bromley et al., 2013), our participants highly valued helping and giving back. However, our participants also defined community as being made up of people contributing to society most often in ways that they themselves were not. More specifically, they spoke of community members as being employed, having families, homes, resources, and no criminal history. Public mental health service users described the ways that they were different from these community members, how they worked to contribute more, and the ways that they felt excluded from and looked down upon by community members. While they often named their neighborhood as community, further discussion included the ways that their personal histories or characteristics marginalized or excluded them, even while they were physically in the community, as described by Ware et al. (2007).

These discussions of marginalization and exclusion require us to challenge our thinking about community and well-being. While understandings of community promote integration and belonging, these same concepts can fragment peoples, not just unite them (Delanty, 2010). As Mulligan (2015) notes, community creates a sense of both insiders and outsiders, and our participants describe experiences of exclusion related to community. Belton (2013) has described the "mythological promise of community" which downplays the tension between community, identity and marginality, and Hudson (2012) notes, "in traditional conceptualizations of community, the multidimensionality of marginalized populations is often unacknowledged" (p. 167). These recent scholars remind us that community is not an apolitical concept and community is of central concern to power relations. "Recasting the notion of community as a political construct highlights how social inequalities are organized via structural principles of communities and are made comprehensible through a language of community" (Collins, 2010, p. 8). However, the political concept of community can therefore also be a catalyst of social justice and powerful principle for social justice initiatives (Collins, 2010; Hudson, 2012) and further work is needed to develop these efforts for people using public mental health services in the community. In order to harness the emancipatory potential of community, it is critical to understand how people experiencing structural disadvantage and marginalization experience and understand the communities they live in and identify with. These qualitative data demonstrate understandings and experiences of community among a particularly stigmatized and disadvantaged population.

These qualitative data also help to elucidate the ways our participants think about subjective social status through their explanations of why they placed themselves on the ladder where they did. These explanations were often complex and involved multiple factors. Specifically, our participants report experiencing multiple types of marginalization. Participants identify the intersection of these barriers and discriminatory practices as causal mechanisms for low community status ladder scores. For mental health service users, community status includes experiences of both inclusion and isolation.

While the mean ladder scores reported in this study are lower than those found within the broader population, the patterns associated with demographic characteristics regarding subjective community status replicate those found by Schnittker and Bacak (2013). History of incarceration, experiences of homelessness, and lower income are associated with lower subjective community status scores in both studies. The subjective reports of community status in this study might reflect lack of community integration among mental health consumers. Objective measures of community integration among mental health consumers living in supported independent housing were found to be low among consumers meeting criteria for poverty and living in disadvantaged communities (Yanos, Stefancic, & Tsemberis, 2012). Poverty is a critical barrier for the subjective and objective community integration of mental health service users.

Community standing also reflected personal and internal factors. While many people defined their community geographically or socially, participants commonly discussed their own changing community status throughout their life course. Personal history, past status, and future status goals factored into the explanations that these mental health service users provided regarding their subjective community status. Thus, when promoting community integration it would be useful to utilize a life course perspective and consider past experiences and stigmatized statuses, rather than focus exclusively on current factors. It is also important to consider how mental health service users conceptualize their future community status. Several participants reported future goals, such as educational experiences and avoiding substance abuse, which they consider as pathways by which they can climb the ladder. Others, however, reflected on their past failures to reach their goals as justification for their low community status.

While our mixed methods examination of the relationships among definitions of community and SSS are exploratory, they suggest that further work is needed to disentangle the multiple sources of exclusion experienced by public mental health service users and the ways in which efforts at community integration shape and define community. There are many important potential implications of these preliminary findings for research, practice, and policy and we address several here. Similar to the limited qualitative findings of others examining how people using mental health services define community, our participants highlight the importance of service-user or peer communities. However, participants who defined community in terms of these mental health or peer communities reported their overall SSS as 4.90, comparatively lower than other community definitions. More work is needed to understand the benefits and meaning of participation in these communities, and the complex relationships among integration in sub-communities and more broadly defined communities, as well as experiences of multiple aspects of stigma (concealment, consciousness, and internalized), social capital, social cohesion, and health and well-being. It is also striking to note that when our participants defined their community in terms of people who work (employed for pay) as opposed to when they define community in terms of people who contribute more broadly (in ways like volunteering or helping others), they are likely to report their position in the community as lower. Given the low rates of paid employment among the public mental health service users in our sample (2% full-time employment and 11% part-time employment; $n = 294$), as well as the many structural barriers to paid work, it is possible that, in addition to the many positive impacts of programmatic efforts to promote employment, there may be unintended consequence of sending messages that full community membership requires paid work in contrast to other ways to contribute to community. These efforts thus might impact the subjective social status of those who are currently not employed, exacerbating experiences of stigmatization, marginalization, and isolation.

There are several limitations to the generalizability of these findings. First, this study sample included service users from busy, urban public mental health outpatient clinics. Further work is needed to understand the experiences of community and subjective community status of people living in non-urban areas. Secondly, there may be important differences in these experiences and perspectives among people using public or safety-net services compared to those using other mental health services. Our participants describe multiple sources of marginalization and experiences of stigma. Third, our exploration of the relationships among community definitions and SSS is limited. Further work is needed to more fully examine these relationships, particularly in light of the finding that people often held multiple definitions of community. Additional work should also examine potential mediators and moderators of these relationships. Finally, understanding of community and subjective community status was not the primary focus of the research protocol. All participants in the study consented to participate in research aimed at increasing understanding of the role of literacy in the lives of people with serious mental illness. While best attempts were made at each clinic to randomize recruitment, there is likely bias introduced into our sample by nature and content of the primary study questions.

CONCLUSION

This examination of how people understand community and think about their place within it demonstrates that people using public mental health services think about community in many of the same ways as the larger population. The roles of place and social relationships are quite strong. However, while the importance of service-user and peer communities, and the potential buffering effects of these communities on our participants' experiences of exclusion from other communities, is evident, many of our participants saw community as composed of people engaged in activities and relationships that they themselves were not. Communities included people who were working, had homes, or had families. Many of our participants reported that these were desires or goals they had for themselves, but their lack of participation in these aspects of community, combined with experiences of multiple stigma related to mental illness, substance use or prior incarceration, contributed to strong feelings of exclusion and lower community status. These were compounded by the multiple stigmatized identities and sources of exclusion associated with race, gender identity, poverty, and living in violent and stigmatized neighborhoods. Our participants provide us with critical reminders that community mental health and calls for community integration must account for the multiple sources of exclusion and marginalization that people using public mental health services experience, as well as examine potential unintended consequences of our efforts to promote social integration. These data help us understand why subjective social status can be as powerful a force as objective social status in understanding health and mental health. Programs and policies aimed at increasing social inclusion for people with serious mental illness and promoting community social capital must take into account service-user beliefs and experiences of exclusion, focusing not only on the stigma of mental illness, but also the many social consequences, and associated stigmas, of living with serious mental illness in the United States.

ACKNOWLEDGMENTS

We would like to thank the entire Literacy Project steering committee, and particularly our Consumer Consulting Group. This manuscript benefits from the insightful contributions of Suzanne Garverich, Tammi Arford, and Christopher Prener, whom we thank. This work is supported by NIMH grant 1R01MH096707-04 (PI: Alisa K. Lincoln).

REFERENCES

Adler, N. E., Epel, E. S., Castellazzo, G., & Ickovics, J. R. (2000). Relationships of subjective social status with psychological and physiological functioning: Preliminary data in healthy, white women. *Health Psychology*, *19*(6), 586–592.

Adler, N., Stewart, J., & the Psychosocial Working Group. (2007). *The MacArthur scale of subjective social status*. Retrieved from http://www.macses.ucsf.edu/research/psychosocial/subjective.php

Adler, N., Singh-Manoux, A., Schwartz, J., Stewart, J., Matthews, K., & Marmot, M. G. (2008). Social status and health: A comparison of British civil servants in Whitehall-II with European- and African-Americans in CARDIA. *Social Science and Medicine*, *66*(5), 1034–1045.

Belton, B. (2013). 'Weak power': Community and identity. *Ethnic and Racial Studies*, *36*(2), 282–297.

Bond, G. R., Salyers, M. P., Rollins, A. L., Rapp, C. A., & Zipple, A. M. (2004). How evidence-based practices contribute to community integration. *Community Mental Health Journal*, *40*(6), 569–588.

Bromley, E., Gabrielian, S., Brekke, B., Pahwa, R., Daly, K. A., Brekke, J. S., & Braslow, J. T. (2013). Experiencing community: Perspectives of individuals diagnosed as having serious mental illness. *Psychiatric Services*, *64*(7), 672–679.

Collins, P. H. (2010). The new politics of community (2009 ASA Presidential Address). *American Sociological Review*, *75*(1), 7–30.
Cook, J. A. (2006). Employment barriers for persons with psychiatric disabilities: Update of a report for the President's commission. *Psychiatric Services*, *57*(10), 1391–1405.
Daker-White, G., Sanders, C., Rogers, A., Vassilev, I., Blickem, C., & Cheraghi-Sohi, S. (2014). A constellation of misfortune: Narrative accounts of adverse life events, chronic illness, and subjective social status. *SAGE Open*, *4*(4), 1–10.
Davis, J. (1956). Status symbols and the measurement of status perception. *Sociometry*, *19*(3), 154–165.
Delanty, G. (2010). *Community* (2nd ed.). London: Routledge.
Draine, J., Salzer, M. S., Culhane, D. P., & Hadley, T. R. (2002). Role of social disadvantage in crime, joblessness, and homelessness among persons with serious mental illness. *Psychiatric Services*, *53*(5), 565–573.
Flaherty, J., & Brown, R. B. (2010). A multilevel system model of community attachment: Assessing the relative importance of the community and individuals levels. *American Journal of Sociology*, *116*(2), 503–542.
Gesler, W. M. (1992). Therapeutic landscapes: Medical issues in light of the new cultural geography. *Social Science & Medicine*, *34*(7), 735–746.
Goe, W. R., & Noonan, S. (2007). The sociology of community. In C. D. Bryant & D. L. Peck (Eds.), *21st century sociology: A reference handbook* (pp. 455–464). Thousand Oaks, CA: Sage.
Goodman, E., Adler, N. E., Kawachi, I., Frazier, L., Huang, B., & Colditz, G. A. (2001). Adolescents' perceptions of social status: Development and evaluation of a new indicator. *Pediatrics*, *108*(2), E31.
Hillery, G. (1955). Definitions of community: Areas of agreement. *Rural Sociology*, *20*, 111–123.
Hudson, K. D. (2012). Bordering community: Reclaiming ambiguity as a transgressive landscape of knowledge. *Affilia: Journal of Women and Social Work*, *27*(2), 167–179.
Hunter, A., & Riger, S. (1986). The meaning of community in community mental health. *Journal of Community Psychology*, *14*, 55–71.
Kilpatrick, F. P., & Cantril, H. (1960). Self-anchoring scaling: A measure of individuals' unique reality worlds. *Journal of Individual Psychology*, *16*, 158–173.
Lamb, H. R., & Bachrach, L. L. (2001). Some perspectives on deinstitutionalization. *Psychiatric Services*, *52*(8), 1039–1045.
Macintyre, S., Ellaway, A., & Cummins, S. (2002). Place effects on health: How can we conceptualise, operationalise and measure them? *Social Science & Medicine*, *55*, 125–139.
Mandiberg, J. M. (2010). Another way: Enclave communities for people with mental illness. *American Journal of Orthopsychiatry*, *80*(2), 170–176.
McLaughlin, K. A., Costello, E. J., Leblanc, W., Sampson, N. A., & Kessler, R. C. (2012). Socioeconomic status and adolescent mental disorders. *American Journal of Public Health*, *102*(9), 1742–1750.
Mulligan, M. (2015). On ambivalence and hope in the restless search for community: How to work with the idea of community in the global age. *Sociology*, *49*(2), 340–355.
Nicklett, E. J., & Burgard, S. A. (2009). Downward social mobility and major depressive episodes among Latino and Asian-American immigrants to the United States. *American Journal of Epidemiology*, *170*(6), 793–801.
Pahwa, R., Bromley, E., Brekke, B., Gabrielian, S., Braslow, J. T., & Brekke, J. S. (2014). Relationship of community integration of persons with severe mental illness and mental health service intensity. *Psychiatric Services*, *65*(6), 822–825.

Paulson, G. (2012). *Closing the asylums: Causes and consequences of the deinstitutionalization movement*. Jefferson, NC: McFarland.

Pescosolido, B. A. (2013). The public stigma of mental illness: What do we think; what do we know; what can we prove? *Journal of Health and Social Behavior*, *54*(1), 1–21.

Rowe, M., & Pelletier, J. (2012). Citizenship: A response to the marginalization of people with mental illness. *Journal of Forensic Psychology Practice*, *12*(4), 366–381.

Schnittker, J., & Bacak, V. (2013). A mark of disgrace of a badge of honor?: Subjective status among former inmates. *Social Problems*, *60*(2), 234–254.

Singh-Manoux, A., Adler, N., & Marmot, M. (2003). Subjective social status: Its determinants and its associations with measure of ill-health in the Whitehall II study. *Social Science & Medicine*, *56*(6), 1321–1333.

Substance Abuse and Mental Health Service Administration. (2006). *From exclusion to belonging: Transforming mental health care in America*. Rockville, MD: Author.

Townley, G. (2015). "It helps you not feel so bad – Feel like you again": The importance of community for individuals with psychiatric disabilities. *Journal of Psychosocial Rehabilitation and Mental Health*, *2*(2), 113–124.

Vassilev, I., Rogers, A., Sanders, C. e., Cherahi-Sohi, S., Blickem, C., Brooks, H., ... Kennedy, A. (2014). Social status and living with a chronic illness: An exploration of assessment and meaning attributed to work and employment. *Chronic Illness*, *10*(4), 273–290.

Ware, N. C., Hopper, K., Tugenberg, T., Dickey, B., & Fisher, D. (2007). Connectedness and citizenship: Redefining social integration. *Psychiatric Services*, *58*(4), 469–474.

Williams, A. M. (2007). The continuing maturation of the therapeutic landscape concept. *Therapeutic Landscapes (Geographies of Health Series)*. Aldershot: Ashgate.

Wolff, L. S., Subramanian, S. V., Acevedo-Garcia, D., Weber, D., & Kawachi, I. (2010). Compared to whom? Subjective social status, self-rated health, and referent group sensitivity in a diverse US sample. *Social Science and Medicine*, *70*, 2019–2028.

Wong, Y. I., Sands, R. G., & Solomon, P. L. (2010). Conceptualizing community: The experience of mental health consumers. *Qualitative Health Research*, *20*(5), 654–667.

Yanos, P. T., Stefancic, A., & Tsemberis, S. (2012). Objective community integration of mental health consumers living in supported housing and of others in the community. *Psychiatric Services*, *63*(5), 438–444.

PART III
CONFRONTING STIGMA AND ITS CONSEQUENCES

REVISITING THE RELATIONSHIPS AMONG COMMUNITY MENTAL HEALTH SERVICES, STIGMA, AND WELL-BEING

Kristen Marcussen and Christian Ritter

ABSTRACT

Purpose – *This chapter examines the effects of mental health services and stigma on changes in self-concept and well-being for individuals with SPMI.*

Methodology/approach – *Data for this chapter come from structured interviews and service data for 140 individuals with severe and persistent mental illnesses. We use structural equation modeling to examine the relationship between perceived and internalized stigma, as well as the relationships among stigma, self-concept (self-esteem and mastery), and well-being (quality of life and functioning).*

Findings – *We find that case management is negatively related to quality of life and psychiatric services are positively related to functioning.*

50 Years after Deinstitutionalization: Mental Illness in Contemporary Communities
Advances in Medical Sociology, Volume 17, 177–206

ISSN: 1057-6290/doi:10.1108/S1057-629020160000017007

Crisis services and assessment are associated with mastery in opposite directions. Internalized stigma is positively associated with self-esteem and mastery, and negatively associated with functioning. We do not find a relationship between services and stigma.

Research limitations/implications – *A limitation to this chapter is the sample size, which prohibits us from examining a full range of services and outcomes. Nonetheless, our findings provide information about how services and stigma impact well-being, and may be used as a starting point for considering strategies for improving services and reducing stigma. Future work should consider pairing outcomes with services to determine their effectiveness.*

Originality/value – *This chapter builds on previous research that examines the relative effects of services and stigma among individuals in community health care by extending measures of both services and stigma, and by examining the relationship between them, in order to better determine their implications for self-concept and well-being.*

Keywords: Mental health services; perceived stigma; internalized stigma; self-concept; quality of life; functioning

The negative consequences of deinstitutionalization have been widely documented in the last 50 years, despite general agreement that increasing community-based programs are a worthy goal in mental health care reform. On the one hand, reform policies emphasized the need to provide individuals transitioning out of long-term hospitalization access to services that would increase their quality of life, integrate them into the community, and positively influence their recovery process. On the other hand, questions persist regarding the availability and effectiveness of community mental health services in the years following the closing of institutions (e.g., Lamb & Bachrach, 2001). Moreover, mental health scholars have found that stigma associated with mental illness and mental health treatment has remained a concern in the time since deinstitutionalization processes began; in many ways growing worse over the years (Link, Phelan, Bresnahan, Stueve, & Pescosolido, 1999; Pescosolido, 2013; Pescosolido et al., 2010).

As such, concerns about the mutual effects of community services and stigma remain an important focus for research that seeks to understand the impact of mental health policies on the lives of individuals living with severe and persistent mental illnesses (SPMI).

In this chapter, we examine the relative effects of services and stigma on the well-being of individuals living with mental illness. In doing so, we reconsider the debate within the sociological literature concerning the positive and negative consequences of labeling mental illness: namely, the potential for services to increase, and stigma to decrease, self-concept and well-being for individuals with SPMI. Specifically, we build on Rosenfield's landmark study (Rosenfield, 1997) that finds that both services and stigma are associated with quality of life, but in opposite ways. Similar to Rosenfield's study, we explore the relative effects of service use and perceived stigma on quality of life, and suggest that self-concept (i.e., self-esteem and mastery) plays an important role in linking both services and stigma to well-being.

Our study also extends Rosenfield's work in a number of important ways. First, we examine the relationships among received services, self-concept, and well-being within the context of a Community Support Program (CSP). CSPs represent a vital link between services and community health centers, and have been described as an important phase in mental health reform following deinstitutionalization and the rise of community health care (Morrissey & Goldman, 1986). Second, drawing on current psychological models of stigma, we extend our focus on stigma to include both perceived (public) stigma and internalized (self) stigma. While previous work in this area has focused on perceived stigma, mental health scholars across disciplines have advanced models of stigma that also demonstrate the impact of internalized stigma on self-concept and well-being. Third, in addition to a general measure of quality of life, we consider daily functioning in our assessment of well-being. Improved functioning is consistent with the goals of psychiatric models of recovery, as well as with the objectives of CSPs. Fourth, while previous studies have focused on the independent effects of services and stigma on well-being (e.g., Marcussen, Ritter, & Munetz, 2010; Rosenfield, 1997), we also explore the relationship between stigma and services. Finally, we use longitudinal data to assess *changes* in self-concept and well-being as a function of service use and stigma. By expanding our conceptualization and measurement of services, stigma, and well-being, we hope to provide a more current and comprehensive examination of the important questions raised about the relative effects of labeling for individuals with SPMI.

BACKGROUND

Deinstitutionalization and Community Mental Health Services

The intended goal of deinstitutionalization was to release and divert individuals from settings such as psychiatric hospitals to alternative facilities in the community, while at the same time developing services for the care of a non-institutionalized mentally ill population that would improve the lives of individuals with SPMI (Lamb & Bachrach, 2001). The transfer of care from hospitals to the community moved forward quite quickly, with the number of institutionalized individuals in state hospitals falling dramatically in the last half of the twentieth century. However, the development of services has progressed far more slowly. It was not until decades after the initiation of deinstitutionalization that attention was paid to expanding and improving community health care services and allocating more money to community-based care (Lamb & Bachrach, 2001). In the meantime, negative outcomes associated with deinstitutionalization policies included increased homelessness and the re-institutionalization of individuals with SPMI into hospitals, jails, and prisons (Lamb, 1997; Mechanic & Rochefort, 1990)

Although there has been a great deal of discussion about the perceived failures of deinstitutionalization with regard to the transition to community services, research has shown that the proposed benefits of these policies have been realized for at least some individuals (Grob, 1994). These benefits include increased quality of life (Forrester-Jones et al., 2002; McGrew, Wright, & McDonel, 1999), a reduction in (or greater adherence to) medication needs (Hobbs, Newton, Tennant, Rosen, & Tribe, 2002), and increased functioning (Priebe, Hoffmann, Isermann, & Kaiser, 2002). In their longitudinal study following the closing of a state hospital, McGrew et al. (1999) found that individuals transitioning from the hospital to the community experienced increased quality of life (with respect to safety and occupation) and level of functioning (with respect to engagement with services). The researchers note that while their findings showed incremental increases in quality of life and level of functioning, they did not suggest high levels of well-being in absolute terms. Nonetheless, these incremental changes were encouraging, suggesting that the lives of individuals with SPMI were somewhat improved by the shift from hospitalization to community services.

Deinstitutionalization and Stigma

Reintegrating individuals with SPMI into communities also had the potential to reduce stigma associated with mental hospitals and psychiatric institutions. According to Corrigan and Penn (1999), familiarity with mental illness in the general public is inversely related to prejudicial attitudes. Unfortunately, researchers have also argued that deinstitutionalization promoted stigma, primarily through fear and hostility that increased when individuals with mental illness were more visible (Brown, 1985). This claim is supported by a series of recent studies showing that public fear of dangerousness and perceptions of violence regarding individuals with mental illness has increased, rather than decreased, over the last several decades (Link et al., 1999; Pescosolido, 2013; Pescosolido et al., 2010).

Goffman's work on total institutions and discredited identities (Goffman, 1961, 1963) considers the effect of asylums on identity processes and self-concept. Goffman described being institutionalized as a process whereby the institutionalized individual experiences a mortification, or death, of their former self (Goffman, 1961). In this process, identities are stripped and regenerated to better reflect societal expectations. Through interactions with family, doctors and staff, and others in the institution, individuals eventually develop a "moral career" as a mental patient (Goffman, 1961). Importantly, being released from the institution does not translate to a release from the status of being mentally ill. Rather, stigma from the public continues to impact the released individual's self-worth and well-being. As such, the experience of institutionalization becomes part of a value system that incorporates cultural stereotypes and negatively impacts self-views (Estroff, 1981). The impact of deinstitutionalization on stigma and self-concept is illustrated in a study conducted by Wright, Gronfein, and Owens (2000), who found that during the two-year period following their release from a state hospital, former patients experienced social rejection, self-deprecation, and decreases in mastery. The authors concluded that the status of former mental patient had a significant and long-term impact on stigma and self-concept.

Debating Labeling: Stigma versus Services

The positive and negative implications of psychiatric labeling and treatment are the focus of a classic debate in the sociological literature.

Drawing on symbolic interactionism and classical labeling theories of deviant behavior, Scheff's (1966) theory of mental illness begins with the notion that being labeled deviant or mentally ill starts a process whereby individuals internalize societal perceptions and stereotypes of mental illness. Through continued interactions that reinforce or reward behaviors associated with the deviant label, the labeled individual ultimately develops a "career" in deviance. With this career comes a deviant self-concept, along with the stigma associated with the label.

Critics of labeling theories of mental illness have argued that stigma resulting from psychiatric labels and hospitalization is exaggerated or non-existent (Gove, 1982; Gove & Fain, 1973; Townsend, 1976). The arguments against the influence of stigma center around three main ideas: first, reactions to mental illness are more likely rooted in the behaviors exhibited by individuals with mental illness than in the label itself; second, stigma is not an inevitable (or even likely) result of psychiatric labels for most individuals with SPMI; and third, when stigma does occur it is likely to be temporary and minor relative to the benefits of treatment (Gove & Fain, 1973). Defenders of this position argue that psychiatric labels are a necessary step toward better communication among medical professionals, and subsequently, better access to services and treatment. Each issue mentioned above has garnered responses from mental health scholars and led to important theoretical developments in labeling theories of mental illness.

Modified Labeling Theory

Link's modified labeling theory (Link, Cullen, Struening, Shrout, & Dohrenwend, 1989) directly addresses issues raised in this classic debate, showing that individuals do in fact respond to the label (more so than behavior) with respect to perceived dangerousness of ex-mental hospital patients (Link, 1987). Link also suggests that the potential for stigma is high among individuals with SPMI, and the effects of stigma on self-esteem are likely to be long lasting (Link, Struening, Rahav, Phelan, & Nuttbrock, 1997). In short, Link's model suggests that socialization processes result in the development of beliefs about how mental illness is viewed in society generally and these beliefs become self-relevant when individuals enter treatment (Link, 1987; Link et al., 1989). Importantly, Link argues that the discrimination can be experienced indirectly, through expectations of how individuals with mental illnesses are perceived in the general population.

Identity Threat
Alternative models of stigma provide further evidence for the connection between stigma and well-being. Under the identity threat model, stigma is tied to group membership. In other words, belonging to a group conveys a social identity that, when perceived as devalued, translates to lower self-esteem and well-being. Here collective (or group) self-esteem is seen as distinct, and in some cases inconsistent with, personal self-esteem. An important aspect of the identity threat model is a focus on in-group and out-group comparisons, where the self-esteem of stigmatized individuals is compared to others who share their social identity (the stigmatized) as well as to those who do and not share the identity (the non-stigmatized). Identity threat processes are also somewhat unique when the identity is concealable, as in the case of mental illness (Quinn, 2006). When concealable identities become known to others, the risk of negative evaluation increases (Quinn, 2006).

Numerous studies have shown the negative implications of devaluation and discrimination, including the association between stigma and self-concept (Rosenfield, 1997), employment (Link, 1982, 1987), and quality of life (Marcussen et al., 2010; Rosenfield, 1997). Longitudinal studies have also addressed Gove's argument about the short-term impact of stigma by showing that stigma is negatively associated with self-concept (Marcussen et al., 2010; Markowitz, 1998, 2001; Wright et al., 2000), life satisfaction (Marcussen et al., 2010; Markowitz, 1998, 2001) and recovery (Corrigan, 2004; Markowitz, 2001) over time. Some of these studies examined the effects of stigma in the context of services, raising questions about the relationships among services, stigma, and well-being.

Stigma, Services and Well-being

Nearly 20 years ago, Rosenfield (1997) examined issues at the heart of the labeling debate by comparing the relative effects of services and stigma simultaneously. She found that services, particularly those that provided economic resources and emphasized empowerment, were positively related to the quality of life of individuals with chronic mental illnesses. Her study also showed that perceived stigma was negatively associated with quality of life. The results of Rosenfield's study indicated that life satisfaction was highest for those who perceived little stigma and have received high-quality services, and lowest among those who perceived high levels of stigma and did not have access to such services. Integral to these relationships, and consistent with modified labeling theory (e.g., Link, 1987; Link et al., 1989), Rosenfield also found that self-concept played a significant role in these processes. Specifically, self-concept mediated the negative relationship between perceived stigma and quality of life, as well as the positive relationship between received services and quality of life.

While Rosenfield's study provided evidence for the connection between stigma, self-concept, and well-being, limitations of the study raised new questions about the precise nature of these relationships. First, the study used cross-sectional data, making it impossible to determine the causal direction of the proposed relationships. This is important, as studies examining stigma among those receiving services have shown the relationship between perceived stigma and self-concept is bi-directional (e.g., Markowitz, 1998, 2001). A second issue in this study was the type of services examined. Similar to other studies examining mental health populations (e.g., Link, Castille, & Stuber, 2008), services in Rosenfield's study were linked to a clubhouse environment. Clubhouses have a somewhat unique mission in that they are consumer run and are focused more so on empowerment than treatment-related services. Clubhouses are also relatively rare, and therefore less likely to be an option for many individuals diagnosed with SPMI. Other studies use samples of individuals in self-help and outpatient groups (e.g., Markowitz, 1998, 2001); however, these studies did not directly examine the impact of particular services on self-concept or well-being. Building on these studies, Marcussen et al. (2010) used longitudinal data to examine the effects of community-based services and stigma on well-being. Their study showed that while services such as counseling had a positive effect on quality of life, others such as inpatient services had a negative effect on quality of life. They also found that while the influence of stigma on quality of life operated through self-esteem and mastery, services had no effect on changes in self-concept.

Taken together these studies show that stigma and services may indeed be a "package deal," as suggested by Link and Phelan (2001). In other words, for mental health scholars the focus has shifted from determining whether services *or* stigma impact quality of life to better understanding the mechanisms that might increase the positive effects of services and decrease the negative impact of stigma. Moving forward, we argue that work-linking stigma, services, and the well-being of individuals with SPMI might benefit from more specific conceptualizations of both stigma and services. In particular, we suggest that focusing on services that are most commonly available to individuals within the community, in conjunction with a broader conception of stigma, can help to expand and clarify what we know about the relationships among services, stigma, and well-being.

Elaborating Services and Stigma

Community Health Services

Community mental health care centers (CMHCs) represented a critical cycle in mental health reform; however, the negative implications of deinstitutionalization were highlighted in their inability to reach and treat individuals. Similar to the institutions that preceded them, CMHCs were insufficiently funded. That fact, combined with changes in policy, led to a shift in their population from individuals with more general mental health needs to individuals in need of critical care (Goldman & Morrissey, 1985). In the late 1970s, in response to criticism surrounding inadequate community mental health care, the National Institute of Mental Health created CSPs. CSPs offer a potentially new cycle in mental health reform, focusing on meeting the needs of individuals with SPMI in community settings (Morrissey & Goldman, 1986). An important feature of CSPs is that they offer an integrated system of physical and mental health care (Goldman & Morrissey, 1985), as well as a system of support among community agencies. In particular, CSPs are designed to provide a full range of mental health care services, including: case management, vocational and supportive living services, psychosocial rehabilitation and counseling services, and crisis care services.

Case management, which involves the organization of services and the monitoring of treatment for individuals living with SPMI in the community (Ziguras & Stuart, 2000), has played a critical role in the community health care cycle of mental health reform. Initially, case management was considered a necessary response to the transitional period from hospital care to community health care, as accessing services proved to be an overwhelming task. More recently, attention has shifted to addressing deficiencies associated with fragmented or non-continuous mental health care. In a meta-review of 44 studies examining the effectiveness of case management on service use and effectiveness, Ziguras and Stuart (2000) found case management was successful with respect to specific outcome domains including family burden, family satisfaction with services, and cost of care. With respect to social functioning and quality of life, some studies have found case management to have little or no effect (see Marshall, Gray, Lockwood, & Green, 2000, for a review), while others concluded that it was associated with reduced symptoms, increased services, reduced dropout rates, and improved social functioning (Ziguras & Stuart, 2000).

In addition to case management, individuals connected to community health care facilities have access to a variety of services, including vocational assistance, residential services, psychiatric services and assessment, crisis intervention, and day treatment. Given the particular needs of consumers, some of these services may be instrumental in terms of recovery, while others may be reflective of ongoing difficulties. In other words, not all services are equally or uniformly instrumental in improving well-being for individuals with SPMI. That said, many studies that examine services do not do so directly, but rather tend to use samples that include individuals who are currently receiving either inpatient or outpatient services in various hospital and community settings. By focusing on services provided by CSPs, including case management, we are better able to explore the potential benefits (and costs) of common types of community mental health care for the quality of life and functioning of individuals with SPMI.

Internalized Stigma

Most sociological studies of stigma focus on a measure of devaluation and discrimination designed by Link and colleagues (e.g., Link, 1987; Link & Phelan, 2001). Referred to as perceived stigma (e.g., Link, 1987; Link & Phelan, 2001), anticipated stigma (e.g., Markowitz, 1998), or public stigma (e.g., Corrigan, 2004), devaluation and discrimination focus specifically on cultural views about the meaning and implications of mental illness. According to Corrigan, Watson, and Barr (2006), *self-stigma* is distinguished from Link's devaluation and discrimination based on three key dimensions: stereotype agreement, self-concurrence, and self-esteem decrement. Each of these characteristics moves beyond the awareness of stereotypes regarding mental illness to an internalization of the stereotypes. That is, individuals may come to agree that the stereotypes are accurate, true about their own experiences with mental illness, and ultimately feel like less of a person as a result of agreement and concurrence.

Similarly, Ritsher, Otilingam, and Grajales (2003) argue that *internalized stigma* encompasses numerous dimensions of stigma (e.g., stereotype agreement, alienation, discrimination experience, social withdrawal, and resistance) all of which capture elements of the internalization process. Studies examining these types of stigma have found different aspects of internalized stigma to be predictive of self-esteem and mastery (e.g., Drapalski et al., 2013; Livingston & Boyd, 2010; Ritsher & Phelan, 2004; Yanos, Roe, Markus, & Lysaker, 2008), social functioning (Yanos, Lysaker, & Roe, 2010), and subjective quality of life (see Livingston & Boyd, 2010, for a review).

Link's modified labeling theory and internalized stigma models argue that individuals with mental illness are adversely affected by negative stereotypes, and that this process results in diminished self-esteem, efficacy, and well-being. The differences between the models lie primarily in the extent to which perceptions of devaluation are seen as accepted by the public in general (public or social stigma) or accepted as one's personal experience (internalized stigma). In some cases, aspects of Link's modified labeling theory are subsumed in measures of internalized stigma. For example, Ritsher et al., (2003) include social withdrawal, discrimination experiences, and alienation as dimensions of internalized stigma. These dimensions are meant to capture feelings, experiences, and responses associated with stigma that are personally relevant. The implications for stigma on self-concept and well-being is generally the same in both theories; however, according to Corrigan and colleagues (e.g., Corrigan, Rafacz, & Rusch, 2011), the most likely scenario is that perceived stigma is mediated by internalized stigma as it affects outcomes such as self-esteem and well-being. Given the implications of internalized stigma on self-concept and well-being, it is likely to undermine the potential positive aspects of mental health services (Ritsher & Phelan, 2004).

Services and Internalized Stigma

As suggested in the studies discussed above, the relationship between services and stigma (in addition to the independent effects that each has on well-being) may be an important direction for research that seeks to better understand their combined effects on self-concept, quality of life, and functioning. While some studies have found stigma to be a barrier to help-seeking and treatment adherence (e.g., Corrigan, 2004; Corrigan, Druss, & Perlick, 2014; Link, Struening, Neese-Todd, & Phelan, 2001), others suggest that the effects of stigma on help-seeking are quite modest (e.g., Clement et al., 2014). Perhaps the more relevant question for research examining the impact of ongoing services on well-being is: to what extent are received services associated with stigma?

For the most part, services have the potential to decrease stigma (particularly, self or internalized stigma) if they encourage empowerment (Corrigan, Larson, & Rusch, 2009; Rosenfield, 1997). A sense of empowerment is positively linked to self-esteem and self-efficacy, and encourages individuals to be more actively engaged in their recovery process. Treatment models that emphasize empowerment services specifically tend to be consumer-operated services such as clubhouses (Link et al., 2001; Rosenfield, 1997), drop-in centers, or peer support and mentoring services (Corrigan et al., 2009). The extent to which CSPs provide these services is less understood. While on the one hand, CSPs share a goal of fostering independence among individuals with SPMI (similar to consumer-operated programs), they also concentrate on services that are designed to assist individuals with symptom management and crisis care (a goal not necessarily consistent with all consumer-operated programs). Given the array of services offered by CSPs, it is possible that some services might be associated with lower levels of internalized stigma based on their ability to empower individuals (e.g., vocational services), whereas others might be associated with higher levels of internalized stigma (e.g., crisis services). A better understanding of the degree to which service use in CSPs promotes or inhibits the internalization of stigma would provide valuable insight into understanding the relationship between services and stigma in the context of community health care.

Research Questions

Previous research has increased our understanding of the relative effects of services and stigma in a community environment, but has also provided additional research questions. First, what types of services affect self-concept, quality of life, and functioning? We explore this question in the context of CSPs that offer a range of services to individuals with SPMI. Second, how does internalized stigma add to our understanding of the relationships among perceptions of devaluation, self-concept, and well-being among individuals who are engaged in community services? Traditional labeling theorists point to both the stereotypes and internalization of labels as part of the development of a career in mental illness (e.g., Scheff, 1966), indicating that both aspects of stigma may be important to consider. Recent research that links the two suggests that the effects of public stigma are mediated by internalized stigma (e.g., Ritsher & Phelan, 2004; Corrigan et al., 2011). We examine these relationships in the context of a model that considers the effects of both services and stigma on well-being. Third, we examine the relationship between services and stigma, focusing particularly on the association between service use and internalized stigma. Though researchers have concluded that services and stigma are a package deal, exploring the link between services and internalized stigma (or stigma experiences) has the potential to extend our understanding of their combined effects on self-concept and well-being.

Based on research discussed above, we expect that stigma will be negatively associated with quality of life and functioning. We also expect that internalized stigma will mediate the relationship between perceived stigma and self-concept, as well as between perceived stigma and well-being. Finally, there is theoretical and empirical reason to believe that self-esteem and mastery represent an important link between stigma and well-being (e.g., Markowitz, 1998; Rosenfield, 1997; Wright et al., 2000). What remain exploratory in this study are the relationships among services, self-concept, and well-being, as well as the relationship between service use and internalized stigma. While Rosenfield (1997) finds services to be positively related to mastery, Marcussen et al. (2010) do not. Further, as discussed above the services associated with CSPs range in terms of their use and goals. Therefore, we do not make specific predictions about these relationships, but we do explore similar pathways for both services and stigma.

METHOD

Data/Sample

Participants in this study came from a sample of randomly identified active clients of a community support center located in a large Midwestern city. The center provides integrated primary and mental health care services. Active clients were defined as those who had received services within the previous 120 days. Of more than 2,500 active clients, 1,500 were randomly selected during the spring of 2012 and sent a letter requesting their participation in the study. Clients who were interested and agreed to participate in the study were scheduled for a face-to-face interview and screening of health indicators. Those who completed all steps were provided small monetary compensation. Institutional review boards at participating universities approved the research, and approval was granted from the research review board at the community health provider agency.

The research team received confirmation of interest to participate in the study from 262 individuals from the group of 1,500 active clients who were originally contacted (17%). Interviews were scheduled and completed with 223 participants (85%), 203 of which completed the full interview. Of these, we were able to collect follow up data 18 months later on 141 individuals. Logistic regression analysis (not shown) indicated that self-esteem was the only study variable associated with attrition from baseline to time 2. Specifically, individuals with higher self-esteem were less likely to participate in the second interview ($p = .046$)

To assess the possibility of selection bias within our sample, we compared the study participants with the balance of all clients of the community mental health center who did not participate in our study either because they were not randomly chosen to be contacted about the study or because they chose not to participate in the interviews ($N = 2{,}168$) on the following factors: gender, age, race, number of units of mental health services used, and the proportion of clients who were Medicaid eligible. The only statistically significant differences between the sample and the broader population of active clients from which it was drawn were a higher proportion of women (sample 60% vs. population 44%; $p < .001$) and a higher proportion of clients who were Medicaid eligible in the study sample (sample 88% vs. population 80%; $p < .001$).

Measures

Service Use

Service use data were collected via the Medicaid database accessed through the county mental health board. We obtained units of nine clinical services received for the nine months preceding the first and the second interviews. The nine services received were: assessment, case management (individual and group), day treatment, psychiatric services (including pharmacologic management), counseling, crisis intervention, residential services, and vocational services. Each service was coded based on standard billable units of time per the Medicaid taxonomy. Counseling, vocational, and case management (individual and group) were measured in 15-minute units. Assessment, crisis intervention, and psychiatric are measured in one-hour units. Day treatment was measured in three-hour units. Residential was measured in 24-hour units. The service data were merged with the interview data.

Perceived Stigma

Perceived stigma was measured using the devaluation and discrimination scale developed by Link and colleagues (Link et al., 1997). The scale consisted of 12-items that capture cultural stereotypes and include questions such as "Most people feel that having a mental illness is a sign of personal failure" and "Most people think less of a person who has a mental illness." Response categories ranged from 1 "strongly agree" to 4 "strongly disagree". All items were coded such that higher scores reflect higher levels of public stigma with a range from 12 to 72. As in previous research, the reliability for this scale was high ($\alpha = .793$).

Internalized Stigma

We examined three central elements of internalized stigma adapted from the Internalized Stigma Mental Illness (ISMI) scale (Ritsher et al., 2003): discrimination experience, alienation, and social withdrawal. We examined these particular dimensions of internalized stigma (and not stereotype agreement and stigma resistance) because they represent internalizations of the various aspects of devaluation and discrimination as measured in public stigma measures, but are at the same time distinct from our measures of perceived stigma and self-concept. The ISMI has been used broadly across disciplines, and has been found to have high validity, internal consistency, and test-retest reliability in various formats (e.g., Ritsher et al., 2003) as well as in multinational studies spanning more than 50 countries (e.g., Boyd, Adler, Otilingam, & Peters, 2014)

Discrimination experience was assessed with four items that measure perceptions that one has been treated differently or poorly as a result of mental illness. Items include "People discriminate against me because I have a mental illness" and "People ignore me or take me less seriously just because I have a mental illness." *Alienation* measures the individual's sense of feeling disconnected or ashamed as a result of mental illness. Alienation has been referred to as an "us and them" divide according to stigma scholars (e.g., Link & Phelan, 2001; Ritsher & Phelan, 2004). This scale included six items, such as "I feel out of place in the world because I have a mental illness" and "People without mental illness could not possibly understand me." *Social withdrawal* measures the extent to which one avoids contact with others due to mental illness. While a component of the ISMI, social withdrawal also overlaps with Link and colleagues' conception of withdrawal as a coping strategy for dealing with stereotypes related to mental illness. This scale had six items, including "I don't talk about myself much because I don't want to burden others with my mental illness" and "Negative stereotypes about mental illness keep me isolated from the 'normal' world". For each scale, items were coded such that high scores indicated higher internalized stigma. Items were summed to create three scales, all of which had high reliability (α = .840, .887, and .869 for discrimination, alienation, and withdrawal, respectively).

Self-Concept

To assess self-concept, we examined both self-esteem and mastery at time 2 (controlling for baseline levels). Self-esteem was assessed with the Rosenberg Self-Esteem Scale (Rosenberg, 1979) and included items such as "I feel that I am a person of worth, at least on equal plane with others" and "I take a positive attitude toward myself." Mastery was measured with a seven-item scale developed by Pearlin and colleagues (Pearlin & Schooler, 1978) and included items such as "What happens to me in the future mostly depends on me" and " I can do just about anything I really set my mind to." Both scales ranged from 1 "strongly agree" to 4 "strongly disagree." Negatively worded items were reverse coded and items were summed to create the two scales ranging from 12 to 40 (time 1) and 10 to 40 (time 2) for self-esteem, and 10 to 28 (time 1) and 9 to 25 (time 2) for mastery. The reliability of the scales were high at both time periods ($\alpha = .898$ and .877) for self-esteem, and ($\alpha = .719$ and .756) for mastery for baseline and time 2, respectively.

Quality of Life

Quality of life was assessed at time 2, controlling for baseline levels with two-item measure adapted from Lehman (1988). Respondents were asked at the beginning and end of the interview "How do you feel about your life in general?" Response categories range from 1 "Terrible" to 7 "Delighted." Consistent with previous research (e.g., Marcussen et al., 2010), the two items were summed to create a single measure of quality of life ($r = .635$).

Functioning

We use four items from the Multnomah Community Ability Scale (MCAS-SR) to assess daily functioning in community settings at baseline and time 2. The MCAS has been increasingly viewed as an important outcome measure for assessing whether individuals with SPMI are making progress with treatment goals such managing symptoms and stress in their everyday lives (Hodges & Wotring, 2000). The MCAS is considered a reliable measure for assessing functioning in this population (O'Malia, McFarland, Barker, Barron, 2002). Here, we used items that focus on mental and physical health issues. Respondents were asked about trouble they have had with physical health, thoughts (relating to symptoms such as seeing or hearing things), with moods, and with handling stress. Responses ranged from 1 "very much" to 5 "not at all" such that high scores indicated higher functioning. Items were summed to create a scale that ranged from 4 to 20 for both time periods ($\alpha = .863$ and .826 for baseline and time 2, respectively).

Controls

In preliminary analysis, we controlled for demographic characteristics that might be related to our mediating and dependent outcomes, including gender, race, age, marital status, employment status, parental status, and level of education. We also controlled for diagnosis, including schizophrenia, bipolar, depressive, and substance abuse disorders. None of the control variables were related to our study variables. To preserve degrees of freedom, they were omitted from the analyses presented.

RESULTS

Descriptive Analyses

As shown in Table 1, our sample was 60% female and 44% nonwhite, with an average age of 50 years old. Nearly 8% of the respondents were married, 12% were employed at least part time, and 59% were parents. The average number of years of education was approximately 12. In terms of diagnosis, half of the sample had a diagnosis of schizophrenia, and 48% had a co-occurring substance abuse disorder. The remaining diagnoses included bipolar disorders (17%) and depressive disorders (29%).

Table 1 also shows the distribution of each of the nine services for the nine-month period prior to time 2 interviews. At the time of the second interview, 93.6% participants had used individual case management in the previous nine months and about 50% had used psychiatric services in the previous nine months. Rate of use for the additional services during the study period is as follows: vocational (25%), assessment (20%), counseling (about 20%), group case management (about 14%), day treatment (10%), residential treatment (about 6%), and crisis intervention (5%). Based on consultations with staff at the county mental health board, as well as a psychiatrist associated with the community health agency that comprises our sample, we are confident that this distribution has face validity and is consistent with the larger population of clients with the agency. Of these prevalence rates and ranges, only the use of psychiatric services was somewhat surprising. While psychiatric services are not required, the rate of use is lower than expected.

Given our sample size and the exploratory nature of the analysis examining these particular services, we conducted preliminary analysis to determine the extent to which each type of service was related to either changes in self-concept and/or changes in well-being. These analyses led us to focus on four services in our multivariate analysis: individual case management (which we refer to as case management in the remaining text), psychiatric services, assessment services, and crisis services. Notably, crisis services were significantly related to our key study variables despite the fact

Table 1. Descriptive Statistics for Sample and Study Variables (N = 140).

	N	Mean (%)	SD	Range
Demographic characteristics				
Female	84	60.00		0–1
Age	140	49.66	9.10	28–72
Nonwhite	56	43.57		0–1
Years of education	140	12.11	2.10	6–17
Employed	17	12.14		0–1
Married	11	7.86		0–1
Children	82	58.57		0–1
Diagnosis				
Schizophrenic disorder	75	50.00		0–1
Bipolar disorders	26	17.14		0–1
Depressive disorders	32	28.58		0–1
Other diagnosis	12	10.71		0–1
Substance abuse disorder	72	47.86		0–1
Mental Health Services				
Case management-individual[a]	131	13.17	48.68	0–302
Psychiatric services[b]	69	1.93	4.53	0–30
Vocational services[b]	35	8.92	40.51	0–365
Assessment[b]	28	.23	.51	0–2
Counseling[a]	27	4.26	12.77	0–68
Case management-group[a]	19	13.17	48.68	0–379
Day treatment[c]	14	2.37	13.87	0–149
Residential services[d]	9	1.44	11.19	0–130
Crisis intervention[b]	7	.88	4.93	0–40
Stigma				
Perceived stigma	140	32.51	5.07	12–47
Internalized stigma				
Discrimination experience	140	10.05	2.32	4-16
Alienation	140	13.89	3.60	6-24
Social withdrawal	140	14.67	3.45	6-24

Note: Means for service use are based on billable units.
[a]15-minute intervals.
[b]60-minute intervals.
[c]24-hour period.
[d]3-day period.

that only 5% of the sample received such services in the preceding nine-month period.

Table 1 also shows the descriptive statistics for our measures of stigma. In Table 2, we present the means and standard deviations for each of these variables at baseline and time 2. We also present *t*-tests and correlations

Table 2. Descriptive Statistics and Comparisons of Self-Concept and Well-Being at Time 1 and Time 2 ($N = 140$).

	Time 1		Time 2		Time 1–Time 2	
	Mean	SD	Mean	SD	*t*-test	*r*
Self-concept						
Mastery	18.52	3.10	16.71	2.61	6.80***	.40***
Self-esteem	28.51	5.01	28.49	5.31	.14	.67***
Well-Being						
Quality of life	6.51	2.57	6.79	2.84	1.41	.64***
Functioning	27.99	12.92	21.11	14.64	7.31***	.65***

Note: *** = p<.001.

comparing these variables at each point in time. As can be seen, self-esteem and quality of life were quite stable over the time periods. Mastery and functioning, on the other hand, were significantly lower at the time of the second interview.

Analytic Strategy

We used structural equation modeling (SEM) for the multivariate analysis. The use of SEM is ideal because we were using a latent construct for internalized stigma and assessing the effects of multiple measures of services, self-concept, and well-being simultaneously. This was especially important given the potential correlation between our mediating variables (self-esteem and mastery) and our well-being outcomes (functioning and quality of life).

We examined three primary sets of relationships. First, we examined the relationship between service use and well-being, with a focus on the mediating effects of self-esteem and mastery. Second, we examined the relationship between perceived stigma and well-being with a focus on the mediating effects of internalized stigma and self-concept. Third, we examined the relationship between service use and internalized stigma. We did not specify a sign for the effect for services on self-concept, stigma, or well-being. We did not make a priori predictions about how specific services or types of services affect these processes.

In all analyses, variables were entered in models as observed variables with the exception of internalized stigma. We used this strategy to preserve degrees of freedom in our relatively small sample. In all structural equation models, we used maximum likelihood estimation. Fit statistics for the final model appear in Fig. 1. As can be seen, the final trimmed model fit the data very well: $\chi^2 = 83.26$ (df = 80, $n = 140$, $p = .380$), GFI = .925, CFI = .968, RMSEA = .017, and SRMR = .128.

The Relationships among Services, Self-Concept, and Well-Being

Fig. 1 shows standardized coefficients for the effect of services (psychiatric services, crisis intervention, assessment, and case management) and perceived stigma on well-being, with internalized stigma, self-esteem, and mastery as mediators. We found three distinct patterns regarding the relationships among services, self-concept, and well-being. First, increased use of psychiatric services has a direct and positive effect on changes in daily functioning ($\beta = .185$, $p < .01$), but is not significantly related to self-concept or quality of life. Second, crisis intervention services has a negative effect, and assessment services has a positive (marginal) effect, on changes in mastery ($\beta = -.201$, $p < .01$ and $\beta = .146$, $p < .10$, respectively). Third, case management has a direct negative effect on changes in quality of life only ($\beta = -.143$, $p < .05$). Though changes in mastery are significantly associated with changes in quality of life, the indirect effects of services (crisis intervention and assessment) on quality of life are not significant. Aside from the direct effects of these two services on mastery, changes in self-concept appeared to be unrelated to the services we examined.

The Relationships among Stigma, Self-Concept, and Well-Being

The second set of relationships we examined was among stigma, self-concept, and well-being. We found that perceived stigma is indirectly related to mastery and functioning (through internalized stigma). We also found the effect of perceived stigma on quality of life is partially mediated by internalized stigma and self-esteem (indirect effect: $\beta = -.113$, $p < .05$; direct effect $\beta = -.144$, $p < .10$). The relationship between perceived stigma and self-esteem is also partially mediated by internalized stigma (indirect effect: $\beta = .122$, $p < .05$). Though the relationship between perceived stigma and self-esteem was reduced when internalized stigma was added to the model, it remained statistically significant ($\beta = .256$, $p < .01$). Finally, the relationship between internalized stigma and quality of life is indirect through self-esteem (indirect effect: $\beta = -.116$, $p < .05$). These findings suggest that internalized stigma plays a central role in the relationship

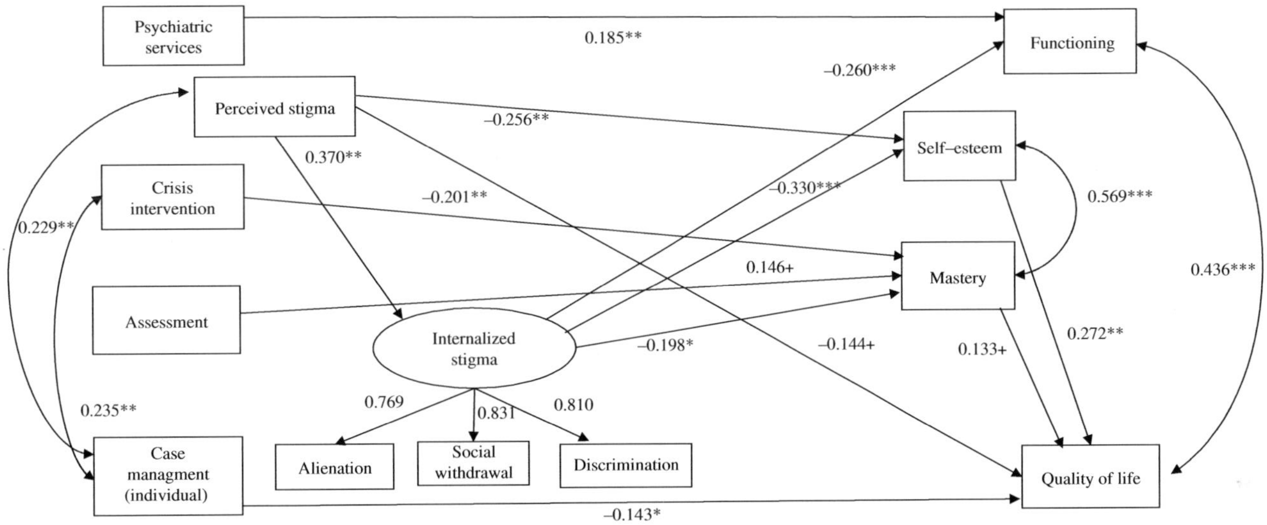

Fig. 1. Standardized Coefficients for Services, Stigma, Self-Concept, and Well-Being. *Notes*: Fit statistics: $X^2 = 83.26$, 80 df, $p = .380$; GFI = .925; CFI = .968; RMSEA = .017; SRMR = .128. Only significant paths are shown. $^{***}p < .001$; $^{**}p < .01$; $^{*}p < .05$; $+p < .10$.

between perceived stigma and self-concept, as well as between perceived stigma and well-being (functioning). Further, self-esteem plays a key role in the relationship between stigma and quality of life, but mastery does not.

The Relationship between Services and Stigma

With regard to final question about the relationship between service use and stigma, we find that service use (based on the four services we examine in our final model) is unrelated to internalized stigma. Although we did not examine the direct relationship between service use and perceived (or public) stigma, it should be noted that correlation between case management and perceived stigma is significant ($r = -.229$, $p < .01$). This finding is suggestive of a relationship between perceived stigma and case management that requires future investigation. Overall, the model presented here suggests that neither internalized stigma nor self-concept mediate the effect of case management, psychiatric services, or crisis services and assessment on well-being.

DISCUSSION

Fifty years ago, deinstitutionalization resulted in a dramatic shift toward community mental health care and services. Decades later, Rosenfield (1997) addressed concerns about the potential impact of psychiatric labels by examining the relative effects of services and stigma on the well-being of individuals with SPMI. Our goal in this study was to revisit these important relationships with an expanded model of both services and stigma, as well as an examination of the relationship between services and stigma.

Our first question focused on the relationships among services, self-concept, and well-being. We build on previous work examining services and well-being in a few ways. First, we included an examination of a range of services available to individuals in a community mental health setting. CSPs are likely more common than specialized or intensive programs such as clubhouses and may be more indicative of types of services available – particularly among those who lack sufficient resources and/or are in greater need of critical care. Second, we used a different mechanism for assessing services than previous research that relied on self-report of services received (e.g., Marcussen et al., 2010; Rosenfield, 1997). By using this measure of service use, we had a more accurate picture of actual services received. We were also able to focus on the quantity of these resources, rather than the use or non-use of each service. Finally, we included case management in this study. Though case management may be characterized as both a service and an organizational structure of services, it has been identified as a focal point for community mental health services following deinstitutionalization.

Overall, we found that only four of the nine services we initially examined were related to either self-concept or well-being. This was somewhat surprising, particularly given the intended goals of services such as vocational training and residential assistance. We also found no unifying pattern with respect to the relationship between service use and well-being in our final model. In other words, the relationships among services, self-concept, and well-being appeared to depend on the type of service and outcome examined.

The strongest relationship between services and well-being was the positive effect of psychiatric services on changes in functioning. Though the content of psychiatric services may vary to some extent across respondents, the key elements of this service include time spent with physicians and nurses, and the management of medication. It makes sense that with increased management of symptoms comes the perception that one is functioning better with respect to symptom control, physical health, and managing stress. Importantly, we did not find these services to be associated with decreases in internalized stigma and/or increases in self-esteem or mastery.

Interestingly, we also found that two of the services we examined were associated with changes in mastery, but in opposite ways. Higher levels of assessment services were positively (though only marginally) associated with mastery, whereas the use of crisis intervention services was negatively associated with mastery. However, we find that neither of these services had a direct effect on either functioning or quality of life. We think the relationship between crisis services and mastery is especially interesting. As we speculate above, it is possible – if not likely – that some services are related to recovery and some may be associated with the early stages of treatment or represent needs for those who have been receiving services for a longer time period. We did not make predictions about services such as crisis intervention because it could be argued that it is positive to have the service available, even if it represents increased need. That said, the relationship between crisis intervention and decreased mastery might suggest that the continuous supervision associated with this particular service reduces one's sense of control, or alternatively that the need for crisis services is stimulated by a decrease in personal control over time.

Finally, we found that case management was negatively associated with quality of life over the study period. This is somewhat surprising, but we believe informative. As discussed above, studies indicate that the effects of case management are somewhat mixed – depending on the type of management used (Marshall et al., 2000; Ziguras & Stuart, 2000). We speculate that too much case management might work against at least one of the goals of community health services, which is to foster independence (Corrigan et al., 2014). Unlike previous research, our work does not compare individuals who have case management to those who do not, but rather we look at the amount of this service they receive. Though we control for previous levels of quality of life and functioning, we suspect there is a relationship between amount of services needed and amount of services received – suggesting that there might some selection of less healthy individuals into more case management. We also wonder, however, if too much supervision might result in individuals feeling as though they are not capable of managing their mental health care, thus reducing their overall assessment of life satisfaction.

Our second goal in this study was to examine the relationships among stigma, self-concept, and well-being. Here, we build on previous work by including both perceived and internalized stigma. Consistent with Rosenfield's 1997 study, our findings indicate that perceptions of devaluation and discrimination are consequential (and detrimental) for self-esteem and quality of life. We also found, as others have, that internalized stigma mediated the relationship between perceived stigma and self-concept. These findings support previous work that identifies a significant relationship between internalized stigma and self-esteem (Drapalski et al., 2013; Livingston & Boyd, 2010; Ritsher & Phelan, 2004; Yanos et al., 2008). They also suggest that internalized stigma plays a key role in the relationship between self-concept (particularly self-esteem) and well-being, above and beyond cultural stereotypes about mental illness.

Our last question concerns the nature of the relationship between services and stigma. We suggested that one way to better assess the impact of services on well-being was to consider whether service use is associated with stigma. We did not find any of the services we examined to be significantly related to internalized stigma. Though we did not offer specific hypothesis (given the variation in services we examined), we find it a somewhat surprising that none of the services were associated with the feelings or experiences of alienation, discrimination, and social withdrawal. The fact that we did not find a relationship between services and internalized stigma in this study may be related to the types of services we examine. It is worth noting that our analyses did reveal a significant negative association between perceived (public) stigma and case management. While we did not examine the relationship between service use and perceived stigma, this pattern raises the question about whether services are potentially related to public stigma. A closer look at this relationship requires a fully longitudinal model that examines stigma and service use over time.

Limitations and Future Directions

This chapter advances our understanding of the relationships among services, stigma, and well-being in the context of community health care; however, we recognize that there are limitations that should be considered when interpreting our results. First, our sample is fairly large for studies of this type, but also has a fair amount of attrition between baseline and time 2. We took steps to compare the information we received about service use in our sample to the broader population of consumers at the CSP, which gives us some confidence that our respondents were comparable in terms of the amount of services they received. Nonetheless, our findings are not necessarily generalizable beyond the study sample.

Additionally, our measure of quality of life, while consistent with some previous studies (e.g., Marcussen et al., 2010), assesses overall life satisfaction rather than satisfaction in various aspects on one's life (e.g., employment, residential situation, social relationships). Similarly, our measure of functioning focuses specifically on health-related aspects of functioning. We think it will be important in future work to examine a broad range of outcomes, particularly in light of our findings which suggest that specific services might be linked to specific outcomes. It makes sense that some services are designed to "match" particular (and sometimes immediate) needs of consumers. Broadening the scope of what is meant by recovery, and including a wider array of recovery-based outcomes, may provide useful information about which services are most beneficial in terms of meeting both individual and community goals.

We also believe that expanding the focus of service use will be important in future work. In our study, we attempted to build on measures of received services by adding a more objective measure of service use. However, we would also suggest that future researchers turn their attention to the content or meaning of these services to the consumer. In particular, it would be important to know the extent to which services provide opportunities for social interaction with peers and members of the community. For services that are more focused on symptom reduction or crisis intervention, it would also be useful to know how satisfied individuals were with the services provided by CSPs, and to what extent the services restored positive functioning and quality of life over time. Understanding service engagement and involvement in supportive activities more generally would provide more complete information about the connections between service use and outcomes such stigma, self-concept, and well-being.

Finally, incorporating stigma resistance or management will be an important step toward determining the ways in which individuals deflect negative perceptions regarding their mental illness. According to Thoits (2011), the relationship between stigma and self-concept is persistent, but often quite modest in light of what labeling and modified labeling theories might predict. Thoits argues that this is due to resistance strategies such as deflecting or challenging stereotypical notions of mental illness. Along those lines, Corrigan and colleagues (e.g., Corrigan et al., 2009; Corrigan & Watson, 2002) describe a process of empowerment and/or righteous anger that mediates the relationship between self-stigma and recovery. Similarly, identity threat models suggest that individuals are active appraisers of their environment and their abilities with respect to coping with discrimination. For instance, individuals who hold a stigmatized social identity might attribute negative feedback to prejudiced attitudes toward their group (rather than make internal attributions) and/or make selective comparisons of their group relative to the dominant out-group in an effort to protect self-esteem (Crocker & Major, 1989). Such resistance or management does not necessarily change public attitudes, but it might reduce the internalization of those attitudes (Thoits, 2011; Thoits & Link, 2015; Marcussen and Asencio (2016). In many ways, these suggestions echo the conclusions and recommendations that Rosenfield made 20 years ago. Services that foster or encourage empowerment are more likely to decrease stigma, increase self-esteem and mastery, and increase functioning and quality of life. Given the somewhat more malleable nature of self-stigma relative to public stigma, we further suggest that services designed specifically to facilitate stigma resistance and/or foster positive social comparisons (and thereby reduce internalized stigma) would play an important role in maximizing the positive effects of CSPs, while at the same time minimizing the negative influence of stigma on self-concept and well-being.

ACKNOWLEDGMENTS

We thank the clients and staff of Community Support Services (CSS) and the Consumer Education Outreach Center for their assistance in research design and data collection. In particular we thank Terrence Dalton and

Frank Sepetauc, from CSS, for their help with logistics and their support of this effort. We also thank Tom Grande and Nick Veauthier of the County of Summit Alcohol, Drug Addiction and Mental Health Services Board for technical assistance. This study could not have been done without their help. Collaborators for this project who contributed to the research design include: Richard E. Adams, Kristin Baughman, Natalie Bonfine, Sara E. Dugan, Mary Gallagher, Kristen Marcussen, Kristin Mickelson, R. Scott Olds, Elizabeth Piatt, and James Werner. This work was supported by the Northeast Ohio Medical University Office of Research and Sponsored Programs (Christian Ritter, PI). Funding for the study is provided by Northeast Ohio Medical University, Christian Ritter (PI).

REFERENCES

Boyd, J. E., Adler, E. P., Otilingam, P. G., & Peters, T. (2014). Internalized stigma of mental illness (ISMI) scale: A multinational review. *Comprehensive Psychiatry*, *55*(1), 221–231. doi:10.1016/j.comppsych.2013.06.005

Brown, P. (1985). *Transfer of care: Psychiatric deinstitutionalization and its aftermath.* London: Routledge.

Clement, S., Schauman, O., Graham, T., Maggioni, F., Evans-Lacko, S., Bezborodovs, N., … Thornicroft, G. (2014). What is the impact of mental health-related stigma on help-seeking? A systematic review of quantitative and qualitative studies. *Psychological Medicine*, *45*(1), 11–27. doi:10.1017/S0033291714000129

Corrigan, P. (2004). How stigma interferes with mental health care. *American Psychologist*, *59*(7), 614–625. doi:10.1037/0003-066X.59.7.614

Corrigan, P., & Penn, D. L. (1999). Lessons from social psychology on discrediting psychiatric stigma. *American Psychologist*, *54*(9), 765–776. doi:10.1037/0003-066X.54.9.765

Corrigan, P. W., Druss, B. G., & Perlick, D. A. (2014). The impact of mental illness stigma on seeking and participating in mental health care. *Psychological Science in the Public Interest*, *15*(2), 37–70. doi:10.1177/1529100614531398

Corrigan, P. W., Larson, J. E., & Rusch, N. (2009). Self-stigma and the "why try" effect: Impact on life goals and evidence-based practices. *World Psychiatry*, *8*(2), 75–81. doi:10.1177/1529100614531398

Corrigan, P. W., Rafacz, J., & Rusch, N. (2011). Examining a progressive model of self-stigma and its impact on people with serious mental illness. *Psychiatric Research*, *189*(3), 339–343. doi:10.1016/j.psychres.2011.05.024

Corrigan, P. W., & Watson, A. C. (2002). The paradox of self-stigma and mental illness. *Clinical Psychology: Science and Practice*, *9*(1), 35–53. doi:10.1093/clipsy.9.1.35

Corrigan, P. W., Watson, A. C., & Barr, L. (2006). The self-stigma of mental illness: Implications for self-esteem and self-efficacy. *Journal of Social and Clinical Psychology*, *25*(8), 875–884. doi:10.1521./jscp.2006.25.8.875

Crocker, J., & Major, B. (1989). Social stigma and self-esteem: The self-protective properties of stigma. *Psychological Review*, *96*(4), 608–663. doi:10.1037/0033-295x.96.4.608

Drapalski, A. L., Lucksted, A., Perrin, P. B., Aakre, J. M., Brown, C. H., DeForge, B. R., & Boyd, J. E. (2013). A model of internalized stigma and its effects on people with mental illness. *Psychiatric Services*, *64*(3), 264–269. doi:10.1176/appi.ps.001322012

Estroff, S. E. (1981). Psychiatric de-institutionalization: A socio-cultural analysis. *Journal of Social Issues*, *37*(3), 116–132. doi:10.1111/j.1540-4560.1981.tb00832.x

Forrester-Jones, R., Carpenter, J., Cambridge, P., Tate, A., Hallam, A., Knapp, M., & Beecham, J. (2002). The quality of life of people 12 years after resettlement from long stay hospitals: Users' views on their living environment, daily activities and future aspirations. *Disability & Society*, *17*(7), 741–758. doi:10.1080/0968759021000068469

Goffman, E. (1961). *Asylums: Essays on the social situation of mental patients and other inmates*. Garden City, NY: Anchor.

Goffman, E. (1963). *Stigma: Notes on the management of spoiled identity*. New York, NY: Simon & Schuster.

Goldman, H. H., & Morrissey, J. P. (1985). The alchemy of mental health policy: Homelessness and the fourth cycle of reform. *American Journal of Public Health*, *75*(7), 727–731. doi:10.2105/AJPH.75.7.727

Gove, W. R. (1982). *Deviance and mental illness*. Beverly Hills, CA: Sage.

Gove, W. R., & Fain, T. (1973). The stigma of mental hospitalization: An attempt to evaluate its consequences. *General Psychiatry*, *28*, 494–500. doi:10.1001/archpsyc.1973.01750340034005

Grob, G. N. (1994). *The mad among us: A history of the care of America's mentally ill*. New York, NY: The Free Press.

Hobbs, C., Newton, L., Tennant, C., Rosen, A., & Tribe, K. (2002). Deinstitutionalization for long-term mental illness: A 6-year evaluation. *Australian and New Zealand Journal of Psychiatry*, *36*, 60–66. doi:10.1046/j.1440-1614.2002.00984.x

Hodges, K., & Wotring, J. (2000). Client typology based on functioning across domains using the CAFAS: Implications for service planning. *The Journal of Behavioral Health Services & Research*, *27*(3), 257–270. doi:10.1007/BF02291738

Lamb, H. R. (1997). The new state mental hospitals in the community. *Psychiatric Services*, *48*(10), 1307–1310. doi:10.1176/ps.48.10.1307

Lamb, H. R., & Bachrach, L. L. (2001). Some perspectives on deinstitutionalization. *Psychiatric Services*, *52*(8), 1039–1045. doi:10.1176/appi.ps.52.8.1039

Lehman, A. F. (1988). A quality of life interview for the chronically mentally ill. *Evaluation Program Planning*, *11*(2), 51–62. doi:10.1016/0149-7189(88)90033-X

Link, B., Castille, D. M., & Stuber, J. (2008). Stigma and coercion in the context of outpatient treatment for people with mental illnesses. *Social Science & Medicine*, *67*(3), 409–419. doi:10.1016/j.socscimed.2008.03.015

Link, B. G. (1982). Mental patient status, work, and income: An examination of the effects of a psychiatric label. *American Sociological Review*, *47*(2), 202–215. doi:10.2307/2094963

Link, B. G. (1987). Understanding labeling effects in the area of mental disorders: An assessment of the effects of expectations of rejection. *American Sociological Review*, *52*(1), 96–112. doi:10.2307/2095395

Link, B. G., Cullen, F. T., Struening, E., Shrout, P. E., & Dohrenwend, B. P. (1989). A modified labeling theory approach to mental disorders: An empirical assessment. *American Sociological Review*, *54*(3), 400–423. doi:10.2307/2095613

Link, B. G., & Phelan, J. C. (2001). Conceptualizing stigma. *Annual Review of Sociology, 27*, 363–385. doi:10.1146/annurev.soc.27.1.363

Link, B. G., Phelan, J. C., Bresnahan, M., Stueve, A., & Pescosolido, B. A. (1999). Public conceptions of mental illness: Labels, causes, dangerousness, and social distance. *American Journal of Public Health, 89*(9), 1328–1333. doi:10.2105/AJPH.89.9.1328

Link, B. G., Struening, E. L., Neese-Todd, S., & Phelan, J. C. (2001). The consequences of stigma for the self-esteem of people with mental illnesses. *Psychiatric Services, 52*(12), 1621–1626. doi:10.1176/appi.ps.52.12.1621

Link, B. G., Struening, E. L., Rahav, M., Phelan, J. C., & Nuttbrock, L. (1997). On stigma and its consequences: Evidence from a longitudinal study of men with dual diagnoses of mental illness and substance abuse. *Journal of Health and Social Behavior, 38*(2), 177–190. Retrieved from http://www.jstor.org/stable/2955424

Livingston, J. D., & Boyd, J. E. (2010). Correlates and consequences of internalized stigma for people living with mental illness: A systematic review and meta-analysis. *Social Science & Medicine, 71*(12), 2150–2161. doi:10.1016/j.socscimed.2010.09.030

Marcussen, K., & Asencio, E. K. (2016, in press). Stigma resistance and the mental illness self-view. In. J. E. Stets & R. T. Serpe (Eds.), *New directions in identity theory and research* (pp. 473–508). New York, NY: Oxford University Press.

Marcussen, K., Ritter, C., & Munetz, M. R. (2010). The effect of services and stigma on quality of life for persons with serious mental illnesses. *Psychiatric Services, 61*(5), 489–494. doi:10.1176/appi.ps.61.5.489

Markowitz, F. E. (1998). The effects of stigma on the psychological well-being and life satisfaction of persons with mental illness. *Journal of Health and Social Behavior, 39*(4), 335–347. doi:10.2307/2676342

Markowitz, F. E. (2001). Modeling processes in recovery from mental illness: Relationships between symptoms, life satisfaction, and self-concept. *Journal of Health and Social Behavior, 42*(1), 64–79. doi:10.2307/3090227

Marshall, M., Gray, A., Lockwood, A., & Green, R. (2000). Case management for people with severe mental disorders. *Cochrane Database System Review*. doi:10.1002/14651858. CD000050.pub2

McGrew, J. H., Wright, E. R., Pescosolido, B. A., & McDonel, E. (1999). The closing of central state hospital: Long-term outcomes for persons with severe mental illness. *Journal of Behavioral Health Services and Research, 26*(3), 246–261. doi:10.1007/BF02287271

Mechanic, D., & Rochefort, D. A. (1990). Desinstitutionalization: An appraisal of reform. *Annual Review of Sociology, 16*, 301–327. doi:10.1146/annurev.so.16.080190.001505

Morrissey, J. P., & Goldman, H. H. (1986). Care and treatment of the mentally ill in the United States: Historical developments and reforms. *The Annals of the American Academy of Political and Social Science, 484*(1), 12–27. doi:10.1177/0002716286484001002

O'Malia, L., McFarland, B. H., Barker, S., & Barron, N. M. (2002). A level-of-functioning self-report measure for consumers with severe mental illness. *Psychiatric Services, 53*(3), 326–331. doi:10.1176/appi.ps.53.3.326

Pearlin, L. I., & Schooler, C. (1978). The structure of coping. *Journal of Health and Social Behavior, 19*(1), 2–21. doi:10.2307/2136319

Pescosolido, B. A. (2013). The public stigma of mental illness: What do we think; what do we know; what can we prove? *Journal of Health and Social Behavior, 54*(1), 1–21. doi:10.1177/0022146512471197

Pescosolido, B. A., Martin, J. K., Long, J. S., Medina, T. R., Phelan, J. C., & Link, B. G. (2010). "A disease like any other"? A decade of change in public reactions to schizophrenia, depression, and alcohol dependence. *American Journal of Psychiatry*, *167*(11), 1321–1330. doi:10.1176/appi.ajp.2010.09121743

Priebe, S., Hoffmann, K., Isermann, M., & Kaiser, W. (2002). Do long-term hospitalised patients benefit from discharge into the community? *Social Psychiatry and Psychiatric Epidemiology*, *37*(8), 387–392. doi:10.1007/s00127-002-0568-1

Quinn, D. M. (2006). Concealable versus conspicuous stigmatized identities. In S. Levin & C. VanLar (Eds.), *Stigma and group inequality: Social psychological perspectives* (pp. 83–103). Mahwah, NJ: Erlbaum.

Ritsher, J. B., Otilingam, P. G., & Grajales, M. (2003). Internalized stigma of mental illness: Psychometric properties of a new measure. *Psychiatry Research*, *121*(1), 31–49. doi:10.1016/j.psychres.2003.08.008

Ritsher, J. B., & Phelan, J. C. (2004). Internalized stigma predicts erosion or morale among psychiatric outpatients. *Psychiatric Research*, *129*(3), 257–265. doi:10.1016/j.psychres.2004.08.003

Rosenberg, M. (1979). *Conceiving the self*. New York, NY: Basic Books.

Rosenfield, S. (1997). Labeling mental illness: The effects of received services and perceived stigma on life satisfaction. *American Sociological Review*, *62*(4), 660–672. doi:10.2307/2657432

Scheff, T. J. (1966). *Being mentally ill: A sociological theory*. Chicago, IL: Adeline.

Thoits, P. A. (2011). Resisting the stigma of mental illness. *Social Psychology Quarterly*, *74*(1), 6–28.

Thoits, P. A., & Link, B. G. (2015). Stigma resistance and well-being among people in treatment for psychosis. *Society and Mental Health*, *74*(1), 1–20. doi:10.1177/0190272511398019

Townsend, P. (1976). *Sociology and Social Policy*. Harmondsworth: Penguin Books.

Wright, E. R., Gronfein, W. P., & Owens, T. J. (2000). Deinstitutionalization, social rejection, and the self-esteem of former mental patients. *Journal of Health and Social Behavior*, *41*(1), 68–90. doi:10.2307/2676361

Yanos, P. T., Lysaker, P. H., & Roe, D. (2010). Internalized stigma as a barrier to improvement in vocational functioning among people with schizophrenia-spectrum disorders. *Psychiatry Research*, *178*(1), 211–213. doi:10.1016/j.psychres.2010.01.003

Yanos, P. T., Roe, D., Markus, K., & Lysaker, P. H. (2008). Pathways between internalized stigma and outcomes related to recovery in schizophrenia spectrum disorders. *Psychiatric Services*, *59*(12), 1437–1442. doi:10.1176/appi.ps.59.12.1437

Ziguras, S., & Stuart, G. (2000). A meta-analysis of the effectiveness of mental health case management over 20 years. *Psychiatric Services*, *51*(11), 1410–1415. doi:10.1176/appi.ps.51.11.141

THE SELF-STIGMA OF PSYCHIATRIC PATIENTS: IMPLICATIONS FOR IDENTITIES, EMOTIONS, AND THE LIFE COURSE

Sarah K. Harkness, Amy Kroska and Bernice A. Pescosolido

ABSTRACT

Purpose – *We argue that self-stigma places patients on a path of marginalization throughout their life course leading to a negative cycle of opportunity and advancement. Mental health patients with higher levels of self-stigma tend to have much lower self-esteem, efficacy, and personal agency; therefore, they will be more inclined to adopt role-identities at the periphery of major social institutions, like those of work, family, and academia. Similarly, the emotions felt when enacting such roles may be similarly dampened.*

Methodology/approach – *Utilizing principles from affect control theory (ACT) and the affect control theory of selves (ACTS), we generate*

50 Years after Deinstitutionalization: Mental Illness in Contemporary Communities
Advances in Medical Sociology, Volume 17, 207–233

ISSN: 1057-6290/doi:10.1108/S1057-629020160000017008

predictions related to self-stigmatized patients' role-identity adoption and emotions. We use the Indianapolis Mental Health Study and Interact, *a computerized version of ACT and ACTS, to generate empirically based simulation results for patients with an affective disorder (e.g., major depression and bipolar disorder) with comparably high or low levels of self-stigmatization.*

Findings – *Self-stigma among affective patients reduces the tendency to adopt major life course identities. Self-stigma also affects patients' emotional expression by compelling patients to seek out interactions that make them feel anxious or affectively neutral.*

Originality/value – *This piece has implications for the self-stigma and stigma literatures. It is also one of the first pieces to utilize ACTS, thereby offering a new framework for understanding the self-stigma process. We offer new hypotheses for future research to test with non-simulation-based data and suggest some policy implications.*

Keywords: Mental health; stigma; affect control theory; affect control theory of selves; life course; social psychology

After President Kennedy signed the Community Mental Health Centers Act of 1963, mental health treatment dramatically shifted from large-scale, in-patient custodial care to predominantly community care and out-patient programs. From this movement, termed deinstitutionalization, practitioners and the public hoped that mental health patients would have the opportunity to more fully engage in the social world and occupy mainstream identities tied to major cultural institutions, like work and family (see Frank & Glied, 2006; Mechanic, 1990 for an overview).

However, recent life course research indicates there to be a number of deleterious sequential outcomes for those diagnosed with mental illness. Although certain life events and their timing may increase the risk of mental health problems (Jackson, 2004), being diagnosed with a mental illness also affects patients' life trajectories. Early-onset mental illness, for example, is generally associated with lower socioeconomic status and less stable family forms (see George, 2013 for an overview). In a particularly telling longitudinal study, patients diagnosed with an affective disorder, like major depression, had significantly lower occupational prestige, were more likely to have either never been married or to have multiple divorces or separations, and to have remained childless than those diagnosed later in life (Turnbull, George, Landerman, Swartz, & Blazer, 1990). Early-onset mental illness is also predictive of recurrent mental health episodes for many disorders (Kim-Cohen et al., 2003).

These life course trajectories are constrained by a number of consequential factors, including stigma: the negative stereotypes, prejudice, and discrimination directed toward the mentally ill (Hinshaw & Stier, 2008; Link & Phelan, 2001; Major & O'Brien, 2005; Pescosolido & Martin, 2007, 2015). Notably, in the decades since deinstitutionalization, stigma toward mentally ill adults and children has not abated (Martin, Pescosolido, Olafsdottir, & McLeod, 2007; Payton, & Thoits, 2011; Pescosolido, 2013; Pescosolido et al., 2008, 2010; Phelan, Link, Stueve, & Pescosolido, 2000; Schnittker, 2008). For example, only about half of Americans report a willingness to work with someone who has major depression or to have someone with major depression marry into their family (Pescosolido et al., 2010).

Those who receive an official mental health diagnosis are also at risk of self-stigmatization, referring to the acceptance of these negative cultural beliefs into patients' views of themselves (Kroska & Harkness, 2006, 2008). Note that self-stigma is distinct from felt stigma (Livingston & Boyd, 2010), whereas the latter pertains to the negative outcomes resulting from the awareness and anticipation of being stigmatized by others, self-stigmatization conceptualizes patients' agreement with negative cultural beliefs and the application of these beliefs to themselves, termed "self-concurrence" (Corrigan, Watson, & Barr, 2006).

Self-stigmatization has deep ramifications for the course of daily interactions for those with a wide spectrum of mental illnesses. Everyday decisions and experiences, even seemingly nominal ones, set the stage for a multitude of consequential outcomes later in life – outcomes ranging from emotional to economic. We propose that mental health patients with higher levels of self-stigma may feel much lower self-esteem, efficacy, and personal agency, making them more inclined to adopt role-identities as peripheral or disengaged members of major social institutions, like those of work, family, and academia. Similarly, the emotions felt when enacting such roles may be dampened, consequently feeding the negative affective components of their disorders. We argue that self-stigma places patients on a path of marginalization throughout their life course leading to a negative cycle of opportunity and advancement, which may also have deleterious consequences for the progression, including possible reoccurrence, of their illnesses.

We utilize principles from affect control theory and the affect control theory of selves to test these predictions. Using the Indianapolis Mental Health Study and *Interact*, a computerized version of these theories (found at http://www.indiana.edu/~socpsy/ACT/interact.htm), we generate empirically based simulation results for those officially diagnosed with an affective disorder (e.g., major depression, bipolar disorder). Our findings have implications for the life course and stigma literature. This is also one of the first studies to utilize the affect control theory of selves, thereby introducing a new theoretical tool to the stigma literature.

STIGMA AND SELF-STIGMA

When individuals receive an official diagnosis of mental illness, they are placed into a stigmatized cultural category. A steady stream of research documents the deleterious effects stigma processes have on patients' life course. Stigma processes resulting from this official label may result in lower earnings and unemployment (Link, 1982, 1987; Link Cullen, Struening, Shrout, & Dohrenwend, 1989, Link, Mirotznik, & Cullen, 1991), constricted social networks (Link et al., 1989), and a greater likelihood of rejection and negative evaluations (Farina & Felner, 1973; Kroska, Harkness, Thomas, & Brown, 2014; Kroska, Harkness, Brown, & Thomas, 2015; Lucas & Phelan, 2012; Mehta & Farina, 1997; Page, 1995; Perry, 2011; Sibicky & Dovidio, 1986; Wright, Gronfein, & Owens, 2000). Patients' experiences of stigma are also linked with increased demoralization (Link, 1987; Markowitz, 1998; Ritsher & Phelan, 2004; Wright et al., 2000), lower self-efficacy (Markowitz, Angell, & Greenberg, 2011; Wright et al., 2000), lower quality of life (Markowitz et al., 2011; Rosenfield, 1997), and self-stigmatization more broadly (Evans-Lacko, Brohan, Mojtabai, & Thornicroft, 2012; Corrigan et al., 2006; Hinshaw & Stier, 2008; Kroska & Harkness, 2006, 2008; Lysaker, Roe, & Yanos, 2006; Markowitz et al., 2011; Vogel, Wade, & Hackler, 2007).

Patients with an official diagnosis may be particularly vulnerable to self-stigmatization's deleterious effects on self-efficacy and self-esteem (Evans-Lacko et al., 2012; Hinshaw & Stier, 2008; Link, 1987; Markowitz, 1998; Markowitz et al., 2011; Ritsher & Phelan, 2004; Wright et al., 2000). Self-esteem gaps, for instance, are uncommon between racial and ethnic minorities and whites (Crocker & Major, 1989; Crocker & Quinn, 2000), yet these gaps are often found between patients and non-patients with the same symptomatology (Link, 1987; Link, Struening, Neese-Todd, Asmussen, & Phelan, 2001). Stier and Hinshaw (2007) argue that many features of mental illness, including the isolation and anxiety arising from stigma (Frable, Pratt, & Hoey, 1998; Pachankis, 2007), put psychiatric patients at a heightened risk for internalizing these negative cultural beliefs.

This is not to argue that self-stigmatization is inevitable on receipt of an official illness label (Thoits, 2011). Awareness of cultural stereotypes does not automatically lead to self-stigmatization (Rusch, Angermeyer & Corrigan, 2005). Corrigan & Watson, 2002 and Corrigan et al. (2009) contend that some patients may actively reject the stigma of the mental illness label and seek empowerment instead. Scambler and Paoli (2008) have advanced the terms "project stigma and deviance" to signify this active rejection of the shame and blame of stigmatization. Similarly, Thoits (2011) discusses challenging and deflecting resistance strategies to stigmatization.

Those who have self-stigmatized, however, are at greater risk for numerous harmful consequences. In addition to lower self-esteem and self-efficacy (Corrigan et al., 2006; Rusch et al., 2006; Wright et al., 2000), Rusch et al. (2005) argue that self-stigma may deter patients from pursuing major life course goals, particularly in the areas of work and independent living. This is an argument that aligns with the research of Link (1987) who found that people who received an official psychiatric diagnosis were more likely to be unemployed than those with comparable symptomatology but without the official label. Exactly how self-concurrent stigmatization affects this process awaits a formal test, however.

Kroska and Harkness (2006, 2008) show that patients' assessments of the cultural beliefs about their group are related to their sense of self (termed self-sentiments), with greater perceptions of stigma (operationalized as low evaluation, potency, and activity ratings of the cultural category "a mentally ill person") negatively related to self-sentiments (measured as the evaluation, potency, and activity of the identity "myself as I really am"). This relationship, however, varies by diagnostic group. In particular, as stigma sentiments decline in evaluation, potency, and activity, the self-sentiments of those with an affective diagnosis (e.g., major depression) tend to also decline in goodness, potency, and activity.

We build on this work by examining the likely interactional consequences of internalizing comparatively high or low levels of stigma for patients with an affective disorder. We predict that higher levels of self-stigma will reduce the likelihood of engaging in major life course roles, thereby partially explaining why many patients have not fully benefitted from deinstitutionalization. In particular, we examine the role-identities and emotions that are most confirmatory and authentic for patients with high and low self-stigma, and the likely compensatory role-identities patients will select if they are compelled to enact an identity requiring higher levels of self-esteem, efficacy, and agency than their self-sentiments warrant.

No data, of which we are aware, directly pertain to issues of role selection and emotionality. Therefore, we draw on the theoretical and empirical components of affect control theory, the affect control theory of selves, and their computer program instantiation, *Interact*, to make empirically based predictions. It is our intent for these predictions to be generative for future research on the interactional consequences of self-stigma.

AFFECT CONTROL THEORY

In any social interaction, people imbue the setting, identities, emotions, and behaviors involved in the encounter with affective meaning – a general feeling or sentiment about these aspects of the interaction. According to affect control theory (hereafter ACT), the affective meanings associated with social events shape individuals' behavior and the behavior others direct toward them (Heise, 1979, 2007; MacKinnon, 1994; Smith-Lovin & Heise, 1988). Identities have a reflexive quality in that individuals monitor and compare the feedback they receive from others to the affective standard, otherwise known as the fundamental sentiment, of the identity they are embodying. Through this comparison process, individuals are able to adjust their behavior to elicit confirmatory responses from others in the social situation. Fundamental sentiments, ACT scholars suggest, represent core societal understandings of situations, actors, and expected actions; they are another way of capturing the elusive constructs of "culture" and, importantly, "stigma" (Kroska & Harkness, 2006, 2008).

ACT researchers measure affective meaning according to assessments of the evaluation (good versus bad), potency (powerful versus weak), and activity (active versus inactive) of identities, roles, emotions, and other features of the interaction. Evaluation, potency, and activity (EPA) comprise the three universal dimensions of meaning Osgood et al. identified in their cross-cultural research (Osgood, May, & Miron, 1975). The evaluation dimension assesses feelings about goodness; the potency dimension gauges perceptions of strength, size, and force; and the activity dimension pertains to considerations of stimulation, speed, age, and keenness (Heise, 2007;

MacKinnon, 1994). Research in 25 cultures has shown that assessments of social concepts, including self-concepts, universally involve responses across these three dimensions (Osgood et al., 1975).[1]

The key insight from ACT is that individuals manage social interactions in an effort to maintain their preexisting, fundamental impression of themselves, the people with whom they are interacting, and other elements of the situation. If something goes amiss during the course of the interaction, individuals are motivated to rectify this by behaving in ways that bring their immediate impressions of the interaction (known as transient sentiments) to align with their fundamental sentiments of the various features of the situation, including their various identity meanings.

Emotions and Affect Control Theory

As we manage our social interactions and enact our self- and role-identities, we feel various emotional outcomes, with certain types of emotions being more commonly felt given the identities we are enacting. Indeed, self-stigmatization may make the experience of negative emotions more likely. According to ACT, emotions provide valuable information aiding individuals in their assessments of events. Through interaction, people develop impressions of themselves and other interactants, and emotions allow individuals to feel that impression viscerally (Heise, 2007). Emotions also signal the difference between the identity an actor intends to enact and the identity others perceive the actor to be enacting, thereby providing information on how fully the event confirmed the fundamental sentiments tied to their identity in the situation. For example, if an adult harangues a child without cause, the adult may feel very bad, impotent, and inactive, consequently experiencing the pang of being ashamed. In this case, the child would feel unpleasant but very active and consequently experience anger or contempt (event simulation from *Interact*). Conversely, if a child does something that causes a display of shock in others, the child may feel embarrassed that her behavior caused such a response. These transient emotions allow interactants to sense how well the interaction is proceeding and guide the determination of who our interaction partners are.

When the identities we enact are perfectly confirmed, we are expected to experience characteristic emotions, which are emotions with an EPA profile that matches the profile of the enacted identity. For example, according to college females, a physician has an EPA profile of 2.48, 2.74, 1.49,[2] which is quite good, extremely potent, and slightly active (Francis & Heise, 2006).

When her physician identity is perfectly confirmed, she would most likely feel a sense of satisfaction, which is similarly extremely good, extremely potent, and slightly active (EPA profile of 2.92, 2.60, 1.07). Conversely, a sick person (EPA profile of −1.21, −1.72, −2.03), which is slightly bad, quite impotent, and quite inactive, would feel a sense of resentment, embarrassment, discouragement, and pessimism if her identity were to be perfectly confirmed (all these emotions have EPA profiles that are similarly bad, impotent, and inactive). Note the similarity between the EPA profile of the identity and characteristic emotion. For identities lower in self-esteem (evaluation), self-efficacy (potency), or activity (e.g., the identities negatively impacted by self-stigma), the emotions people will want to feel (as they are the most confirmatory) will be similarly dampened.

Affect Control Theory of Selves

The roles mental health patients select directly shape their life course trajectories. Self-stigmatization may constrain the roles considered feasible or comfortable for patients to enact, thereby setting them on a path of disengagement from dominant institutions, like work and family, as the life course and stigma literature suggests (George, 2013; Link, 1982, 1987; Link et al., 1989, 1991; Turnbull et al., 1990). But which role-identities are patients most willing and comfortable adopting? The affect control theory of selves (hereafter ACTS) theorizes the interrelationship between selves, role-identities, and social institutions to answer this question (MacKinnon & Heise, 2010). According to the theory, individuals seek to enact identities that most closely align with their fundamental self-sentiments (i.e., the EPA ratings of "myself as I really am"). Self-evaluation corresponds to self-esteem and self-worth; self-potency aligns with feelings of self-efficacy and empowerment; and self-activity taps feelings of liveliness achieved through personal agency (MacKinnon, 2015). Role-identities that are similar in meaning to an actor's self-sentiments create a feeling of self-actualization – a role experience that feels true to one's self.

Identities farther away affectively to fundamental self-sentiments create a sense of inauthenticity compelling people to inhabit compensatory identities in the opposing affective direction to offset this inauthenticity. For example, a woman who has neutral self-sentiments (0.00, 0.00, 0.00) who is constrained to enact an identity that is much higher affectively, like a teacher (2.85, 2.43, 1.63), will likely select a subsequent identity like victim (−2.60, −2.39, −2.18) or pessimist (−2.13, −2.39, −1.11) to balance her identity enactments (results from *Interact*). Thus, individuals can iteratively confirm their self-sentiments with opposing role-identities that roughly evenly encircle the fundamental self-sentiments' fulcrum. These ACTS processes are modeled similarly to those underlying ACT (Heise, 2007; MacKinnon & Heise, 2010).

A number of external factors may compel individuals to enact identities that are not immediately self-actualizing. The need for employment and other structural constraints may force individuals to select role-identities associated with the institutions of education and work, for instance. Each institutional setting likewise affects the type of identities that can be invoked given their suitability for that environment. Finally, influential others may impose identities on an individual.

MacKinnon and Heise (2010) provide several tests of ACTS propositions, showing, for example, that the distances between college students' self-sentiments and their EPA ratings of 58 identities are negatively and significantly correlated with the students' rating of how much those identities describe them. Notably, they also use data estimated from published records to demonstrate sociopaths' self-sentiments predict the types of identities they adopted.

EMPIRICAL PREDICTIONS

Because greater levels of stigma may reduce self-evaluation, self-potency, and self-activity in affective patients (Kroska & Harkness, 2006, 2008), we predict that stigmatized patients will want to adopt role-identities that are similarly dampened, as these are more self-actualizing. The overall implication is that self-stigma produces self-sentiments that are not high enough in goodness (self-esteem) and power (self-efficacy) to comfortably seek out identities that are part of major life course transitions, such as an employee, someone's date, a spouse, or a parent, which have quite high cultural EPA profiles.[3]

Hypothesis 1. Self-stigma will reduce the tendency to adopt role-identities associated with major life course transitions.

Additionally, the negative self-sentiments arising from self-stigma should impact patients' characteristic emotions, according to ACTS. Self-stigma reduces affective patients' self-evaluation, self-potency, and self-activity, which should then compel them to seek out identities that generate emotions similarly low on evaluation, potency, and activity. Thus, self-stigma may have deleterious consequences for illness progression and treatment to the extent these more negative emotions feed the depressed or anxious components of their disorder.

Hypotheses 2a–2c. Self-stigma will reduce the (a) evaluation, (b) potency, and (c) activity of characteristic emotions.

When patients are forced to enact identities that are higher in goodness, potency, and activity than their self-identities, ACTS predicts that they will be compelled to offset the resulting feelings of inauthenticity by adopting identities that are even lower in goodness and potency than their self-sentiments, such as an introvert, grouch, or bum (result from *Interact*, Francis & Heise, 2006). Thus, if self-stigmatized patients must occupy identities that are higher in goodness, power, and activity than their self-sentiments, they may seek out offsetting identities that could be deleterious to their well-being and place them even further away from beneficial life course identities noted above.

Hypotheses 3. Self-stigma will increase the likelihood of adopting more marginalized compensatory role-identities.

METHODS

Data

We test these hypotheses with self-sentiments data collected from psychiatric patients who were recently diagnosed with an affective disorder. These data came from wave 1 of the Indianapolis Network Mental Health Study. All respondents were making their first major contact with the mental health system in a large-scale private and public hospital in Indianapolis. To be included in our sample, patients must have been officially diagnosed with an affective disorder, including bipolar disorder, cyclothymia, dysthymia, or major depression. Individuals fitting study criteria were asked to participate through a rolling recruitment beginning in January 1990. Data were collected within three months of the initial hospital contact (response rate for the full sample is 66.4 percent). We have complete data for 93 affective patients.

Independent Variable: Self-Stigmatized Self-Sentiments

Patients provided the EPA rating of their self-sentiments, "myself as I really am," with seven-point semantic differential scales. The evaluation scale was anchored with "good" versus "bad," potency with "powerful" versus "powerless," and activity with "fast, noisy" versus "slow, quiet." The middle point was marked "neutral," and the points on each side were marked "slightly," "quite," and "extremely" and were coded with values ranging from −3 to +3. The direction of the adjectives was randomized across stimuli.

To ascertain the level of stigma patients perceive others have toward the mentally ill, patients also were asked to rate the evaluation, potency, and activity of the stimulus, "a mentally ill person"[4] with the same semantic differential scales. These ratings, termed stigma sentiments (Kroska & Harkness, 2006, 2008), were then used to produce self-sentiment EPA profiles for affective patients with high and low levels of perceived stigma. We used equations developed in a previous study (Kroska & Harkness, 2008) to generate predicted EPA profiles for patients with both high and low self-stigma. Specifically, we regressed patients' self-sentiments on their stigma sentiments, controlling for symptom severity (measured with the Global Assessment of Functioning scale), gender, age, race, and education (see Kroska & Harkness, 2008 for more details on model specification and the reported equations). We used these equations to generate predicted values for patients with high stigma sentiments (1 sd below the mean EPA rating of "a mentally ill person") and low stigma sentiments (1 sd above the mean EPA rating of "a mentally ill person").[5] The resulting EPA profile for highly self-stigmatized patients is 0.03, −0.53, −0.27, or neutral in evaluation, slightly impotent, and neutral in activity. Patients with lower levels of self-stigmatization have a self-sentiments profile of 1.56, −0.05, 0.09 – an identity that is quite good and neutral in potency and activity.

Analytic Approach: Interact

We used various features of *Interact* to test each hypothesis using the Indiana EPA dictionary (Francis & Heise, 2006). This dictionary contains cultural EPA ratings of 500 identities and 300 emotions generated from a sample of Indiana University students in 2002 and 2003. Though these data come from a convenience sample of Indiana University students, these ratings gauge overall cultural semantic (EPA) meanings to which we have all been socialized (Heise, 2010; see also Romney, Weller, & Batchelder, 1986).[6] As such, dictionaries from one country show remarkable stability and consensus over time (Heise, 2007), as do large-scale stratified samples from one time period (Ambrasat, von Scheve, Conrad, Schauenburg, & Schroder, 2014).

Dependent Variables: Self-Actualizing Identities, Compensatory Identities, and Characteristic Emotions

Hypotheses 1 and 3 were tested with *Interact's* "Explore a Self" feature using the lay, business, academe, and family institutional concept gates as these feature major life course role-identities (see Heise, 2013 for more information). We entered the self-sentiment EPA profile for affective patients with high and low self-stigma to generate the *self-actualizing* role-identities found in the dictionary to test Hypothesis 1. Self-actualizing identities have EPA profiles that are no more than a .75 eigenvalue distance away from their self-sentiments.

To identify compensatory identities, we first selected a "sustaining identity" provided by *Interact*. Sustaining identities are ones predicted to be feasible for individuals to enact yet far enough away from their self-identities' semantic meaning to feel uncomfortable or distressing (up to an eigenvalue distance of 1.75 away from self-sentiments). This compels the selection of *compensatory identities* to balance role enactments around self-identities. Sustaining identities were chosen nearest the edge of *Interact's* sustaining identity boundary range for each of the evaluation, potency, and activity dimensions. Note, patients might be forced to engage in role-identities that are outside these boundaries, which would prompt the selection of an even more severe compensatory identity, as predicted by ACTS. What we offer here is a more conservative test of hypothesis 3 in that we are only examining identity selection processes within the narrower range around patients' self-identities. *Interact* then produced the EPA profiles and labels of the resulting compensatory identities patients would likely select to test Hypotheses 3.

Hypotheses 2a–2c were tested using the "Feeling Effects" function of *Interact* by entering the self-sentiments of high and low self-stigmatized patients to generate the *characteristic emotions* most likely felt when either type of patients' self-sentiments are perfectly confirmed. Characteristic emotions have EPA profiles that are the most similar to the patients' self-sentiment EPAs as found in the *Interact* dictionary.

RESULTS

Hypothesis 1: Self-Actualizing Identities

Are highly self-stigmatized patients less likely to find role-identities associated with major life course stages self-actualizing (Hypothesis 1)? Table 1 displays the most self-actualizing role-identities as predicted by *Interact* for patients with both high and low self-stigma. These identities are arranged by major social institutional categories, including everyday lay identities. In every category, there are more self-actualizing identities available for the low self-stigma patients than the high self-stigma patients. This is especially true for identities related to the family, as none are predicted to be confirmatory for highly stigmatized patients. This indicates that occupying family-oriented role-identities would potentially be a source of stress for those with higher levels of self-stigma. Self-actualizing family identities for low self-stigma patients suggest strong engagement with this institution, including the roles of homemaker, housewife, and daughter-in-law.

Indeed, confirmatory identities for high self-stigmatized patients are removed from close interaction with others. For instance, their predicted

Table 1. Self-Actualizing Identities for High and Low Self-Stigmatized Affective Patients by Social Institution.

High Stigma Lay	Low Stigma Lay	High Stigma Academe	Low Stigma Academe
Stranger	Guest	Egghead	Student teacher
Passerby	Visitor		Classmate
Underdog	Neighbor		
Baldy	Asian American		
	Assistant		

Business	Business	Family
Yes-man	Receptionist	Guest
Subordinate	Small businessman	Homemaker
Temporary worker	Secretary	Housewife
Spendthrift	Novice	Houseguest
Tenant	Apprentice	Daughter-in-law
	Assistant	House husband
		Half brother

Note: Generated using the female 2002–2004 Indiana *Interact* dictionary; High self-stigma EPA: 0.03, −0.53, −0.27; Low self-stigma EPA: 1.56, −0.05, 0.09.

lay identities include being a stranger or merely a passerby, and their business identities indicate that these patients would be most comfortable in low-power or temporary positions like subordinate or temporary worker. Conversely, low self-stigma patients are predicted to be more engaged and active in both these arenas, with identities like guest, visitor, neighbor, small businessman, apprentice, and assistant listed as possible actualizing identities. This is even true in the academic institution, with student teacher and classmate as actualizing identities for low self-stigma patients; egghead is the only identity that is confirming for a highly self-stigmatized patient, which is an identity rated as merely neutral across EPA dimensions (−0.46, −0.02, −0.36). These patterns suggest, as predicted by Hypothesis 1, that high self-stigma among affective patients reduces the tendency to adopt role-identities associated with important life course stages. Indeed, self-stigma reduces the overall number of role-identities that would be comfortable for these patients to adopt, which, in turn, may narrow their network contacts and intimate sources of social support.

Hypotheses 2a – 2c: Characteristic Emotions

Self-stigma also dampens the characteristic emotions patients experience (see Table 2). High self-stigma patients feel only slightly good and neutral in potency and activity when their self-identities are confirmed (0.88, −0.39, 0.29). Emotions in the *Interact* dictionary that are similar to the characteristic emotions of high stigma patients include feeling anxious, repentant, contrite, and shocked, while their most confirmatory emotion is to feel no emotion at all. The average reported emotion that is similar to high self-stigma patients' characteristic emotion is 0.23, 0.08, 0.06, and overall fairly neutral, much like their self-sentiments. The only characteristic emotion reported for highly stigmatized patients that is above zero in evaluation and potency is contented (1.86, 1.07, 0.56), though this is close to the boundary of possible characteristic emotions (this boundary is a Euclidian distance of 2.00 from the characteristic emotion; distance of 1.71). This is seconded by eagerness, which is not quite as positive as contented (0.96, 0.60, 1.72; distance of 1.70).

The characteristic emotion for patients with lower levels of self-stigma is much higher in evaluation and potency (1.93, 0.15, 0.55, compared to 0.88, −0.39, 0.29 (reported above)), as predicted by Hypothesis 2a and 2b. The tenor of the emotions similar to this characteristic emotion are also much more positive, including emotions such as charmed, eager, moved, passionate,

Table 2. Characteristic Emotions for High and Low Self-Stigmatized Affective Patients.

Characteristic Emotion EPA	High Stigma		Low Stigma	
	0.95, 0.38, 0.50		1.93, 0.34, 0.55	
	Similar emotions	Euclidian distance	Similar emotions	Euclidian distance
	No emotion	0.98	Contented	0.92
	Awe-struck	1.08	Awe-struck	1.06
	Repentant	1.17	Charmed	1.46
	Anxious	1.23	Nostalgic	1.53
	Contrite	1.44	Eager	1.59
	Lovesick	1.47	Humble	1.78
	Shocked	1.54	Sentimental	1.80
	Nostalgic	1.68	Moved	1.80
	Remorseful	1.69	Passionate	1.87
	Eager	1.70	Thankful	1.88
	Contented	1.71	At-ease	1.94
	Lustful	1.78		
	Indignant	1.92		
	Contemptuous	1.95		

Note: Generated using the female 2002–2004 Indiana *Interact* dictionary; High self-stigma EPA: 0.03, −0.53, −0.27; Low self-stigma EPA: 1.56, −0.05, 0.09.

thankful, and at-ease. The average of these emotions is also much higher in evaluation and potency, though similar in activity, than those of high self-stigma patients (2.03, 1.15, 0.03, compared to 0.23, 0.08, 0.06 (reported above)). The activity dimension, though higher for low self-stigma patients, is not as differentiated as the other two affective dimensions. Overall, these results lend support for Hypotheses 2a and 2b.

Hypothesis 3: Sustaining and Compensatory Identities

The results thus far demonstrate that high self-stigma patients are predicted to be less likely to select identities allowing them to engage fully with social institutions, while being comfortable engaging in roles that make them feel fairly affectively neutral. They may, however, experience structural and relational constraints forcing them to take on role-identities that are not self-actualizing. Table 3 displays the role-identities that, though not self-actualizing, are somewhat sustaining for both high and low self-stigma

Table 3. Self-Sustaining Identities for High and Low Self-Stigmatized Affective Patients by Social Institution.[a]

High Stigma Lay	Low Stigma Lay	High Stigma Business	Low Stigma Business	High Stigma Academe	Low Stigma Academe	High Stigma Family	Low Stigma Family
Stuffed shirt	Elder	Interviewee	Shop clerk	Trainee	Schoolgirl	Mama's boy	Brother-in-law
Lackey	Blonde	Lackey	Laborer	Malingerer	Schoolmate	Spinster	Cousin
Pauper	Innocent	Trainee	Applicant	Applicant	Applicant	Orphan	Stepchild
Malingerer	Traveler	Pauper	Flight attendant	Pupil	Trainee	Stepson	Half-sister
Nut	Passerby	Apprentice	Employee	Has-been	Pupil	Illegitimate child	Bridesmaid
Pedestrian	Pedestrian	Malingerer	Office boy	Grind	Protégé	Foster child	Son-in-law
Sponger	Redhead	Applicant	Interviewee	Ignoramus	Workmate	Stepparent	Stepson
Asian American	Chum	Salesclerk	Salesclerk	Questioner	Aide	Daughter-in-law	Stepparent
Half-wit	Vacationer	Office boy	Trainee	Truant	Alumnus	Divorcée	Stepdaughter
Toady	Brunette	Toady	Client	Schoolgirl	Consultant	Stepmother	Stepbrother
Windbag	Handyman	Novice	Co-worker	Clock watcher	Tutor	Half-sister	Stepfather
Redhead	Advisor	Secretary	Union member		Questioner	Stepchild	Sister-in-law
Beginner	Nut	Has-been	Protégé		Roommate	Ex-husband	Foster child
Miser	Female	Bootlicker	Tenant		Colleague	Half brother	Mama's boy
Bootlicker	Computer expert	Union member	Workmate		Lecturer	Stepbrother	Uncle
Old geezer	Hombre	Laborer	Shopkeeper		Advisor	Ex-wife	Stepmother
Ignoramus	Underdog	Shop clerk	Traveler		Scholar	Old maid	Little sister
Punk	Girl	Clock watcher	Right-hand man		Graduate student	Stepfather	Granddaughter

Mental case	Beginner	Receptionist	Server		Undergraduate	Stepsister	Mother-in-law
Foe	Stranger	Foe	Aide				Aunt
			Consultant				Bridegroom
			Merchant				Father in law
			Worker				Stepsister
			Saleslady				Grandchild
			Vacationer				Matriarch
			Customer				Foster father
			Waitress				Nephew
			Handyman				Grownup
			Advisor				Tot
			Spendthrift				
			Computer expert				
			Waiter				
			Temporary worker				

Note: Generated using the female 2002–2004 Indiana *Interact* dictionary; High self-stigma EPA: 0.03, −0.53, −0.27; Low self-stigma EPA: 1.56, −0.05, 0.09.

[a]Sustaining identities listed in order from those most to least similar to self-sentiments.

patients and are still feasible for patients to enact without too great of an affective strain. The enactment of these sustaining identities, however, compels people to select compensatory identities to balance their role enactments around their self-sentiments, with Hypothesis 3 predicting the resulting compensatory identities of high self-stigma patients will be more marginalized.

Again we see that low self-stigma patients have more role-identities available from which to choose. This is especially the case within the business, academic, and family institutional domains. High self-stigma patients' sustaining identities tend to be on the periphery of the social world, as was the case with their predicted self-actualizing identities. In the academic domain, sustaining identities for high self-stigma patients include, for instance, an ignoramus, truant, and clock watcher. Conversely, protégé, alumnus, tutor, colleague, lecturer, advisor, scholar, and graduate/undergraduate student are sustaining identities for low self-stigma patients. Within the family, high self-stigma patients again tend to be on the periphery with identities involving never having been married, being an illegitimate or foster child, and being someone's step-relation or ex-spouse, which are findings aligning with those of Turnbull, George, Landerman, Swartz, and Blazer (1990) as mentioned previously. Also of note, of the lay identities reported, "mental case" is predicted to be sustaining for high-self-stigma patients ("nut" is expected to be sustaining for both high and low self-stigma patients).

To test Hypothesis 3, we selected sustaining identities with the highest evaluation, potency, and activity to identify the compensatory identities patients would most likely select to offset this identity imbalance. This allows us to address the question: If patients must enact identities that are more positive than their self-identities, what are the compensatory role-identities patients might next select to counteract this increase in evaluation, potency, or activity? For high self-stigma patients, possible sustaining identities with the highest evaluation are receptionist, schoolgirl, pupil, secretary, and office boy (average evaluation rating of 1.41) and represent identities associated with business and academia. When high self-stigma patients enact any of these sustaining identities, they are expected to offset that increase in goodness by subsequently enacting an identity like ignoramus, miser, truant, or divorcée (average evaluation rating of −1.33), which are much lower in evaluation. These are also identities mostly associated with the lay and family spheres, suggesting that while the self-esteem straining role-identities are associated with professional institutions, the informal and family lives of high stigma patients may be particularly impacted by their compensatory role selection. Occupying an identity that is overly high in evaluation can therefore have wide-ranging effects in patients' lives.

Sustaining identities with the highest potency ratings include questioner, stepbrother, stepfather, stepmother, and stepparent more generally (average potency rating of 0.58). Engaging in these identities would prompt high self-stigma patients to soon after behave as a subordinate, half-wit, has-been, or lackey (average potency rating of −1.19), which are also much lower in potency. Further, these stepparent identities are the only type of parental identities reported for high self-stigma patients, and even they would be somewhat affectively straining. Stepparent (0.64, 0.30, 0.12) is also considerably lower in goodness, potency, and activity than the parent identity (2.89, 2.73, 1.73), so the enactment of the affectively neutral stepparent role would likely indicate somewhat of a detachment from the family.

Moving on to the activity dimension, stepsister and schoolgirl have the highest activity ratings (average activity rating of 0.78; schoolgirl is also higher in evaluation as already noted). To compensate for enacting these role-identities, high-stigma patients might select the roles of follower, dummy, clock watcher, malcontent, malingerer, or divorcée to counteract the increase in activity (average activity rating of −1.21). Overall, these compensatory identities tend to again demonstrate a lack of engagement with mainstream institutions and are much lower in evaluation, potency, and activity than even the patients' self-identities.

The compensatory identities for low self-stigma patients are not nearly as extreme or negative. None of the reported identities are too positive to cause compensatory identity strain. A few, however, stress the bounds of potency, with grownup, computer expert, graduate student, scholar, and advisor being the most extreme for these patients (average rating potency of 1.48). Enacting these identities would prompt compensatory identities like pupil or office boy (average potency rating of −0.84). For activity, the waiter, waitress, nephew, and little sister roles are at this boundary (average activity rating of 1.51). Compensatory identities for these role-identities include being a librarian, retiree, elder, or senior citizen (average activity rating of −1.49), indicating that one would prefer to engage in work-related roles with lower activity (i.e., librarian), or that eventually being seen as an elder or senior citizen would be preferable as low stigma patients retire and move into their next life course stage. Exploring the reported sustaining identities a bit further, interacting as a granddaughter (2.46, 0.70, 0.73), an identity that is slightly higher in both evaluation and activity than their self-sentiments, may prompt these patients to subsequently enact identities like trainee, interviewee, applicant, or temporary worker (average evaluation rating of 1.00; average potency rating of −0.17). These compensatory identities still offer beneficial engagement with social institutions (work in particular), while allowing for low self-stigma patients to iteratively confirm their self-identities. In sum, these results suggest that self-stigmatization prompts greater comfort in receding from the social world and support Hypothesis 3.

CONCLUSION

In the decades since deinstitutionalization, the treatment landscape for mental health patients has changed drastically, yet the stigma associated with being mentally ill has, at best, remained steadfast. Stigma, and the processes it engenders, can dramatically alter patients' life chances and opportunities both by affecting the reactions of the non-labeled toward patients, and, notably for this study, patients' perceptions of themselves. This latter process of self-stigmatization brings many deleterious consequences for the mentally ill, including reducing self-esteem and self-efficacy, and altering treatment pathways (Corrigan et al., 2006; Fung, Tsang, & Corrigan, 2008; Kroska & Harkness, 2006, 2008; Lannin, Vogel, Brenner, & Tucker, 2014; Rusch et al., 2006, 2009; Tsang, Fung, & Corrigan, 2009; Wright et al., 2000).

By drawing on ACT and ACTS, this study adds to this body of research by suggesting that self-stigmatization also constrains the role-identities that patients are comfortable occupying. For stigma theories, notably modified labeling theory (Link, 1987; Link et al., 1989), these findings add to the list of processes perpetuating mental health problems by highlighting how self-stigma affects the withdrawal process through role selection.

As predicted, individuals with high self-stigma have fewer self-actualizing and sustaining role-identities available than those with low self-stigma; the small number that are self-actualizing, like stranger or temporary worker, are far more negative and impotent than the life course identities adopted by most adults, such as employer, spouse, or parent. In addition, self-actualizing identities for high self-stigma patients involve disengagement or at least a peripheral relationship with the roles comprising these major social institutions, especially those of the family. By contrast, many of the role-identities that are self-actualizing for those with less self-stigma are fairly beneficial in that they involve positive engagement with various major institutions.

Identities that bring social support and build opportunities are not self-actualizing, nor in many ways self-sustaining, for those with high levels of self-stigma. When these patients are forced to engage in identities that are too good or potent for their diminished self-sentiments, the results suggest they will then be more likely to adopt identities that are even more negatively evaluated and impotent to bring their role-identities back in alignment with their stigmatized selves. These results suggest that some of the life course differences among patients may be in part due to variations in self-stigma.

Self-stigmatization similarly dampens the affective nature of patients' interactions when acting as themselves. Greater levels of self-stigma compel patients to seek out interactions that make them feel anxious or affectively neutral or blunted. Emotions like these may feed affective disorders, making treatment more difficult for those with high levels of internalized stigma, as the work of others has suggested (Fung et al., 2008; Kim-Cohen et al., 2003; Rusch et al., 2009; Tsang et al., 2009). Critically, this emotional outcome is a product of higher self-stigmatization and not a consequence of the various disorders' symptoms or other qualities of their interactions.

It is our intent for these predictions to be generative for future research on the interactional consequences of self-stigma. It is important to note, however, that though these findings are based in *Interact* simulations, *Interact* results are empirically derived, based in years of theory testing, and have empirical support (Schröder & Scholl, 2009; Wiggins & Heise, 1987). These results speak to the cultural scripts of interaction based on ACT and ACTS principles, offering a set of predictions on which to build subsequent research on self-stigmatization in daily interaction.

With deinstitutionalization, patients have more freedom to occupy many mainstream identities tied to cultural institutions, such as spouse, parent, and worker. Yet those who use mental health services and subsequently experience high self-stigma are placed on a trajectory of marginalization in multiple life domains. Without reductions in the cultural stigma tied to mental illness, however, we predict that they are unlikely to adopt mainstream identities because their self-stigma tends to produce self-sentiments that inhibit those pursuits.

These results do suggest some particularized avenues for intervention, however. Policies and programs that increase patients' self-esteem and self-efficacy, even for those with lower levels of internalized stigma, should have a beneficial impact on patients' self-sentiments and, thereby, their emotions and role-identity selection. Programs targeting educational and employment assistance and community involvement may afford the foundational support needed for patients to successfully navigate the work, family, and lay spheres of their social lives. Successful role encounters across these domains may provide the leverage needed to counteract some of the deleterious effects of self-stigma.

NOTES

1. There may be additional dimensions within a specific culture, but these three are found universally.

2. EPA profiles are interpreted as follows: −4.3 is the worst/most impotent/most inert that anything can be; −3.0 is extremely bad/powerless/inactive; −2.0 is quite bad/powerless/inactive; −1.0 is slightly bad/powerless/inactive; 0.0 is neutral; neither bad nor good/powerless nor powerful/inactive nor active; +1.0 is slightly good/powerful/active; +2.0 is quite good/powerful/active; +3.0 is extremely good/powerful/active; +4.3 is the best/most potent/most active that anything can be.

3. EPA profiles according to female college freshman (Francis & Heise, 2006): employee = 1.88, 0.05, 0.84; date = 2.64, 1.87, 1.48; spouse = 2.75, 1.90, 1.39; parent = 2.89, 2.73, 1.73.

4. Others have measured self-concurrent self-stigma with the Self-Stigma of Mental Illness Scale (SSMIS) (Corrigan et al., 2006, 2012; Watson, Corrigan, Larson, & Sells, 2007). This scale includes questions such as, "Because I have a mental illness, I am {dangerous; unpredictable; to blame for my problems; unable to take care of myself}." Measuring self-stigma with evaluation, potency, and activity, as we have done, is a less direct way of ascertaining stigma beliefs, and thereby less susceptible to social desirability and researcher bias, while being a parsimonious way to represent meaning attached to self-identities and cultural beliefs about the mentally ill (Kroska & Harkness, 2006).

5. Higher EPA ratings indicate that the target is better, more potent, and more active. High stigma beliefs are therefore indicated with lower EPA ratings.

6. We use the female EPA dictionary for these analyses, as *Interact* is presently not programmed for researchers to simultaneously use the combined female and male dictionary. The results from the male dictionary are substantively the same as those reported here and are available on request.

ACKNOWLEDGMENTS

We would like to thank the editor of this volume, Brea L. Perry, and the anonymous reviewers for their incisive feedback on this chapter.

REFERENCES

Ambrasat, J., von Scheve, C., Conrad, M., Schauenburg, G., & Schroder, T. (2014). Consensus and stratification in the affective meaning of human sociality. *Proceedings of the National Academy of Sciences, 111*(22), 8001–8006. doi:10.1073/pnas.1313321111

Corrigan, P. W., Larson, J. E., & Rusch, N. (2009). Self-stigma and the 'why try' effect: Impact of life goals and evidence-based practices. *World Psychiatry, 8*(2), 75–81.

Corrigan, P. W., Michaels, P. J., Vega, E., Gause, M., Watson, A. C., & Rusch, N. (2012). Self-stigma of mental illness scale – short form: Reliability and validity. *Psychiatry Research, 199*(2012), 65–69. doi:10.1016/j.psychres.2012.04.009

Corrigan, P. W., & Watson, A. C. (2002). The paradox of self-stigma and mental illness. *Clinical Psychology: Science & Practice, 9*(1), 35–53. doi:10.1093/clipsy.9.1.35

Corrigan, P. W., Watson, A. C., & Barr, L. (2006). The self-stigma of mental illness: Implications for self-esteem and self-efficacy. *Journal of Social and Clinical Psychology, 25*(9), 875–884. doi:10.1521/jscp.2006.25.8.875

Crocker, J., & Major, B. (1989). Social stigma and self-esteem: The self-protective properties of stigma. *Psychological Review, 96*(4), 608–630. doi:10.1037/0033-295X.96.4.608

Crocker, J., & Quinn, D. M. (2000). Social stigma and the self: Meanings, situations, and self-esteem. In T. F. Heatherton, R. E. Kleck, M. R. Hebl, & J. G. Hull (Eds.), *The social psychology of stigma* (pp. 153–183). New York, NY: Guilford Press.

Evans-Lacko, S., Brohan, E., Mojtabai, R., & Thornicroft, G. (2012). Association between public views of mental illness and self-stigma among individuals with mental illness in 14 European countries. *Psychological Medicine, 42*, 1741–1752. doi:10.1017/S0033291711002558

Farina, A., & Felner, R. D. (1973). Employment interviewer reactions to former mental patients. *Journal of Abnormal Psychology, 82*(2), 268–272. doi:10.1037/h0035194

Frable, D. E., Pratt, L., & Hoey, S. (1998). Concealable stigmas and positive self-perceptions: Feeling better around similar others. *Journal of Personality and Social Psychology, 74*(4), 909–922. doi:10.1037/0022-3514.74.4.909

Francis, C., & Heise, D. (2006). *Mean affective ratings of 1,500 concepts by Indiana University undergraduates in 2002–2003* (computer file). Retrieved from http://www.indiana.edu/~socpsy/ACT/interact.htm

Frank, R. G., & Glied, S. A. (2006). *Better but not well: Mental health policy in the U.S. since 1950*. Baltimore, MD: Johns Hopkins University Press.

Fung, K. M., Tsang, H. W., & Corrigan, P. W. (2008). Self-stigma of people with schizophrenia as predictor of their adherence to psychosocial treatment. *Psychiatric Rehabilitation Journal, 32*(2), 95–104. doi:10.2975/32.2.2008.95.104

George, L. K. (2013). Life-course perspectives on mental health. In C. S. Aneshensel, J. C. Phelan, & A. Bierman (Eds.), *Handbook of the sociology of mental health* (2nd ed., pp. 585–602). New York, NY: Springer.

Heise, D. R. (1979). *Understanding events: Affect and the construction of social action*. Cambridge: Cambridge University Press.

Heise, D. R. (2007). *Expressive order: Confirming sentiments in social actions*. New York, NY: Springer.

Heise, D. R. (2010). *Surveying cultures: Discovering shared conceptions and sentiments*. Hoboken, NJ: Wiley.

Heise, D. R. (2013). *Interact guide*. Retrieved from http://www.indiana.edu/~socpsy/public_files/InteractGuide.pdf

Hinshaw, S. P., & Stier, A. (2008). Stigma as related to mental disorders. *Annual Review of Clinical Psychology*, *4*, 367–393. doi:10.1146/annurev.clinpsy.4.022007.141245

Jackson, P. B. (2004). Role sequencing: Does order matter for mental health? *Journal of Health and Social Behavior*, *45*(2), 132–154. doi:10.1177/002214650404500202

Kim-Cohen, J., Caspi, A., Moffitt, T. E., Harrington, H., Milne, B. J., & Poulton, R. (2003). Prior juvenile diagnoses in adults with mental disorder: Developmental follow-back of a prospective-longitudinal cohort. *Archives of General Psychiatry*, *60*(7), 709–717. doi:10.1001/archpsyc.60.7.709

Kroska, A., & Harkness, S. K. (2006). Stigma sentiments and self-meanings: Exploring the modified labeling theory of mental illness. *Social Psychology Quarterly*, *69*(4), 325–348. doi:10.1177/019027250606900403

Kroska, A., & Harkness, S. K. (2008). Exploring the role of diagnosis in the modified labeling theory of mental illness. *Social Psychology Quarterly*, *71*(2), 193–208. doi:10.1177/019027250807100207

Kroska, A., Harkness, S. K., Brown, R. P., & Thomas, L. S. (2015). Gender, status, and psychiatric labels. *Social Science Research*, *54*, 68–79. doi:10.1016/j.ssresearch.2015.06.021

Kroska, A., Harkness, S. K., Thomas, L. S., & Brown, R. P. (2014). Illness labels and social distance. *Society and Mental Health*, *4*(3), 215–234. doi:10.1177/2156869314521431

Lannin, D. G., Vogel, D. L., Brenner, R. E., & Tucker, J. R. (2014). Predicting self-esteem and intentions to seek counseling: The internalized stigma model. *The Counseling Psychologist*, *43*(1), 64–93. doi:10.1177/0011000014541550

Link, B. G. (1982). Mental patient status, work, and income: An examination of the effects of a psychiatric label. *American Sociological Review*, *47*(2), 202–215.

Link, B. G. (1987). Understanding labeling effects in the area of mental disorders: An assessment of the effects of expectations of rejection. *American Sociological Review*, *52*(1), 96–112.

Link, B. G., Cullen, F. T., Struening, E., Shrout, P. E., & Dohrenwend, B. P. (1989). A modified labeling theory approach to mental disorders: An empirical assessment. *American Sociological Review*, *54*(3), 400–423.

Link, B. G., Mirotznik, J., & Cullen, F. T. (1991). The effectiveness of stigma coping orientations: Can negative consequences of mental illness labeling be avoided? *Journal of Health and Social Behavior*, *32*(3), 302–320.

Link, B. G., & Phelan, J. (2001). Conceptualizing stigma. *Annual Review of Sociology*, *27*, 363–385.

Link, B. G., Struening, E. L., Neese-Todd, S., Asmussen, S., & Phelan, J. C. (2001). Stigma as a barrier to recovery: The consequences of stigma for the self-esteem of people with mental illnesses. *Psychiatric Services*, *52*(12), 1621–1626.

Livingston, J. D., & Boyd, J. E. (2010). Correlates and consequences of internalized stigma for people living with mental illness: A systematic review and meta-analysis. *Social Science and Medicine*, *71*(12), 2150–2161. doi:10.1016/j.socscimed.2010.09.030

Lucas, J. W., & Phelan, J. C. (2012). Stigma and status: The interrelation of two theoretical perspectives. *Social Psychology Quarterly*, *75*(4), 310–333. doi:10.1177/0190272512459968

Lysaker, P. H., Roe, D., & Yanos, P. T. (2006). Toward understanding the insight paradox: Internalized stigma moderates the association between insight and social functioning, hope, and self-esteem among people with schizophrenia spectrum disorders. *Schizophrenia Bulletin*, *33*(1), 192–199. doi:10.1093/schbul/sbl016

MacKinnon, N. J. (1994). *Symbolic interactionism as affect control*. Albany, NY: State University of New York Press.

MacKinnon, N. J. (2015). *Self-esteem and beyond*. New York, NY: Palgrave Macmillan.

MacKinnon, N. J., & Heise, D. R. (2010). *Self, identity, and social institutions*. New York, NY: Palgrave Macmillan.

Major, B., & O'Brien, L. T. (2005). The social psychology of stigma. *Annual Review of Psychology*, *56*, 393–421. doi:10.1146/annurev.psych.56.091103.070137

Markowitz, F. E. (1998). The effects of stigma on the psychological well-being and life satisfaction of persons with mental illness. *Journal of Health and Social Behavior*, *39*(4), 335–347.

Markowitz, F. E., Angell, B., & Greenberg, J. S. (2011). Stigma, reflected appraisals, and recovery outcomes in mental illness. *Social Psychology Quarterly*, *74*(2), 144–165. doi:10.1177/0190272511407620

Martin, J. K., Pescosolido, B. A., Olafsdottir, S., & McLeod, J. D. (2007). The construction of fear: Modeling Americans' preferences for social distance from children and adolescents with mental health problems. *Journal of Health and Social Behavior*, *48*(1), 50–67. doi:10.1177/002214650704800104

Mechanic, D. (1990). Deinstitutionalization: An appraisal of reform. *Annual Review of Sociology*, *16*(27), 301–327.

Mehta, S., & Farina, A. (1997). Is being 'sick' really better? Effect of the disease view of mental disorder on stigma. *Journal of Social and Clinical Psychology*, *16*(4), 405–419. doi:10.1521/jscp.1997.16.4.405

Osgood, C. E., May, W. H., & Miron, M. S. (1975). *Cross-cultural universals of affective meaning*. Urbana, IL: University of Illinois Press.

Pachankis, J. (2007). The psychological implications of concealing a stigma: A cognitive-affective-behavioral model. *Psychological Bulletin*, *133*(2), 328–345.

Page, S. (1995). Effects of the mental illness label in 1993: Acceptance and rejection in the community. *Journal of Health and Social Policy*, *7*(2), 61–68. doi:10.1300/J045v07n02_05

Payton, A. R., & Thoits, P. A. (2011). Medicalization, direct-to-consumer advertising, and mental illness stigma. *Society and Mental Health*, *1*(1), 55–70. doi:10.1177/2156869310397959

Perry, B. L. (2011). The labeling paradox: Stigma, the sick role, and social networks in mental illness. *Journal of Health and Social Behavior*, *52*(4), 460–477. doi:10.1177/0022146511408913

Pescosolido, B. A. (2013). The public stigma of mental illness: What do we think; what do we know; what can we prove? *Journal of Health and Social Behavior*, *51*(1), 1–21. doi:10.1177/0022146512471197

Pescosolido, B. A., Jensen, P., Martin, J. K., Perry, B. L., Olafsdottir, S., & Fettes, D. L. (2008). Public knowledge and assessment of child mental health problems: Findings from the National Stigma Study – Children. *Journal of the American Academy of Child & Adolescent Psychiatry*, *47*(3), 339–349. doi:10.1097/CHI.0b013e318160e3a0

Pescosolido, B. A., & Martin, J. K. (2007). Stigma and the sociological enterprise. In W. R. Avison, J. D. McLeod, & B. A. Pescosolido (Eds.), *Mental health, social mirror* (pp. 307–328). New York, NY: Springer Press.

Pescosolido, B. A., & Martin, J. K. (2015). The stigma complex. *Annual Review of Sociology, 41*. doi:10.1146/annurev-soc-071312-145702

Pescosolido, B. A., Martin, J. K., Long, J. S., Edina, T. R., Phelan, J. C., & Link, B. G. (2010). 'A disease like any other'? A decade of change in public reactions to schizophrenia depression, and alcohol dependence. *American Journal of Psychiatry, 167*(11), 1321–1330. doi:10.1176/appi.ajp.2010.09121743

Phelan, J. C., Link, B. G., Stueve, A., & Pescosolido, B. A. (2000). Public conceptions of mental illness in 1950 and 1996: What is mental illness and is it to be feared? *Journal of Health and Social Behavior, 41*(2), 188–207.

Ritsher, J. B., & Phelan, J. C. (2004). Internalized stigma predicts erosion of morale among psychiatric outpatients. *Psychiatry Research, 129*(3), 257–265. doi:10.1016/j.psychres.2004.08.003

Romney, A. K., Weller, S. C., & Batchelder, W. H. (1986). Culture as consensus: A theory of culture and informant accuracy. *American Anthropologist, 88*(2), 313–338. doi:10.1525/aa.1986.88.2.02a00020

Rosenfield, S. (1997). Labeling mental illness: The effects of received services and perceived stigma on life satisfaction. *American Sociological Review, 62*(4), 660–672.

Rusch, N., Angermeyer, M. C., & Corrigan, P. W. (2005). Mental illness stigma: Concepts, consequences, and initiatives to reduce stigma. *European Psychiatry, 20*(2005), 529–539. doi:10.1016/j.eurpsy.2005.04.004

Rusch, N., Corrigan, P. W., Wassel, A., Michaels, P., Larson, J. E., Olschewski, M., et al. (2009). Self-stigma, group identification, perceived legitimacy of discrimination and mental health service use. *British Journal of Psychiatry, 195*(6), 551–552. doi:10.1192/bjp.bp.109.067157

Rusch, N., Holzer, A., Hermann, C., Schramm, E., Jacob, G. A., Bohus, M., et al. (2006). Self-stigma in women with borderline personality disorder and women with social phobia. *Journal of Nervous and Mental Disease, 194*(10), 766–773. doi:10.1097/01.nmd.0000239898.48701.dc

Schnittker, J. (2008). An uncertain revolution: Why the rise of a genetic model of mental illness has not increased tolerance. *Social Science & Medicine, 67*(9), 1370–1381. doi:10.1016/j.socscimed.2008.07.007

Schröder, T., & Scholl, W. (2009). Affective dynamics of leadership: An experimental test of affect control theory. *Social Psychology Quarterly, 72*(2), 180–197. doi:10.1177/019027250907200207

Scambler, G., & Paoli, F. (2008). Health work, female sex workers and HIV/AIDS: Global and local dimensions of stigma and deviance as barriers to effective interventions. *Social Science & Medicine, 66*(8), 1848–1862. doi:10.1016/j.socscimed.2008.01.002

Sibicky, M., & Dovidio, J. F. (1986). Stigma of psychological therapy: Stereotypes, interpersonal reactions, and the self-fulfilling prophecy. *Journal of Counseling Psychology, 33*(2), 148–154. doi:10.1037/0022-0167.33.2.148

Smith-Lovin, L., & Heise, D. R. (Eds.). (1988). *Analyzing social events: Advances in affect control theory*. New York, NY: Gordon and Breach Scientific.

Stier, A., & Hinshaw, S. (2007). Explicit and implicit stigma against individuals with mental illness. *Australian Psychologist, 42*(2), 106–117. doi:10.1080/00050060701280599

Thoits, P. (2011). Resisting the stigma of mental illness. *Social Psychology Quarterly, 74*(1), 6–28. doi:10.1177/0190272511398019

Tsang, H. W. H., Fung, K. M. T., & Corrigan, P. W. (2009). Psychosocial and socio-demographic correlates of medication compliance among people with schizophrenia. *Journal of Behavior Therapy and Experimental Psychiatry*, *40*(1), 3–14. doi:10.1016/j.jbtep.2008.02.003

Turnbull, J. E., George, L. K., Landerman, R., Swartz, M. S., & Blazer, D. G. (1990). Social outcomes related to age of onset among psychiatric disorders. *Journal of Consulting and Clinical Psychology*, *58*(6), 832–839. doi:10.1037/0022-006X.58.6.832

Vogel, D. L., Wade, N. G., & Hackler, A. H. (2007). Perceived public stigma and the willingness to seek counseling: The mediating roles of self-stigma and attitudes toward counseling. *Journal of Counseling Psychology*, *54*(1), 40–50. doi:10.1037/0022-0167.54.1.40

Watson, A. C., Corrigan, P. W., Larson, J. E., & Sells, M. (2007). Self-stigma in people with mental illness. *Schizophrenia Bulletin*, *33*(6), 1312–1331. doi:10.1093/schbul/sbl076

Wiggins, B., & Heise, D. R. (1987). Expectations, intentions, and behavior: Some tests of affect control theory. *The Journal of Mathematical Sociology*, *13*(1–2), 153–169. doi:10.1080/0022250X.1987.9990030

Wright, E. R., Gronfein, W. P., & Owens, T. J. (2000). Deinstitutionalization, social rejection, and the self-esteem of former mental patients. *Journal of Health and Social Behavior*, *41*(1), 68–90.

THE "DIGNITY OF THE SICK": MANAGING SOCIAL STIGMA BY MENTAL PATIENTS IN THE COMMUNITY☆

Nana Tuntiya

ABSTRACT

Purpose – *The chapter revisits the concept of social stigma viewed from the perspective of mental patients integrated in the community based on the example of Geel, Belgium that historically utilized a family care model for a significant number of patients with severe mental illness.*

Methodology/approach – *Interpretive analysis of data presented in ethnographies on the Geel colony by Roosens (1979) and Roosens and Van de Walle (2007), showcasing 30 patients' case studies in addition to research-based author narratives.*

Findings – *This study demonstrates that chronic mental patients tend to reject the sick role and the stigma associated with it by trying to*

☆The "dignity of the sick" expression in the title is attributed to Esquirol, as cited by Dr. J. Moreau (de Tours) in Roosens and Van de Walle (2007, p. 27).

50 Years after Deinstitutionalization: Mental Illness in Contemporary Communities
Advances in Medical Sociology, Volume 17, 235–260

ISSN: 1057-6290/doi:10.1108/S1057-629020160000017009

influence their social image and how their status is being defined in the community. They appear to be active managers, not passive recipients of societal attitudes, and, furthermore, functional members of the community. By forgoing exemption from social roles carried by their significant impairment, mental patients continue to be contributing members of their host families, and in some cases develop into caregivers themselves completing the circle of role reversal.

Research limitations – *The current analysis utilizes secondary data and therefore is restricted by the information included in the primary research.*

Originality/value – *The findings allow us to develop a deeper understanding of the social status chronic mental patients acquire in the community, and how it is influenced by the dynamics of social stigmatization and remedial work these social actors are compelled to perform. Additionally, the study contributes to the inclusion of the chronic patients' perspective in research.*

Keywords: Chronic mental illness; stigma; sick role; family care; Geel

The social stigma associated in public perception with mental illness has been a topic central to the Sociology of Mental Health for a number of years. It gained particular significance with the rise of community treatment programs after the deinstitutionalization movement put them at the forefront of the psychiatric practice. Stigmatization inhibited patients' integration in the community, compromised the success and the implementation of the outpatient programs, and negatively affected the emotional and psychological well-being of current and former patients, as well as their families. It also prevented many others from seeking help in the first place due to the difficulties they might encounter post-treatment.

Given the importance of this topic for successful reintegration of patients in the society, and for the smooth functioning of community alternatives to hospital treatment, it is essential to understand the stigmatization process from the standpoint of the people who are affected by it, namely, patients themselves. Yet, the vast majority of relevant studies focus on patients as objects of prejudice, rather than subjects of social process involved in defining their status in the community, and full-fledged social actors. This study intends to explore patients' social interactions from this vantage point through the interpretive analysis of two studies published by Roosens (1979) and Roosens and Van de Walle (2007), containing collectively 30 patients' case studies, and research-based author narratives that summarize the results of extensive ethnographic fieldwork spanning almost three decades.

FROM OBJECTS TO SUBJECTS

The lack of genuine subjective representation of patients' point of view has been acknowledged in previous research. Karp (1966) gave the following assessment: "The essential problem with nearly all studies of depression is that we hear the voices of a battalion of mental health experts (doctors, nurses, social workers, sociologists, psychologists, therapists) and never the voices of depressed people themselves." (p. 11). Jeannette Pols echoed his statement calling for a wider inclusion of "patient perspective" in relevant research. She noted: "Patients did not appear in research texts as subjects-who-know, but rather as objects-that-are-known by medicine." (2005, p. 204). Similarly, Major and O'Brien found that: "Traditionally, members of stigmatized groups have been portrayed as passive victims of others' negative stereotypes, prejudicial attitudes, and discriminatory behaviors... We close by noting that one of the major insights of a social psychological perspective on stigma is the tremendous variability across people, groups, and situations in responses to stigma." (2005, pp. 411–412).

In spite of these calls for a more patient-centered research, ethnographic studies in mental health are few and far between. Newton et al. (2000) fault the general lack of legitimacy of qualitative inquiry in the medical field and insufficient funding. The time commitment involved in conducting fieldwork observations or interviews plays its role also, as well as complexities involved in collecting data from mental patients, especially if they are non-verbal (Newton et al., 2000; Pols, 2005). In Roosens' (1979) study, 10.2 per cent of patients were either completely or largely non-verbal, and 21.2 per cent were not interested in verbal expression, speaking only in response. Thorne et al. confirm in their extensive metastudy of qualitative research in the area of chronic illness that "diseases that influence verbal communication ... are disproportionally unpopular research topics" and in particular people "with chronic psychological or psychiatric disorders unrelated to physical illness" seldom become the subjects of these studies (Thorne et al., 2002, pp. 444, 443).

These types of challenges in reflecting the viewpoint of the severely mentally ill motivate scholars to search for creative ways to collect data on this population. For instance, Newton et al. stress the value of contextual information in participant observation and "tapping of non-verbal data": "Relevant, but unexpected, findings emerge from social situations which open up further areas for inquiry" (Newton et al., 2000, pp. 484, 489–490). Pols (2005) argues that attempts at representing patients' perspective imply their readiness to develop a narrative about own experiences, to verbalize it, and to have the ability to deal with the interview situation, which might be uncomfortable or threatening to some people. Instead she suggests studying enacted appreciations, in other words, observing which actions people take thereby demonstrating their preferences through verbal or non-verbal means. This approach allows for patients' subjectivity to be taken into account regardless of their verbal or cognitive skills within the constraints of their material and social environment. In our research, we will be guided by the general understanding that people's behavior can be an important expression of their subjectivity if we remain mindful of the opportunity structure or health limitations of particular individuals and the influence of others in their immediate environment. In the community setting that provides different avenues for self-realization, patients manifest their perspective by signaling which activities they participate in or rather avoid, so the analysis of real-life situations can reveal something about their inner world they might not otherwise be able or be willing to articulate. With this goal in mind, this study intends to tap into the wealth of ethnographic data presented in the original monograph on the Geel Colony by Roosens (1979) and his later work in cooperation with Van de Walle (2007), to get a glimpse of the lived experiences of chronic mental patients immersed in the community.

Far from being a newcomer in mental health practice, the town of Geel, Belgium boasts hosting the original (and the first known) model of community treatment for chronic mental patients that goes back centuries. It takes its roots in a religious cult that brought large numbers of sufferers to the area on their pilgrimage trips. The community provided temporary housing and care, which later developed into a boarding system for patients and became an integral part of the Belgian Mental Health Care.

Geel Colony (or Kolonie, as the hospital that supervises the program was traditionally referred to) hardly resembles today its original structure and goals. The program is based on a system of family care and is unique in a number of important ways. The first and the foremost difference of this community from its counterparts throughout the world is the high density of patients in the population,[1] and their remarkable level of integration in the local social networks. It is assisted by a level of awareness of the local population that helps maintain a smooth functioning program while avoiding disruptions to social order. Over the course of eight centuries, the community lived side by side with severely mentally ill, as the program was utilized as a low cost alternative in long-term care for chronic patients. This historic model evolved into an environment of high tolerance towards the patients, allowing them to freely interact with other residents, and be included in the daily life of the community, but did not succeed in fully erasing prejudice and stigmatization (Roosens, 1979). This unusual combination gives us a singular opportunity to observe people with severe mental illness being truly integrated in residential networks instead of remaining largely isolated as often happens in other examples of community placements (Ootes, Pols, Tonkens, & Willems, 2013). It also provides a unique example of deinstitutionalization, not only because of its remarkable authentic history, but also because of the unusual blend of community treatment and close hospital control and supervision, which continuously updates and develops the program in response to socioeconomic and therapeutic needs. The medical staff provides initial screening and selection of patients, matching clients with prospective families, as well as ongoing consultations and home visits after the placements are made. Throughout the program operation, the hospital serves as an organizing force as well as informational and crisis resource for families and patients, offering short stays for the boarders in need of medical attention or while the host family is on out-of-town trips.

Roosens' research[2] highlights this interesting and instructive case in the history of deinstitutionalization. Perhaps the most important benefit of his work is the comprehensive nature of data it represents. Among diverse publications on the Geel system that appeared in press since approximately the middle of the 19th century, Roosens' and Roosens and Van de Walle's inquiries stand out in capturing the most subtle and diverse expressions of what Goffman calls "patient's daily circles" (1971, p. 337), spanning work, leisure (friendships), and family life, in addition to interactions with health care. Roosens did his first round of investigations in Geel as part of The Geel Family Care Research Project, developed by Professor Leo Srole. He focused on the interaction of boarders and Geel residents and later published his observations in an illuminating account "Mental Patients in Town Life: Geel – Europe's First Therapeutic Community" (1979). The variety of methods that were employed in the larger study (with the help of mostly local investigators) that also informed his book, range from participant observation in local bars, public events, and at church services, to interviewing foster families, religious and community leaders, medical staff, and patients themselves. The scope of these explorations was systematic and all-encompassing. During this project, conducted between July 1966 and August 1975, the total population of the host families (approximately, 1,000) was interviewed about boarders' social contacts. Additional 1,000 interviews with host families were conducted on patients' religious practices, 87 interviews with the committee members of religious associations, and observational visits (106) completed in bars, a movie theater, and other public venues (Roosens, 1979). The second inquiry, conducted by Roosens in two phases – in 1999–2000 and 2005–2006 with a broader theme of foster families, consisted of 108 and 19 family visits, respectively, as well as over 50 interviews with psychiatrists, social workers, employees of the workshops and patient centers. This allowed Roosens to add a valuable longitudinal dimension to his report on Geel. The depth of these observations prompted Oliver Sacks to remark in the forward to Roosens' and Van de Walle's manuscript: "These nineteen case studies are exemplary in their richness and detail, and constitute primary material of enormous value." (2007, p. 11). This chapter intends to analyze the information they supplied.

In the following section, we will review theoretical concepts that help understand boarders' status in the community. They will be discussed in conjunction with the information specific to Geel, such as the attitudes of the locals, historically developed practices, and the arrangements of the program itself. This comprises a necessary theoretical background for our analysis and situates patients and their behavior within their proper social, cultural and historic context. As Pols (2005) contends, the clients' appreciations are enacted inside the framework of specific material environment that restricts or enables their actions, and also are being co-produced by others. Therefore, consideration of the social milieu is the key part of the analysis that ensures deeper understanding and interpretation.

THE SICK ROLE AND STATUS CONUNDRUM

The social science literature defines the stigmatization process as power dynamics between a group that sets the rules and a group that complies (or not) with them. However, life doesn't fit into neat little boxes developed by theoreticians. In Geel, the power group representing "the norm" in the patients' immediate environment is the caregivers, who have the authority to monitor patients' behavior, and in some cases issue punishments in the form of withdrawing privileges, or even sending them back to the hospital. The host families set the rules. But they are also the people who share life with the patients, eating at the same table, helping them in the times of crises, socializing together, and developing a lasting bond that resembles familial ties much more than a simple client-provider relationship. Likewise, the community as a whole embraces the patients and gives them the sense of belonging, yet remains vigilant to the violations in their behavior serving as a mechanism of social control.

The prejudiced attitudes that Roosens admits are still to some degree a part of the picture in this community of tolerance and inclusion, presume a division into an in-group and out-group camps (Falk, 2001). In Geel though, the tables are turned and the patients' out-group, the family, is also their in-group acquired through closeness and bonding, while the other boarders, who are supposed to be their in-group, are in some cases resented, avoided, or otherwise treated as an out-group. The ambiguity of this situation might further motivate patients to employ the means accessible to them in order to influence their social standing and to emphasize their "insider" status.

As Roosens reminds us, the separation between the "sick" and the "healthy" is always preserved, and normalization of "guests" does not imply their ultimate return to a dominant group. Having been defined chronic, they are viewed within the boundaries of the illness continuum, although as unique individuals. Similar to Dudley's observations about another stigmatized group, mentally challenged, "there appears to be no established portal to normal living" or "methods for delabeling them" (1983, p. 78) once the categorization is made. This ensures boundary maintenance, one of the essential elements in reproduction of inequality (Schwalbe et al., 2000). Patients' illness therefore has a major impact on how society perceives their social standing. Since stigmatization occurs when one of the groups in the society is accorded a lower status compared to others, the variables that contribute to defining status in a particular way are of the utmost interest to us.

When guests arrive in Geel, there is no ambiguity of their status. They are a part of a known group the community developed a certain relationship with over the centuries of co-existence. Hence, if there is stigma attached to their position, it would be predetermined by their group membership and quite independent from the nature of their specific condition.

It seems necessary now to consider the role of prejudgment in the formation of prejudice. Allport (1954) stresses the commonality of prejudgment, and maintains it turns into prejudice only when irreversible in the face of new information. Still other researchers warn that "automatic categorization facilitates prejudice" (Fiske, 2005, p. 38). In spite of pre-assigned group membership, Geel residents reserve their judgment about the boarders until their personal qualities are assessed. The notion that "every boarder is different" (Roosens, 1979, p. 38) adds an individual dimension to this classification and allows some degree of influence on patient's social standing.

The sociological literature views mental illness as one of the severe stigma generating designations in the society (Falk, 2001; Goffman, 1974; Hinshaw, 2007; Link & Phelan, 1999; Scheff, 1984). Its labeling power has not been reduced by medicalization (Payton & Thoits, 2011) or the acceptance of the genetic and chemical imbalance explanations of the disease (Pescosolido, 2013). The role of contact in deflecting stigmatizing attitudes turned out to be not as straightforward as originally expected (Pattyn, Verhaeghe, & Bracke, 2013). Recognizing the need for better understanding of factors that might contribute to stigma reduction and stigma formation we turn our attention to the particular aspects that influence the perception of patients' overall status.

The labeling power of mental illness is strongly connected to society's attitudes toward illness in general.[3] A loss of productivity and potential dependency constitute social costs of sickness and are often viewed as undesirable or even dysfunctional by individuals and society at large. Falk ventures a view that stigma of mental illness becomes individuals' "master status" (2001, p. 50). Although others disagree with this categorization (Lucas & Phelan, 2012; Thoits, 1985), few would question the impact of the diagnosis on the status of its recipient. Thomas Scheff deems the consequences severe enough to equate medical judgment by a psychiatrist with "making a legal decision" (1984, p. 82) due to its influence on person's reputation. While Falk (2001) treats mental illness as a social role, Gordon (1966) further connects status and role to social identities of participants in social exchange. Accordingly, mental patients enter social interactions carrying characteristics related to their specially defined status.

One concept often used in medical sociology to reflect this special status is the sick role. Developed by Parsons within the framework of the functionalist perspective as an analytical construct applicable predominantly to acute physical illness, it transcendents the original model due to its usefulness in defining the position sick individuals acquire in the society, and the expectations and consequences attached to it. Parsons' theory has been criticized for its limitations and inapplicability to all types of illnesses (Lipman & Sterne, 1969; Varul, 2010), for lack of empirical validation (Gordon, 1966), or for losing its relevance after a shift of focus in sociology from illness to health (Burnham, 2012), among other things. However, the Parsonian model continues to be utilized in discussions of illness behavior or health care consumption (Cockerham, 1981; Shilling, 2002; Williams, 2005), and has been applied to mental illness and chronic conditions (Glenton, 2003; Kassebaum & Baumann, 1965; Lipman & Sterne, 1969; Perry, 2011; Pescosolido, Boyer, & Lubell, 1999).

Parsons' theory deals with the process of acceptance of the sick role, and the assumptions this position entails, for instance the responsibility to take steps toward recovery, to seek professional help, and to conform to medical advice and procedures. There is also an expectation, even an obligation, to give up the usual responsibilities (Parsons, 1966) and focus on healing and recuperation. Parsons points out "a moral connotation" in the expression encouraging the ill individuals "that they *ought* to stay in bed" (Parsons, 1966, p. 437), however reluctant they might be. The key entrance into the sick role requires professional legitimation of the disease. The boarders in Geel are past that entrance point since their diagnosis of chronic mental illness implies the medical legitimation of their condition had occurred at some point prior to their transfer to family care. Moreover, by declaring their condition chronic, the society largely relieves them from the responsibility to get well (although the recovery might still occur), but not from the need for compliance with the medical care system. Patients satisfy the latter condition by their participation in the family care program. Therefore, the core axis of sick role expectations for colony residents remains as shown on Fig. 1.

Thomas Scheff contends: "Sociologically, a status is defined as a set of rights and duties." (1984, p. 212). For boarders in Geel, the exemption from everyday obligations would be considered both a right and a duty of an individual. Ruth Wu adds that "Learning the sick role requires in essence the relinquishment of the rights and duties of normal adult responsibilities and entails a desocialization process." (1973, p. 168). This swap of

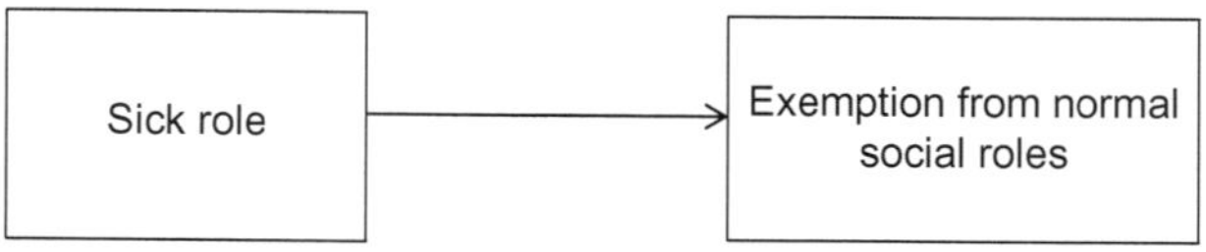

Fig. 1. Patients' Role Expectations.

normative expectations is not a straightforward process. Not only the sick role demands are determined in many ways by cultural and socio-demographic factors, but they also depend on the nature and the severity of the illness, as well as the prognosis for recovery (Gordon, 1966; Kassebaum & Baumann, 1965; Parsons, 1966; Segall, 1976). Pescosolido et al. stress "Parsons's focus on the importance of the community as the adjudicator of the sick role" (Pescosolido et al., 1999, p. 443). Here, we shall remember that boarders in Geel were traditionally expected to participate in the daily life of the household by doing chores or help on the farms, which adds a level of complexity to role expectations stipulated in the theory. Generally, there is no agreement either in the literature or in the society as a whole on the extent of the exemption from the responsibilities the sick role grants, in particular in regard to chronic, untreatable, or mental illness (Crossley, 1998; Gordon, 1966; Segall, 1976; Stewart & Sullivan, 1982). This is additionally complicated in respect to boarders due to overlapping of mental illness diagnosis and the chronic nature of their condition. Kassebaum and Baumann also warn of "a threshold, beyond which the strain on interaction produced by illness outweighs the norm" (1965, p. 25). This implies that the level of exemption is determined by the amount of support the community and the caregivers are prepared to provide. Ruth Wu on the other hand argues that "The exemption accorded the sick may extend beyond the actual disability" (1973, p. 167), while Lipman and Sterne go even further suggesting that society forces aging or untreatable people to disengage by "involuntary ascription" of terminal sick role regardless of whether the ensuing dependency is legitimate or even desired by an individual himself (1969, pp. 198–199).

The Parsonian model is invoked here as a means to provide a theoretical framework for the discussion of boarders' status and of variables that influence it. The medical legitimation of the sick role, in particular, for a condition classified as chronic, leads to increased dependency and stigmatization, although the extent of the exemption from social roles is not clearly determined. The disagreement in the literature on the factors that define patients' social standing, and the expectations for their behavior, underscores the importance of studying Geel as a "natural experiment" (Roosens, 1979, p. 20) that allowed real people affected by severe mental illness to select their preferred level of engagement in daily activities and to negotiate their status in the community. Our analysis of boarders' social interactions and behaviors presented in the following section indicates that they (a) resist stigmatization; (b) reclaim some social roles; and (c) attempt to be grouped with "normal" citizens. The consideration of the context remains an important part of the discussion as particular characteristics of the Geel community and the attitudes of its members carry the potential to influence patients' environment and opportunity structure.

INDEPENDENCE AND RECIPROCITY

There are two quite different images of the Geel Colony that transpire from the Roosens (1979) and Roosens and Van de Walle (2007) books. One is care organized along the more traditional lines, where patients spend most of their time with foster families, and the hospital serves as a supervising force, and a provider of essential services. A quarter of a century later, and after an official merge of family care with the hospital, forming OPZ (Openbaar Psychiatrisch Zorgcentrum or State Psychiatric Care Center), Geel presents a picture of a more centralized system, where medical professionals play an increasingly important role in providing patients with employment and leisure opportunities, in educating foster parents, and insisting on using medical rather than folk terminology. As a result, boarders spend a significant amount of time under staff supervision in workshops, wellness center, or on out-of-town trips, when previously they would have been largely within a family circle (Roosens & Van de Walle, 2007, p. 123). The initial skepticism of Geelians toward psychoactive drugs is also replaced with a more appreciative attitude, resulting in patients often being on regular medication, in sharp contrast with a situation Roosens found earlier. While the role of professionals increased, the number of boarders sharply declined reflecting both the changes in the Belgian mental health care system that now provides diverse opportunities for community placements in different locales, and also developments in Geel itself where traditional farming is being replaced by plentiful industrial opportunities and the upwardly mobile residents are choosing a dual career couple mode. The Geel community has evolved and, as an authentic system, the Geel Colony evolved with it too, absorbing the latest socioeconomic and scientific developments. What hasn't changed, though, is the tolerance of the community toward the patients enabling them to participate in family life and neighborhood events and integrate in different ways in the larger social milieu.

In his first account, Roosens (1979) points out that almost no clients of the Geel Colony are locals. The Geel residents are referred to the Colony only in exceptional cases. From this standpoint, all boarders used to be outsiders in this community and had no special ties or support networks that could influence their rank or give an advantage compared to other patients. More recently Geel became a center of regional rather than national or international care (Roosens & Van de Walle, 2007, p. 40), largely eliminating this insider-outsider dynamic. Medical staff started holding regular briefings with the host families, treating them more like partners in providing services to clients, however the release of patient information is still kept to a minimum, giving the newcomers to the system "a fresh start" (Roosens & Van de Walle, 2007, p. 107) uninhibited by their previous medical or personal history. Neither do Geelians feel a need to seek out the "learned explanations" of boarders' conditions or research them out before inviting clients to share life in their family. "Nobody benefits from dragging up the past" (Roosens & Van de Walle, 2007, p. 107) and patients are given a chance to invent – and reinvent – themselves and to fit in, drawing on all the available resources. Geelians subscribe to the philosophy that "there are normal dimensions in every single patient that one can build on or that can be maintained" (2007, p. 27). This encourages a gradual "mental promotion" (in Dr. Cuvelier's expression) of patients in the family when during their first year they do "things that belong to the 'role of the sick person'" and during the second year "more and more actions appear that one associates with a 'normal role'" (1979, pp. 182–183). The freedoms progressively unfold after consultations of host families and a district nurse and based on what individuals can handle. In this sense, boarders have an ability to potentially shape their networks and image in deliberate ways. Also, the choices they make would be indicative of personal preferences within the obvious health and social constraints.

The main avenues of community participation for colony patients consist of Church attendance, visits to the host family's relatives or neighbors, patronizing local bars, presence at public events and celebrations, small errands or shopping trips, playing sports, going to the movies, clubs or the wellness center, and visits with their own family members. According to Goffman, "The patient does not construct his own avenues of access; he merely uses excessively devices available to anyone in his position. To appreciate this fact, we must look at the community as a system of fences and gates, a system for regulating the formation and growth of social relationships." (1971, p. 373). In agreement with this view, Roosens notes that formal social life other than rare volunteer opportunities for religious or charitable organizations is almost entirely closed to boarders. The social meaning of this prohibition is not lost on them. He stresses the popularity of patient participation in the Association of the Sacred Heart and the high importance they attach to this membership in spite of few social benefits it accords them.[4] As essentially the only opportunity for organizational participation available to them, the membership's symbolic value surpasses the actual social gains. In a similar fashion, boarders are upset with liturgical changes that undermine their ability to "sit next to other members … and outwardly act alike" (Roosens, 1979, pp. 147–148). This underscores a special significance of fitting in and "be like everybody else" the boarders seem to consistently elect. This tendency is apparent in the small vignettes of behavior Roosens provides from Sunday mass when the three young boarders "glance nervously around them to watch what the others do and try to follow what is going on" (1979, p. 102). Another guest "looks around in all directions. He tries to follow closely what others do: kneeling, sitting, standing up" (1979, p. 103).

These examples are not confined to observations at Church services. For instance, a patient "borrows books from the public library like his foster parents, but does not read them." (Roosens & Van de Walle, 2007, p. 99). Similar attitudes also influence more personal life choices, such as selecting a companion: "One feels it is important to have a boyfriend or a girlfriend for social reasons, in order to feel like everybody else." (Roosens & Van de Walle, 2007, p. 38). There is a clear degree of patients' conformity observed in Geel generally. A telling incident at the parade, when one of the boarders gets carried away and starts marching in the street in front of the bandleader, demonstrates how aware the guests are of the possible reaction to their actions: "At those times, however, he looks shyly about him to see whether anyone who might stop him from doing this has noticed him. One move or word from the bandleader suffices for him to quickly resume his place along the sidewalk. There too, he glances about him once in a while to see whether someone is planning to expel him from this privileged place." (Roosens, 1979, p. 98). This person apparently not only perceives his own violation, but predicts potential repercussions from the society, and swiftly implements corrective action. Overall, only a small number of people associated with the colony try to attract attention at public events. The majority of them "recede into the background, like 'normal' spectators." (Roosens, 1979, p. 99). It is worth noting that the threatening sanction society might implement in case of violations in guests' behavior is sending them back to the hospital, which is uniformly perceived as a severe consequence, incidentally highlighting patients' evaluation of hospital versus community care.

Shared definitions of the appropriate social behavior and "cultural agreement regarding the rule-breaking" (Thoits, 1974, p. 223) are often discussed in relation to stigma and self-labeling. Less often, though, the possibility is addressed that internalizing cultural norms can prepare individuals to shape their own behavior to appear more in agreement with the acceptable standard. Schwalbe et al. discuss the concept of "identity codes," stating that: "To know the code is to know how to elicit the imputation of possessing a desired kind of self" (Schwalbe et al., 2000, p. 424). It appears that boarders in Geel are quite attuned to the rules and "the code," which gives them the tools to form their image in a more desirable way. The information illustrating boarders' activities and choices that have relevance to how their social image may be formed in the community will be organized along specific themes.

Outward Signs of Respectability

The Colony used to issue boarders special clothes that marked them as belonging to the system. This practice was abandoned long ago, which is widely perceived as an improvement in their condition due to poor quality of fabric and overall stigmatizing effect. A foster father comments in this regard: "Compared to the past, they are now 'ladies and gentlemen'" (2007, p. 70), an evaluation clearly related to social status. Able to better blend in, patients often become indistinguishable from other residents. This opens up more social opportunities, such as visiting cafes or restaurants in the town center. Data suggests many boarders care about their appearance and dress up going out on weekends. There are examples of patients buying their own furniture or a nice TV set. Another indication it matters to patients how community perceives them is the pleasure they derive from the positive publicity, when acknowledged in the paper as the most loyal customer of a local museum, or being profiled in a documentary on the Geel colony. As we can observe, boarders invest efforts in arranging their physical surroundings and appearance in a positive way, which improves their image.

Social Relations and Rituals of Social Exchange

Guests form connections with the host family and their relatives, often developing a special bond with the children. They take them to school, play, or help with homework. The authors observe: "Dozens of foster parents we visited told us that they and their children were as good as raised by boarders. Time and again they stressed how remarkably well patients and children get along. … Once the children and grandchildren have attached to the guest, it is virtually impossible to send him/her away." (Roosens & Van de Walle, 2007, p. 115). Patients visit grown up children of the foster family in their own homes, and in some cases maintain connections with families they stayed with previously. Contacts with their family of origin are almost never discouraged, but as a general rule do not happen very often.

Some of the boarders view themselves as adopted children, and it is not unusual for them to refer to their foster parent as "mother," "mama," or "mum." They receive an equivalent attitude in response: "It is striking that so many foster mothers compare patients with children, often young children." (Roosens & Van de Walle, 2007, p. 113). They occasionally present themselves in this category in the larger community as well, for instance when patients go from door to door singing during winter holidays for treats and money. This activity is customarily performed by children, yet it attracts almost one out of five guests (19.1%, see Roosens, 1979, p. 87).

Many clients socialize with neighbors or shopkeepers while running errands and get quite involved in local social networks. They seek company of other patients as well and many have a girlfriend or a boyfriend, or even two, with the increased benefits of companionship and status. Others, though, reject the company of peers for "No true friendship to be had there" (Roosens & Van de Walle, 2007, p. 78). Preference is clearly given to contacts with people not associated with the colony: 269 (19.7%) patients visit neighbors not involved in foster care as opposed to 56 (4.1%) who choose to stop by at the homes of other patients (Roosens, 1979, p. 89). Roosens concludes: "In Geel the mobile patients do not form a closed group. The figures cited show that the large majority of the boarders prefer to go where they meet 'normal' Geelians. Grouping among patients or the development of closed networks involving only patients are exceptional." (1979, p. 92).

Boarders like to gift small things to their foster parents on birthdays or other occasions, and bring souvenirs from their trips to children and grandchildren in the family. They give gifts to their girlfriends or boyfriends following usual exchange rituals. Although by law they are not supposed to be engaged in paid employment, they receive small amounts of money allowing them a measure of independence and an ability to make their own purchases. Ootes et al. point out the importance of gift-giving as a vehicle of social inclusion, which allows a client the opportunity "to give back" (Ootes et al., 2013, p. 142). Boarders find more ways to do their share in social relationships and to reciprocate their caregivers or "lend a helping hand" to other members of the community. They might throw a party or treat foster parent or other patrons with drinks in a bar, visit a lonely neighbor or buy a fancy leash for befriended dog, thereby initiating different kinds of positive social exchanges. Parties are given in their honor also, marking birthdays or anniversaries of staying in the family, when they are given plenty of gifts by host parents and neighbors. Authors contend: "All these celebrations are a means to, and an expression of integration. Birthday parties in particular stress social equality: everybody has a birthday, no special talents or merits are required. Presents, whether big or small, whether they are on the giving or receiving end, play a significant role in the boarders' lives." (Roosens & Van de Walle, 2007, p. 111).

The above information demonstrates that guests are able to forge various types of social connections within host families and beyond, often initiating positive social exchanges and participating in the life of the larger community, however giving preference to non-patient contacts.

Time Structuring and Lifestyle

A significant amount of time daily boarders spend at work, which in recent years is offered by hospital organized workshops. In addition, they do chores, such a cooking or cleaning, household shopping, tender the garden and help with farm work. They attend Sunday mass, soccer games, movie theater, and visit local bars or go dancing on weekends. Some go for walks or on a bike ride provided the permission from the colony. Not all of them chose social activities, but a large percentage of them are involved in sports, fishing club or Klimop, patients' social hub, and participate in various competitions. Evidence suggests that a number of guests avoid hospital organized activities and clubs and are quite outspoken in their rejection of these venues.

In contrast, trips organized by the colony proved to be immensely popular with the patients. They provide a social outlet and some independence from the host family. Significantly, guests pay for their travel (as well as the membership in sports clubs) with their own money. Many of them go on annual trips to Spain, France or the Belgian coast. This evidence implies that even though boarders generally prefer "non-patient" activities, they take advantage of organized ones whenever the alternatives are not open to them.

Social Engagement and Responsibilities

One of the major tradeoffs that come with the acquisition of a sick role is real or perceived dependency. Its antithesis is independence or self-sufficiency, valuable culturally acknowledged concepts, if unattainable in its full sense for every single member of the population. Dependency is socially sanctioned for ill individuals, but in case of chronic conditions carries the possibility to define a persons' status long term. Many boarders require assistance in their daily activities, cannot read, write, or count money. However, they develop strategies to overcome their own limitations and to effectively complete tasks they choose to take on. Many boarders like to do shopping for the family. If it is hard for one of them to make shortcuts without getting lost, the guest will return to the center of town after every errand to simplify his route. And if a boarder likes to choose his own boots, and incidentally buys a pair several sizes too large, he will wear it anyway. Independence is more important than the exact fit.

Lipman and Sterne define independence "in terms of the fulfillment of one's reciprocal social obligations" (1969, p. 195). From this standpoint many boarders are on a path of acquiring this quality. In some cases they effectively run the household, take care of the garden, or manage their own business, sourcing help from neighbors when needed. Reportedly, there were cases of boarders successfully running a farm. The important thing, however, is not the magnitude of achievement, but the very act of taking responsibility over any task and completing it, which brings one that much closer to autonomy and gives their efforts social recognition.

Boarders might assert their sense of control in small matters like having a specific chair at the table, disallowing anybody to enter their room or to touch certain belongings, to interfere in their garden work or other activities, or insisting on going to sleep last in order to personally lock all the doors and windows in the house. It is common to hear host parents say that the clients would not take orders from anybody and do "as they please." In some cases their requirements carry underlying status implications, for instance when one sates that he "does everything here" (Roosens, 1979, p. 55) or permanently claims the best seat in the house. Although data suggests that patients are aware of the host family expectation for help with the workload of running the household, foster families have a limited influence on their guests, as is apparent in cases they are reluctant to pitch in. When they do take on responsibilities, boarders take pride in their contribution.

Roosens contends that "two or three out of every 10 patients are involved in the local community in one way or another" (1979, p. 88). In spite of few cases of boarders' volunteering for different associations, and taking initiative to help neighbors, the majority of their activities are centered around host family and their children. It is one more way to "give back" and take charge of the duties that help organize the household and enable clients to become a part of a family unit. The responsibilities occasionally involve taking care of ailing or aging caregivers. As patients in some cases spend 40 or 50 years in the same family, they grow old together with their foster parents and become "co-dependent in their old age" (Roosens & Van de Walle, 2007, p. 77). Their work helps the former caretakers to get through rough periods of incapacity and in some cases allows them to continue living independently. A self-described "guardian angel" of his host mother says: "I put her to bed and only then dare I leave. The dog will bark if I am needed." (Roosens & Van de Walle, 2007, p. 77). Here the reciprocity of attachment has combined with the reciprocity of care, giving a new dimension to the level of responsibilities the boarders are willing to take upon themselves. These data suggest that patients often assert their independence and control in matters of different magnitude, and are willing to take on responsibilities and to pitch in, which benefits their status and a sense of agency.

Individual Expression and Points of Pride

As unique individuals, boarders develop their own interests, such as collecting, listening to music, playing sports, or other hobbies. Fishing contests are popular as well as soccer games. Some engage in entrepreneurial activity, for instance, breeding rare species of rabbits and hamsters, or re-selling cigarettes for profit. Others assemble postcards, watches, CDs, clocks, books or magazines, or obtain a radio or bicycle collection, and proudly display them to visitors. They take pictures while traveling, go dancing, or participate in local events, for instance, Saint Dimpna's procession. The opportunities open in the community allow them to pursue personal hobbies and assert their own uniqueness.

Distancing from Own Group

Gerhard Falk noted that "Sociologists have known for some time that stigmatized persons engage in downward comparisons with other stigmatized persons because it helps them feel better about their own situation." (2001, p. 117). Schwalbe et al. call this type of identity work aimed at deflecting stigma "defensive othering" (Schwalbe et al., 2000, p. 425). There are many examples of patients engaging in this protective behavior through verbal assertions or avoiding the company of other colony fellows. Their statements could be further divided into two different categories: those carrying negative evaluations of peers and those seeking to reject the relationship with a group as a whole. We find plenty of examples of all three types of identity work among persons from the colony. Roosens and Van de Walle give this overall assessment: "Some patients in our sample are very aware of their being stigmatized in one way or another. They try very hard to escape it. Some, for instance, refuse to visit the patients' social club and do not want to be seen with what they consider the really disturbed or mentally retarded … Some do not want to be associated with the Geel foster care system at all. They see themselves as regular, 'normal' foster children who have nothing to do with the mental institution." (Roosens & Van de Walle, 2007, p. 34).

Major and Vick contend: "One way in which targets of prejudice may distance themselves from a devalued ingroup is to *deny membership in the stigmatized group*." (2005, p. 146). The following statements from the text illustrate that the patients employ this strategy: one is "adamant he is 'not a guy from the Colony'…, hates being reminded of this and represses the idea" (2007, p. 74), another claims "he is *not* ill" (1979, p. 46), yet a different boarder "doesn't want to be associated with the OPZ at all, and doesn't attend any event organized by the Hospital. 'Not my thing!'" (2007, p. 73). The list can go on and on.

Fieldwork notes seem to confirm this also. Patients waiting for the Sunday afternoon movie keep their distance from the mentally challenged to avoid being identified with that group. And probably the most vivid illustration of the purposeful nature of their separation is that patients frequently pay for a balcony seat at the movies while they can visit the show for free if seated in the patient designated area. They do this "so as not to be identified with 'the people from the *Kolonie*.'" (Roosens, 1979, p. 106). There is additional evidence of some guests being against host family plans to "adopt" another boarder. One openly stated: "I do not want a loony in this house! I am not a loony!" and a different patient has sent the prospective client "out of the house by means of a broom" (Roosens & Van de Walle, 2007, pp. 101, 84).

In summary, the boarders engage in the community in a number of ways, they pursue their interests and build connections, participating to the extent they prefer and feel comfortable with. Many have limitations or simply "do not wish to go out, even if they are capable of doing so" (1979, p. 84), as Roosens found. This does not mean boarders are content with the implied dependency of a sick role. On the contrary, the choices they make appear to lead to increased involvement and independence. They take on obligations and return attachment and care, thereby fulfilling the most important requirement foster families have for them – the reciprocity of a bond. Gradually building evidence of their independence and responsibility patients counter negative stereotypes and improve their image in the community.

RESILIENCE MESSAGE

The conclusions we can derive from our analysis of two ethnographies on the Geel colony can be summarized in Fig. 2.

Our overview of the literature presented in the theoretical background section ("The Sick Role and Status Conundrum") leads to expect that the achieved medical legitimation of boarders' condition combined with the severity of the diagnosis and unfavorable prognosis for recovery would generate stigmatizing attitudes and a perception of their dependency. Being relieved from the responsibility to move toward recovery, chronic patients qualify for social role exemption as long as it does not contradict community and guardians' tradition-based assumption they should be contributing members of the household. Our reading of Roosens' and Roosens' and Van de Walle's accounts allows us to see that boarders resist stigma-related categorization of chronic illness, attempt to selectively associate with non-patients and do not usually take advantage of sick role exemption. In other words, they act "as *motivated* (i.e., strategic) agents attempting to make sense of their world and to protect their identities from threat." (Major & Vick, 2005, p. 140). In saying so, we recognize that this type of behavior aimed at increased social inclusion is observed among patients who opt for social interaction. The ethnographies document boarders' social encounters or views, and might not always represent the perspective of guests that withdraw from close contacts outside family environment or from verbal communication. Additionally, they were preselected on specific criteria to participate in the program.

The present analysis of this unique case of deep integration of boarders in the community suggests that despite severe mental illness, patients in

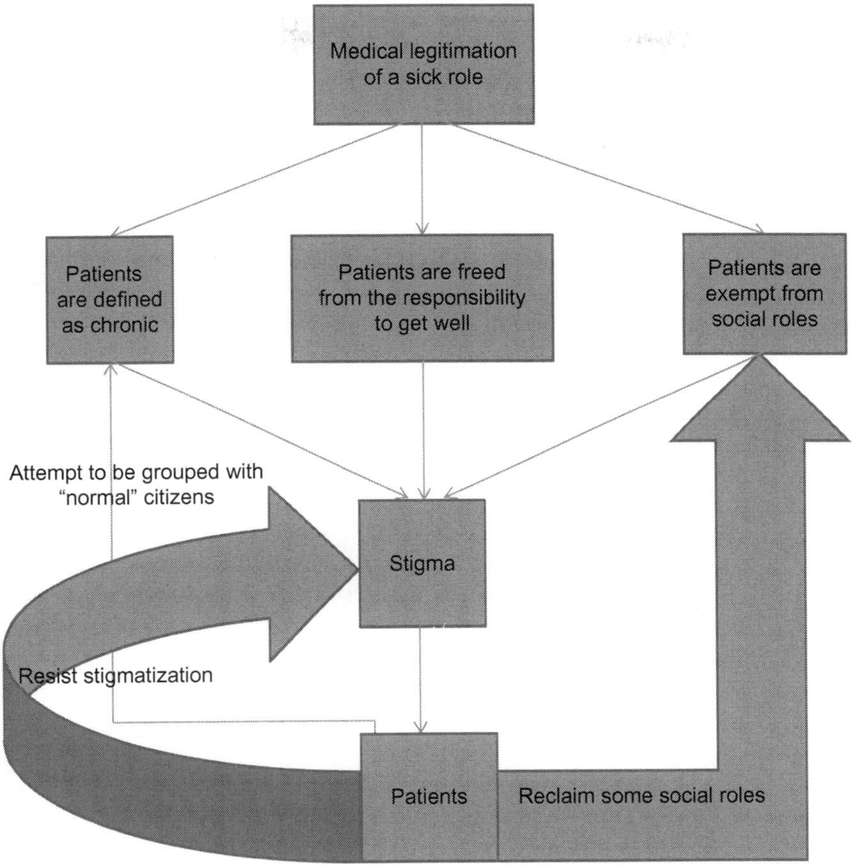

Fig. 2. Summary Model.

Geel gradually advance toward social adaptation and make efforts to defy stigmatizing categorization. They exhibit preference for association with residents who are not connected to the colony. In doing so, they demonstrate high awareness of the rules as well as the factors defining their identity in the community, and are willing to conform to social expectations. Independence and reciprocity are two main channels of status improvement open to patients, the former being an antithesis of dependency associated with sick role, the latter providing evidence of being a good agent of social exchange (valuable, dependable, responsible), capable to return affection and to share life with the host family.

Personal qualities and efforts help determine clients' status and make a difference in how host families and the community perceives them. Patients are accepted as individuals, not stigma or diagnosis carriers, which curiously co-exists with stereotyping them as colony people. In this respect, we can refer to Goffman's notion of personal identity. He maintained that "the whole problem of managing stigma is influenced by the issue of whether or not the stigmatized person is known to us personally" and described a strategy people employ to overcome stigma by moving "on to a more 'personal' plane where in fact their defect will cease to be a crucial factor" (Goffman, 1974, pp. 55, 52). Hence, incorporating patients into family and neighborhood networks encourages seeing them as individuals rather than members of a distant group. We find indirect evidence for this view in Perry's (2011) recent research on the impact of stigma on support networks, when the more pronounced symptoms had increased support for patients in core networks, but made them more vulnerable in peripheral ones, implying that once a personal relationship is attained, the negative impact of illness diminishes. That is why reciprocal personal bond plays such a crucial role in establishing a connection between a boarder and his host family as Roosens and Van de Walle observe: "If no emotional ties develop, other inconveniences which are usually disregarded in a harmonious relationship come to the fore and turn into obstacles one is no longer willing to overcome. When, on the contrary, a mutual warm relationship evolves, foster parents are prepared to go to great lengths to accommodate their guests." (2007, p. 115).

One of the limitations of the current analysis is the secondary nature of data it utilizes. As such it is restricted by the types and the scale of the information the original authors chose to include. We have to rely on observations of the primary researchers, who were not necessarily concerned with our specific research goals. On the other hand, the observations that were recorded are less likely to be biased by personal opinions or expectation of the investigators. The diverse and growing literature on secondary analysis of qualitative data indicates that in spite of the complexity and the limitations involved in assessing data recorded for different purposed and by different researchers, generating the "interpretation of interpretations" (Thorne, Jensen, Kearney, Noblit, & Sandelowski, 2004, p. 1348), the ability to look at existing data with a new set of research goals in mind or across different social groups and settings has a potential to expand knowledge development and to allow the investigation of topics with limited data accessibility. To partially offset these limitations, the conclusions of the present study are strongly supported by the many examples found in the text, and additionally corroborated by sociological theory and research that explain related social phenomena.

It is important to remember that the expressions of patients' subjectivity cannot be used as an approximation of their personal intentions, values, or motives. The choices they make or the behavior patterns they exhibit serve as an indication of their preferences, while we can only speculate what thought process led them to select a certain course of actions. In the course of this study, it became apparent that one of the important dimensions of stigmatization is not given enough attention by sociologists – the overlapping of factors that might potentially impact individual's status, such as mental illness, chronic nature of one's condition, advanced age, retardation, or being non-communicative. Any of these combinations might occur in real life and are found in Geel. Perhaps, future research will bring more light on the independent effects of these categories on prejudice against the affected people in a similar fashion that can be found in other sub-fields of our discipline, for instance, in research tracing independent influence of co-occurring race, gender, ethnicity, and immigrant status.

Concluding our study of two most thorough accounts of this unique example of incorporating severely mentally ill in residential networks and an unusual model of deinstitutionalization practice that merged hospital and community services in one collaborative system, it seems fitting to once again remember the goal of this study, that is to get a glimpse of the patients' perspective on their world defined in many ways by public attitudes and perceptions of mental illness. Allport emphasized that perseverance and redoubling of efforts to counter prejudiced attitudes is the "response most highly approved in our culture" (1954, p. 156). In spite of the shift to a more optimistic perspective on chronic illness that stresses courage and coping instead of the burden of illness (Thorne et al., 2002, p. 441), patients' ability to shape symbolic realities is still not in the spotlight of research. This might be one of the causes of Bury's criticism of our discipline: "a sociological approach needs to recognize the positive actions people take, as well as the problems they face." (1991, p. 451).

Stigma experience is quite possibly unique in any given community. Even more so it would be true about Geel, where history, traditions, and economic realities merged in an inimitable combination. Roosens and Van de Walle (2007) believe that future research would need to answer what types of stigma exist in this community, as some of the restrictions on boarders' participation could be explained by practical realities of living with severely handicapped people, and residents' views, although tolerant, are shaped by the long experience of being confronted with predominantly chronic conditions which highlights the contrast between health and illness. They note that "*Total* integration or *total* social absorption remains an illusion … What makes Geel remarkable is not the blurring of the normal/abnormal boundary, but the recognition of the clients' human dignity to the extent that life in a family and wider community is given an honest chance every single day." (2007, pp. 118–120). These ethnographic accounts are a notable testament to human resilience and adaptation from both, boarders and host families, points of view. As Goffman (1974) reminds us, stigma affects all people at different times and no one is immune to it. In the end, the boarders in Geel are just like everybody else, trying to make it from day to day using whatever resources are available to them and coping with the cards life dealt them.

NOTES

1. 1,300 patients were integrated in the community of 30,000 Geelians at the time of the first study (Roosens, 1979). Their number diminished to 549 by the start of the initial phase of the Roosens' research in 1999 (Roosens & Van de Walle, 2007).
2. Although the second study by Roosens "Geel Revisited: After Centuries of Mental Rehabilitation" (2007) is co-authored by Lieve Van de Walle, he carried out all the fieldwork in preparation to writing the book, as specifically stated in the author credits.
3. The treatment of theoretical perspectives on stigmatization is not meant to be exhaustive. In particular, the process of stigma development is outside the scope of this paper. Due to the space limitations, only the aspects of theories that relate directly to shaping the status and role of mentally ill in the community will be discussed.
4. The organization's goal is to encourage participation in regular religious practices, which allows patients to attend the monthly mass and be counted there as members. The membership is not a prerequisite for mass attendance, and therefore provides few, if any, social advantages as Roosens (1979) describes.

REFERENCES

Allport, G. W. (1954). *The nature of prejudice*. Reading, MA: Addison-Wesley Publishing Company.

Burnham, J. C. (2012). The death of the sick role. *Social History of Medicine*, *25*(4), 761–776.

Bury, M. (1991). The sociology of chronic illness: A review of research and prospects. *Sociology of Health & Illness*, *13*(4), 451–468.

Cockerham, W. C. (1981). Medical sociology. *International Review of Modern Sociology*, *11*(1–2), 231–250.

Crossley, M. (1998). 'Sick Role' or 'Empowerment'? The ambiguities of life with an HIV positive diagnosis. *Sociology of Health and Illness*, *20*(4), 507–531.

Dudley, J. R. (1983). *Living with stigma: The plight of the people who we label mentally retarded.* Springfield, IL: Charles C. Thomas Publisher.

Falk, G. (2001). *Stigma: How we treat outsiders.* Amherst, NY: Prometheus Books.

Fiske, S. T. (2005). Social cognition and the normality of prejudgment. In J. F. Dovidio, P. Glick., & L. A. Rudman (Eds.), *On the nature of prejudice: Fifty years after Allport* (pp. 36–53). Malden, MA: Blackwell.

Glenton, C. (2003). Chronic back pain sufferers – Striving for the sick role. *Social Science and Medicine*, *57*, 2243–2252.

Goffman, E. (1971). The insanity of place. In *Relations in public* (pp. 335–390). New York, NY: Basic Books.

Goffman, E. (1974). *Stigma. Notes on the management of spoiled identity.* New York, NY: Jason Aronson.

Gordon, G. (1966). *Role theory and illness: A sociological perspective.* New Haven, CT: College & University Press.

Hinshaw, S. P. (2007). *The mark of shame: Stigma of mental illness and an agenda for change.* New York, NY: Oxford University Press.

Karp, D. A. (1966). *Speaking of sadness: Depression, disconnection, and the meanings of illness.* New York, NY: Oxford University Press.

Kassebaum, G. G., & Baumann, B. O. (1965). Dimensions of the sick role in chronic illness. *Journal of Health and Human Behavior*, *6*(10), 16–27.

Link, B. G., & Phelan, J. C. (1999). Labeling and stigma. In C. S. Aneshensel & J. C. Phelan (Eds.), *Handbook of the sociology of mental health* (pp. 481–494). New York, NY: Kluwer Academic/Plenum Publishers.

Lipman, A., & Sterne, R. S. (1969). Aging in the United States: Ascription of a terminal sick role. *Sociology and Social Research*, *53*, 194–203.

Lucas, J. W., & Phelan, J. C. (2012). Stigma and status: The interrelation of two theoretical perspectives. *Social Psychology Quarterly*, *75*(4), 310–333.

Major, B., & O'Brien, L. T. (2005). The social psychology of stigma. *Annual Review of Psychology*, *56*, 393–421.

Major, B., & Vick, S. B. (2005). The psychological impact of prejudice. In J. F. Dovidio, P. Glick, & L. A. Rudman (Eds.), *On the nature of prejudice: Fifty years after Allport* (pp. 139–154). Malden, MA: Blackwell.

Newton, L., Rosen, A., Tennant, C., Hobbs, C., Lapsley, H. M., & Tribe, K. (2000). Deinstitutionalization for long-term mental illness: An ethnographic study. *Australian and New Zealand Journal of Psychiatry*, *34*, 484–490.

Ootes, S. T., Pols, A. J., Tonkens, E. H., & Willems, D. L. (2013). Opening the gift: Social inclusion, professional codes and gift-giving in long-term mental healthcare. *Culture, Medicine, and Psychiatry*, *37*, 131–147.

Parsons, T. (1966). *The social system.* New York, NY: The Free Press.

Pattyn, E., Verhaeghe, M., & Bracke, P. (2013). Attitudes toward community mental health care: The contact paradox revisited. *Community Mental Health Journal*, *49*, 292–302.

Payton, A. R., & Thoits, P. A. (2011). Medicalization, direct-to-consumer advertising, and mental illness stigma. *Society and Mental Health*, *1*(1), 55–70.

Perry, B. L. (2011). The labeling paradox: Stigma, the sick role, and social networks in mental illness. *Journal of Health and Social Behavior*, *52*(4), 460–477.

Pescosolido, B. A. (2013). The public stigma of mental illness: What do we think; what do we know; what can we prove? *Journal of Health and Social Behavior*, *54*(1), 1–21.

Pescosolido, B. A., Boyer, C. A., & Lubell, K. M. (1999). The social dynamics of responding to mental health problems. In C. S. Aneshensel & J. C. Phelan (Eds.), *Handbook of the sociology of mental health* (pp. 441–460). New York, NY: Kluwer Academic/ Plenum Publishers.

Pols, J. (2005). Enacting appreciations: Beyond the patient perspective. *Health Care Analysis*, *13*(3), 203–221.

Roosens, E. (1979). *Mental patients in town life: Geel – Europe's first therapeutic community*. Beverly Hills, CA: Sage.

Roosens, E., & Van de Walle, L. (2007). *Geel revisited: After centuries of mental rehabilitation*. Antwerp: Garant Publishers.

Scheff, T. J. (1984). *Being mentally ill: A sociological theory*. New York, NY: Aldine Publishing Company.

Schwalbe, M., Godwin, S., Holden, D., Schrock, D., Thompson, S., & Wolkomir, M. (2000). Generic processes in the reproduction of inequality: An interactionist analysis. *Social Forces*, *79*(2), 419–452.

Segall, A. (1976). The sick role concept: Understanding illness behavior. *Journal of Health and Social Behavior*, *17*(2), 162–169.

Shilling, C. (2002). Culture, the "Sick Role" and the consumption of health. *British Journal of Sociology*, *53*(4), 621–638.

Stewart, D. C., & Sullivan, T. J. (1982). Illness behavior and the sick role in chronic disease: The case of multiple sclerosis. *Social Science and Medicine*, *16*, 1397–1404.

Thoits, P. A. (1985). Self-labeling processes in mental illness: The role of emotional deviance. *American Journal of Sociology*, *91*(2), 221–249.

Thorne, S., Jensen, L., Kearney, M. H., Noblit, G., & Sandelowski, M. (2004). Qualitative metasynthesis: Reflections on methodological orientation and ideological agenda. *Qualitative Health Research*, *14*, 1342–1365.

Thorne, S., Paterson, B., Acorn, S., Canam, C., Joachim, G., & Jillings, C. (2002). Chronic illness experience: Insights from a metastudy. *Qualitative Health Research*, *12*(4), 437–452.

Varul, M. Z. (2010). Talcott Parsons, the sick role and chronic illness. *Body & Society*, *16*(2), 72–94.

Williams, S. J. (2005). Parsons revisited: From the sick role to ...? *Health: An Interdisciplinary Journal for the Social Study of Health, Illness and Medicine*, *9*(2), 123–144.

Wu, R. (1973). *Behavior and illness*. Englewood Cliffs, NJ: Prentice-Hall.

PART IV
BIOMEDICALIZATION IN THE ERA OF COMMUNITY MENTAL HEALTH

BORDERLINE PERSONALITY DISORDER AND THE BIOMEDICAL MISMATCH

Sandra H. Sulzer, Gracie Jackson and Ashelee Yang

ABSTRACT

Purpose – *To examine how clinicians navigate providing treatment to Borderline Personality Disorder (BPD) in the context of the DSM 5, deinstitutionalization, and the biomedical model.*

Methodology/approach – *We conducted 39 interviews with mental health providers in the United States in a two-year period preceding and following the release of the DSM 5. Using Constructivist Grounded Theory, we analyzed the data for themes that emerged.*

Findings – *Clinicians faced pressures from insurance companies, the DSM categories, and their professional training to focus on biomedical treatments. These treatments, which emphasized pharmaceuticals and short courses of care, were ill-suited to BPD, which has a strong evidence base recommending long-term therapeutic interventions. We term this contradiction a "biomedical mismatch" and use Gidden's concept of structuration to better understand how clinicians navigate the system of care. Providers ranged in their responses to the mismatch: some*

50 Years after Deinstitutionalization: Mental Illness in Contemporary Communities
Advances in Medical Sociology, Volume 17, 263–290

ISSN: 1057-6290/doi:10.1108/S1057-629020160000017011

championed biomedicine, others were complicit, and a final group behaved as activists, challenging the paradigm. The sum of the strategies had downstream effects which included crisis reinstitutionalization and a discourse of untreatability. Ultimately, we discuss how social factors such as gender bias, stigma, and trauma are insufficiently represented in the biomedical model of care for BPD.

Originality/value – *BPD fits poorly within the biomedical underpinnings of the current system. Accordingly, it illuminates the structuration of health care and where the rules of care break down. More precisely, deinstitutionalization was designed to remove patients from long courses of inpatient care. Many patients with BPD have failed to experience this outcome, with some patients now cycling through long courses of short-term crisis reinstitutionalization instead of having effective outpatient care over long periods. This unintended consequence of deinstitutionalization calls for a more biopsychosocial response to BPD.*

Keywords: Borderline personality disorder; DSM 5; institutionalization; mental health; insurance providers; biomedicine

INTRODUCTION

The biomedical model has been the main mode of thinking about medicine for physicians since the middle of the 19th century. Biomedicine focuses on physical processes in the body, such as the biochemical, pathological, and physiological. It treats diagnosis as an objective process, rather than a socially influenced negotiation between clinician and patient (Annandale, 1998). Psychiatry has had a contested relationship with the biomedical model, being "of two minds" about the etiology and treatment of mental illness, torn between biomedicine (biopsychiatry), and a psychodynamic history (Luhrmann, 2001; Orr, 2010). Psychiatry was founded with an emphasis on symbolism and psychodynamic thinking, characterized by practitioners such as Sigmund Freud and Carl Jung. As the 20th century wore on, the biomedical model of medicine became more dominant in non-mental health fields. Consequently, psychiatry struggled to maintain legitimacy as a medical subfield, and thus faced pressure to biomedicalize (see Kirk & Kutchins, 1992; Luhrmann, 2001; Orr, 2010; Whooley, 2010).

In modern psychiatry, the biomedical focus translates into efforts to alter the biochemistry of the brain, primarily with pharmaceuticals (see

Abraham, 2010). This orientation particularly emerged with the invention of Haldol and Thorazine in the 1950s, and has been buttressed by SSRI's and other more recent additions to the pharmaceutical arsenal of psychiatrists (Conrad, 2007; Conrad & Schneider, 1980; Horwitz & Wakefield, 2012; Karp, 2007; Metzl, 2009).

The advent of these medications was an important component of the push to deinstitutionalize those suffering from mental illness in favor of a community-based model. Instead of long-term stays spent in (often inhumane) institutions, many patients could now be released into their communities, as long as they adhered to drug regimens and regular check-ins with healthcare providers on an outpatient basis. In this new context, institutionalized care shifted to shorter term stays focused on crisis situations, such as self-harm or threats to others (Kelly, 2009; Metzl, 2009). And yet, despite the introduction of these medications, and even as patients were being routed into biomedically oriented community care, psychiatry struggled to fit neatly within a deinstitutionalized biomedical model. Not all mental health conditions were treatable with pharmaceutical interventions, nor was the etiology of many conditions entirely understood. Furthermore, an important component of deinstitutionalization had also been the increasingly visible anti-psychiatry movement, which questioned not just "imprisonment" within asylums, but psychiatry itself (see Szasz, 1961).

Facing professional backlash, psychiatrists too were negotiating their legitimacy as providers of modern medicine. By increasingly biomedical standards, the field of psychiatry could no longer claim a medical background. Without medical credibility in their field, psychiatrists could not distinguish themselves from other mental health providers such as clinical psychologists, social workers, or counselors (Horwitz, 2002; Orr, 2010; Whooley, 2010). This lack of professional legitimacy, the increase of medication-based treatments, and the deinstitutionalization movement set the stage for the revisions of the Diagnostic and Statistical Manual (DSM) third edition (American Psychiatric Association [APA], 1980).

The DSM-III was designed to create a structure and provide billing codes wherein insurance companies could be billed for the treatment of a catalogue of mental health conditions (Miller, Bergstrom, Cross, and Grube, 1981). In principle, this was a necessary step in the deinstitutionalization process, as a network of community care would require many more providers to submit for reimbursements. The DSM provided a standard language for clinicians to communicate with insurers and attempted to legitimize mental health care as being more similar to other forms of medical care. It would provide clinicians with a reliable and exhaustive list of diagnoses, shifting away from the field's earlier psychodynamic approach (See APA, 1950, 1968, 1980). In turn, psychiatrists could be seen in a more scientific light, by basing diagnoses on symptoms that were supposedly explained by biology (Horwitz, 2002; Kirk & Kutchins, 1992; Whooley, 2010; Whooley & Horwitz, 2013). The inclusion of behavioral observations of symptoms in the DSM was also supposed to make generalizable research possible, using uniform diagnostic criteria (Spitzer, Williams, & Skodol, 1980). However, this formative relationship between insurance companies and the creation of diagnostic categories also sparked controversy and created ongoing pressures for clinicians (see Whooley, 2010).

Scholars disagree about the extent to which the intention of the DSM was to cater to insurance company billing requirements, but today, it is difficult to contest the relationship between the DSM and insurers (see Godderis, 2011; Orr, 2010; Whooley, 2010). A dental health condition not defined in the DSM can generally not receive reimbursement for medical care. And as the DSM came to influence the work of not only clinicians, but also insurance and pharmaceutical companies, and researchers in the field, society's understanding of mental disorders became increasingly biological (Kirk & Kutchins, 1992). Within this framework, disorders that could not be explained by biological symptoms received less credibility in the field, leading to less reimbursement by insurance companies, and less research for alternative treatments (Whooley, 2010).

Of particular note in terms of conditions failing to receive credibility were Axis II disorders. Axis I was reserved for mood disorders, while Axis II was for the more "characterological" conditions. Personality disorders on this Axis were implicitly categorized as untreatable, primarily because personalities themselves were arguably not biochemical disorders, but rather, immutable characteristics of personhood. Whooley (2010) has suggested Axis II conditions were a carry-over from psychodynamic psychiatry and treated by clinicians as if they were not suited for biomedicine. By categorizing a patient as an Axis II or personality disorder, "psychiatrists create a group of patients who fall outside the authority of the DSM" (Whooley, 2010, p. 459). As the DSM-III provided codes for insurance billing, this effort to medicalize a greater range of human conditions also offered an apparent "out" for insurance companies: mood disorders were treatable, whereas personalities, arguably, were not (Kutchins & Kirk, 1987). This Axial system was removed from the most recent edition, DSM 5 (APA, 2013a). According to the task force "there is no fundamental difference between disorders described on DSM-IV's Axis I and Axis II, DSM 5 has shifted to a single axis system" (APA, 1994, 2013a, 2013b, p. 2). Yet for the decades of the DSM-III and IV, Axis II disorders occupied black sheep status as arguably life-long personality characteristics, and therefore not plausibly treatable mental health conditions.

THE CASE OF BORDERLINE PERSONALITY DISORDER

Borderline Personality Disorder (BPD), was one of these Axis II disorders. Originally, it described patients who did not respond to treatment within psychoanalysis. The first time this concept appeared in writing was 1938, when Adolph Stern found that a subset of his patients did not respond to therapeutic intervention. This group was described in relation to other groups – at the border of psychosis and neurosis (Stern, 1938). Historically then, this was a group defined by their failure to respond to conventional treatment.

In 1980, BPD was included in the DSM-III (APA, 1980). The 1980 definition of BPD was distinct from the earlier psychoanalytic conceptualizations of the disorder, because, like other conditions of the DSM-III, it focused on observable behaviors in an effort to fit it more clearly within an objective medical taxonomy (see Brown, 1990). Despite consisting of observable behaviors that were objectively verifiable, BPD was placed on the new Axis II which housed it and other personality disorders. The current DSM 5 defines BPD as "A pervasive pattern of instability of interpersonal relationships, self-image, and affects, and marked impulsivity," as evidenced by patients meeting five of nine subsequent criteria (APA, 2013a, 2013b). Aside from small wording changes, it is nearly identical to the DSM-IV definition, and has not changed substantially from the 1980 definition. The only major shift has been the removal of Axes.

BPD represents an interesting case to examine how clinicians today navigate a biomedical model when faced with a condition that does not fit well within the rules. It flies in the face of all markers of biomedicalization; it is non-responsive to pharmaceuticals, requires person-intensive treatments, has no clear biochemical etiology, has been plagued by stigma among mental health professionals, and occupies the Axis II.

Different from conditions like schizophrenia, BPD is generally not responsive to pharmaceuticals (Bateman, Gunderson, & Mulder, 2015; Zanarini, 2004). Although enough evidence has suggested that BPD can be effectively treated using therapist interventions, such as Dialectical Behavioral Therapy and Mentalization Based Therapy (Bateman & Fonagy, 2008; Clarkin, Levy, Lenzenweger, & Kernberg, 2007; Linehan, 1993; Linehan et al., 2006; Oldham, Skodol, & Bender, 2005), it is also noted that long-stay units specializing in treating BPD are few and far between (Avery, Francois, Martins, Park, & Roth, 2012). The treatment of BPD is person-intensive, but shows no evidence of having an underlying biochemical imbalance.

The stigmatization of BPD also contributes to the difficulty of treatment. Past research has suggested that BPD may not have ever achieved fully medicalized status and that patients themselves are considered non-medically, morally deviant (Sulzer, 2015b). The behaviors codified in the BPD diagnostic criteria are also behaviors typically categorized as "difficult" in mental health settings (Fiore, 1988; Kelly & May, 1982; Koekkoek, van Meijel, & Hutschemaekers, 2006; Luhrmann, 2001; Nehls, 1998, 1999; Schwartz & Goldfinger, 1981). In many cases the category of "borderline" itself is directly linked to the stereotypes of "difficult patients," much more so than other mental health illness like schizophrenia (Gallop, Lancee, & Garfinkel, 1989; Manning, 2000; Treloar, 2009). BPD thus occupies a unique space of being untreatable with dominant biomedical approaches, undesirable among clinician who could provide person-intensive and effective treatments, and yet not being a mysteriously untreatable condition. If psychiatry at large has been working toward professional legitimation through biomedicalization, BPD is a prime example of a condition that may be deeply problematic for providers. Scholars have called for a more structural consideration of how patients with BPD fare in this system (Koekkoek, 2015; Sulzer, 2015a). This leads to our central inquiry: *Given the current clinical landscape of the DSM 5, the insurance system and the biomedical model, how do clinicians navigate providing clinical care of Borderline Personality Disorder in the United States?*

METHODS

Taking an inductive, grounded theory approach (Charmaz, 2006), the research group conducted 39 in-depth interviews with clinicians working in the United States. On average, interviews were approximately one hour per respondent, ranging from 30 minutes to three hours. Questions were semi-structured, with an emphasis on the diagnostic process and the influence of the DSM in this encounter.

To include a diverse sample of respondents, clinicians were first recruited based on purposive sampling that focused on gender, and profession. After early difficulties securing sufficient interviews, we utilized snowball sampling (Morgan, 2008; Small, 2009). Snowball sampling was primarily used to increase the number of respondents who met purposive criteria and to leverage professional networks. No more than two clinicians were used from a single referral, and each clinician was interviewed one time. The sample of 39 clinicians included 24 women and 15 men. There were 16 psychologists, 8 psychiatrists, 12 licensed clinical social workers, and 4 licensed professional counselors. These clinicians practiced in a wide range of settings including public hospitals, private practices, and university campus health. Clinicians represented eleven states: Wisconsin, New York, Maryland, New Jersey, North Carolina, Mississippi, Pennsylvania, Alaska, Illinois, Texas, and Minnesota. We initially sampled purposively by gender and profession, anticipating possible variation due to the gender bias in diagnosis and differing professionalization practices (see Wirth-Cauchon, 2001). The strength of our strategy was a wide range of perspectives, and ultimately sample saturation, which is the gold standard in grounded theory. However, we acknowledge this means our sample may not be representative. Interviewing concluded once the data became saturated, meaning that no additional information was learned from subsequent interviews. Thus, the most relevant themes and findings should be represented in the data.

The data was collected from 2011 to 2014. The study was approved by the University of Wisconsin Madison Institutional Review Board (IRB) and the University of North Carolina Chapel Hill IRB. All interview participants voluntarily gave written or verbal consent prior to the beginning of the interview in accordance with the guidelines of respective IRB rulings. Further questions about the purpose of the study were addressed following the completion of the interview.

RESULTS

This study uncovered the implicit rules clinicians were following to treat BPD. We found that the biomedical model served as the primary clinical framework, yet we also learned clinicians utilized a variety of strategies to navigate the mismatch between biomedicine and the needs of their patients. A small minority agreed with the appropriateness of a biomedical approach for patients, while others disagreed but were complicit, and still others engaged in activist efforts against the model's fit. After discussing biomedical domination and mismatch, as well as how providers navigated contradictions, we will review implications for patients including crisis reinstitutionalization, and a discourse of untreatability.

BIOMEDICAL DOMINATION – THE ROLE OF STRUCTURATION IN MENTAL HEALTH CARE

The first major finding of our research was that providers, through their discussion of medications, generally agreed that biomedicine dominated their provision of mental health care. The prioritization of conditions that had a "clear" chemical or biological etiology infused all aspects of their professional experience: treatment preferences, professional education, and reimbursement practices.

A useful frame for describing this phenomenon is Giddens' concept of structuration (1984). This theory suggests that systems are grounded in the activities of situated actors. The actors draw on rules, and by following them (or not) in a variety of contexts those actors (re)produce (or not) the social system. Utilizing the concept of structuration, the biomedical model provides the structure from within which clinical actors go about their daily activities. It directs and guides their expectations for how a clinical encounter should proceed, and how they should respond to patients. In this case, the rules are about how clinicians are supposed to identify who qualifies as a patient and how patients should be treated utilizing the guidelines of insurance companies, DSM definitions, professional training expectations, and workplace norms. Structuration may also break down in situations where the rules do not fit with the situation at hand.

Giddens' model helps us to separate out the actors (clinicians) working across multiple contexts and settings from the structure that they are reproducing. Because these clinicians are drawing on social rules, we can understand their behavior best by determining what underlying and implicit rules are guiding their actions. In this case, it is particularly important to understand that clinicians do not necessarily conceptualize their choices with any given patient as being part of some larger system of care; in fact, they may have little sense at all of the structure they are helping to recreate. This is because the "rules implicated in the production and reproduction of social practices are only tacitly grasped by actors: they know how to 'go on'"

(Giddens, 1984, pp. 22–23). Providers know how to do their jobs, which is not the same as knowing how the performance of their job reinforces patterns of care for patients who have historically not fit well within the system. Across many contexts and many providers, the structure emerges because "repetitive activities, located in one context of time and space, have regularized consequences, unintended by those who engage in those activities, in more or less 'distant' time-space contexts" (Giddens, 1984, p. 14). In this way, the individual choices of disparate clinicians help to maintain (or dismantle) the structure that determines care, whether or not they realize how interconnected all of their actions really are. In this case, structuration helps to explain how actors may perpetuate and extend a biomedical model for patients.

When considering the individual choices of disparate clinicians in our sample, they consistently pointed to the reality that medications were the primary tools of their trade. As one clinician explained in her interview, "if you go to a psychiatrist, you gonna get a pill. It's kind of like, you go to a hair, you know, you go to a barber shop, you gonna get a haircut." Providers also explained that more educational time in their curriculums was devoted to conditions that were readily treatable with medications. A clinical social worker who has practiced for more than 11 years recalled her experience, "I think one of the reasons why people know so much about depression is there are so much medications on depression." Thus, the connection between medication and mental health is a rule of the biomedical model of care that is openly acknowledged by clinicians.

BIOMEDICAL MISMATCH

Although the biomedical model seemed to dominate mental health care, BPD consistently failed to fit within biomedical expectations. At one time, this lack of fit seemed to suggest a promising alternative vision for how mental health care in America might become more psychosocially managed. For example, Theodore Million believed that the redefinition of BPD in the DSM-III was revolutionary since it moved away from a disease model into one that considered social context and duration (Millon, 1983). Unfortunately, as deinstitutionalization proceeded, this potential shift was not fully realized, resulting in a biomedical mismatch for conditions like BPD.

Providers in our sample frequently argued that the biomedical model did not fit well with the needs of their BPD patients. One psychologist who had been practicing for more than a decade made it clear that the current biomedical model was problematic in dealing with borderline patients.

> I think the tendency for psychiatrists to want to medicate X symptom … I personally think it's a disservice to the vast majority of individuals that are suffering from borderline personality disorder, because quite often they get slapped with the label of bipolar and they are taking this heavy duty medicine and quite often an anti-psychotic, that more than likely they don't really need and has time and time again shown to be ineffective. I think that's problematic.

This provider pointed out that persons with BPD are frequently medicated, despite empirical evidence that these medications are not effective, and may cause additional harms, a finding also validated in the scientific literature (Bateman et al., 2015; Zanarini, 2004).

It was not just psychiatrists in our sample who felt that patients with BPD were overly medicated due to a biomedical structure. Many of the providers in our sample were trained in social work or psychology, and they still felt tied to the larger model of treatment via medication. At the same time, they also sensed that BPD was quite different. As a licensed professional counselor mentioned, "I know that medication is gonna be really important … for the bipolar and some of the self-regulation are really important for that. For borderline, we really need to be looking at skills that somebody didn't get, that enable them to manage intensive emotions." This larger finding that BPD did not fit well within the biomedical model of treatment-by-medication was echoed across the majority of interviews.

Providers generally felt that BPD was distinct and needed different tools than other conditions. A clinical social worker believed that "BPD is not impacted or treated successfully with just regular treatment-as-usual. And the research is very clear that the treatment-as-usual does not work with borderline." Another licensed professional counselor stated that BPD was "different than anything else that we have, you know, in the Diagnostic Statistical Manual in terms of … how to handle the symptoms, the type of work you have to do with the client, um, is different than anything else we have." The finding that BPD does not respond to medications is consistent across scientific research (Bateman et al., 2015; Gunderson, Morey, & Stout, 2004; Ingenhover, Lafay, Rinne, Passchier, & Duivenvoorden, 2010; Lieb, Vollm, Rucker, Timmer, & Stoffers, 2010; Zanarini, 2004). Under a biomedical rule set however, this leaves providers in a position of seeing patients who they are unable to effectively treat *if they follow the rules*. If medications and a biomedical approach are not appropriate, then how do providers navigate the person-intensive care required for BPD?

PERSON-INTENSIVE PERSONALITY DISORDERS

The place for personality disorders generally, and BPD specifically, in once-a-week therapy sessions, or 20-minute visits with psychiatrists, as conditions that do not respond to medication, remains contested. Even as scientifically validated treatments for BPD, such as Dialectical Behavioral Therapy (DBT), have been growing in recognition and availability for decades, many clinicians have expressed reluctance to treat this particular disorder in the context of outpatient resources (see Sulzer, 2015b). DBT does not require advanced technology for testing or therapy, but it is labor-intensive on the part of clinicians. It includes weekly one-on-one patient sessions, a skills group, and for the clinician to have an hour of supervision for each hour of therapy. Additionally, clinicians often have extended calling hours, during which patients may call without limit (see Linehan, 1987). While there is an evidence base suggesting that a resource-intensive approach is most effective, it is difficult to provide in many community settings due to resource limitations (Bateman & Fonagy, 2008; Clarkin et al., 2007; Linehan, 1993; Oldham et al., 2005).

"Resource limitations" seem to be caused primarily by the reluctance of insurers (particularly private) to fund non-pharmaceutical and non-short-term therapies. This pressure from insurance companies makes sense within a biomedical model wherein other mental health conditions are treated primarily as if they are physical ailments. A clinical social worker who had worked in both public and private settings explained that in her understanding, "[insurance] did not reimburse for services that were to treat any Axis II." One early career psychiatrist explained the tensions between coverage and care:

> If it gets into the policies and the, you know, coverage stuff. Even at the public hospital where I was working, we were lucky in that we had kind of extra time because we were fellows or we interned. We weren't like overbooked. So we could spend longer with them in terms of actually sitting and talking with them until we got a clear picture of patterns and stuff, whereas most of the professionals that are hired on after our level of training, they don't have that amount of time. You know? .... I think it gets worse when they leave psychology and get into psychiatry because then they're even more crammed for time, they put them in 15 minute increments.

One provider gave a description of what her practice was like in the context of an HMO, rather than a public hospital:

> We're only going to treat Axis I here at the HMO, and Axis II we're not even going to talk about that ... you listen even to the language. Nobody is a therapist, you're a provider. And you are uhm, you're limited to you know, there's great pressure if they announce that you've got twenty visits a year to the subscribers, but they, in reality, any therapist that sees them more than 4.8 visits, the average number of visits per client per year, gets over 4.6 or 4.8, or something like that? They're called in on the carpet. You know, that have to limit, you know, so they're doing a lot of bandaid work. And for some people who are good clinicians, they're probably able to work with people with more severe problems for a little while, and then put them on hold and then come back and get them so they're able to extend the therapy for many years, but a few visits a year.

The primary concern of insurance companies in determining reimbursements seemed to revolve around the amount of time a therapist spent with any given patient. A clinical social worker who found a significant amount of success in treating BPD patients reported:

> My experience with insurance companies is that they call me up and beg me to try to take somebody who's tried to kill themselves, slit her wrists for a third time, and they don't have anybody out-patient to see her, so they look within a 20 mile radius ... and they'll be like "will you see her? Please, please?" They'll ask me to see her and you know, three months later, she's not suicidal or finishing up school or has a job, is doing okay. And they're like "why are you seeing her twice a week?" and they hassle me.

The pressure against providers spending ongoing time with patients seemed universal. Overall, insurance companies seemed to place barriers on providing outpatient care, and clinics seem to have fallen in-step by limiting the length of appointment times to maximize billing. At the same time, providers agreed that person-intensive resources were necessary. A newly licensed psychologist said simply: "It can be treated, with, unfortunately, a lot of time and energy." Another licensed professional counselor offered an itemization of why patients with BPD, particularly those receiving state-of-the-art DBT require so much time from providers.

> They need to be in a DBT program and that requires an authorization of 52 individual sessions a year and 52 group sessions a year at least. And then preferably at a higher rate because these clients across the board typically require more ... highly trained therapists and more clinical time and attention .... A part of the program is telephone conversation with them for all the week. You know, clients are emailing or texting me throughout the week, and if you get 4 cases of Borderline, your attention holds all the week.

How then do clinicians strategize within this mismatch of resources versus needed care? Some use the rules of BPD, not biomedicine, to guide their care, perhaps even behaving as activists. Others were biomedically complicit by relying on alternative coding. A final group championed biomedicine, and the removal of patients with BPD from their purview. After reviewing each strategy, we will explain how the sum of these strategies created a new structural response: crisis reinstitutionalization and a discourse of untreatability.

ACTIVIST CLINICIANS

A minority of clinicians actively worked to provide the level of care they felt patients needed, despite the biomedical rules. As one social worker explained, "I would rather throw the sink at you and give you whatever you needed to keep you out of the hospital, rather than see you at the hospital every five minutes." She links the consequences of failing to provide intensive resources to later inpatient resource utilization, which will be discussed more in-depth as one of the outcomes of the poor fit of BPD within the biomedical model. The strategies for tackling this varied from policy level interventions to daily bureaucratic doggedness.

One provider shared that she was involved with Mental Health Parity Initiatives, and reported that her and colleagues would "send [insurance company] letters and send them to clarify, you know, we don't think you're in compliance with the Parity Bill, and then you know, like eight months later the insurance company will get back to us." She said to-date, her group had been unable to secure positive responses from insurance companies with regard to providing personality disorder treatment. She reported companies claimed to be in compliance, in the absence of any government agency operating as a watchdog to their behaviors.

Another provider tackled the issue on a case-by-case basis, behaving as an activist in his own clinic. He would intentionally use the BPD diagnosis on insurance forms and actively fought each instance an insurance company tried to deny treatment. He said "I don't understand why any clinician would lose the war. I mean the insurance companies can't claim to be more authoritative than the practice guidelines ... besides Dialectical Behavioral Therapy, there are a bunch of other therapies that have been shown in controlled studies to be helpful with these patients." He also reported having sufficient staff persons available to manage the many cycles of faxes necessary to achieve his aims.

These providers however, were relatively unique. Far more providers engaged in activities that implicitly validated the biomedical model. They utilized psychiatric workarounds (see Whooley, 2010) to provide the care they thought was appropriate, without meaningfully disrupting the structural rules of the mental healthcare system.

THE BIOMEDICALLY COMPLICIT

The DSM 5 removed the axial system, which had relegated personality disorders to an Axis II status, separate from mood disorders such as depression or anxiety. However, the overwhelming majority of providers we interviewed a year after the release of DSM 5 were either primarily using the DSM-IV definitions or were unaware of the implications of the removal of the axial system. Most clinicians explained that they were unfamiliar with the changes present in the DSM 5 because their institution had not yet transitioned to using the DSM 5 for billing purposes.

As a result, providers continued to use a simple, yet effective strategy for increasing their ability to provide care to patients with BPD. They used alternate codes on insurance paperwork to bill for sessions. They constructed a *reimbursable patient*. For example, a provider may code something as Major Depressive Disorder, instead of BPD to avoid problems with coverage. A clinical social worker pointed out, "I know there're a number of therapists out there that a couple of things they give diagnoses that they can bill longer and that may or may not be completely accurate." Another directly said "I'm going to avoid a personality disorder diagnosis on the insurance form if I legitimately can, if there's enough other stuff going on, because you never know whether the insurance is going to cover personality disorder." One psychologist explained "I don't put Borderline on the insurance claim. Because it's a kiss of death. At least it used to be. And I've just kept the practice, I think most therapists do this, they, there's a euphemism there, or uh you put the personality disorder not otherwise specified. It's a political thing when you're dealing with diagnoses." Another said "if I have to give them a bill for insurance, I will write PTSD or depression or anxiety." Another did this with the participation of the patient "Sometimes I will, with a client's permission, change their diagnosis to something that sounds more serious. And then they can get more sessions." In this way, actors were participating in some of the rules of biomedical diagnosis set forth by the arrangement between insurance companies and the DSM, and yet they were also subverting them. These findings were consistent with past research on how psychiatrists in particular navigate the intrusion of insurance companies into their professional realm. The clinician "determines the treatment and compensation he thinks a patient deserves and applies the necessary code to achieve these ends" (Whooley, 2010, p. 460).

While the removal of the axial system might cause a sea-change in the long run, it has not been effective in the short run at altering the common practices surrounding Axis II reporting to insurance agencies. These providers ultimately are following the larger rules of the biomedical model: they continue to use the DSM to bill insurance companies to be compensated for care. Their form of protest is nearly impossible to clinically document for any given patient and creates the illusion of some amount of autonomy from the biomedical rules.

The long-term issues with this are not entirely clear. This behavior supports implicit continued discrimination against patients with BPD, by behaving *as if* it is accurate that the condition is untreatable, simply because insurance companies are reluctant to reimburse for appropriate and necessary care. But it also demonstrates where the rules break down for biomedicine. Providers in this group have allowed their behaviors to be shaped to a relatively large extent by insurance company demands, and they generally do not try to fight the refusal to provide care. And yet, their practices show that in the case of BPD, when the rules break down, providers find a workaround.

BIOMEDICAL CHAMPIONS

Still other providers, the smallest group in the sample, did not find biomedicine at large, or care options for BPD to be problematic. Rather, they played an active role themselves in routing patients out of are, citing a "lack of fit" with the resources at hand. While the routing of patients with BPD out of care has been discussed at greater length elsewhere (see Sulzer, 2015b), some key examples will demonstrate how the most biomedically oriented of our sample saw the issue as lying with patients, not the mental health care system.

A well-established psychiatrist who managed an inpatient ward explained how the biomedical-based insurance plays a role in the treatment process by saying:

> Psychiatrist: Our county doesn't generally like to fund people that have a primary diagnosis of Borderline Personality Disorder, just feeling like they are better served in other resources. They are more likely to find somebody that has, acutely manic or acutely psychotic. And I don't really disagree with that.
>
> Interviewer: What's the logic behind that?
>
> Psychiatrist: The logic behind that is that there are other facilities that aren't as intense and as expensive as the hospital to provide short-term safety and kind of uhm management 'til they can resume the outpatient care.

Another provider who disagreed with this mindset, nonetheless explained her helplessness to counteract it. This psychologist shared "if I see someone who has a personality disorder, a Borderline Personality Disorder, and they just attempted [suicide] and there are more signs and I think they should go to the inpatient center of the state hospital, then the psychiatric team for example would be like 'no that's not helpful for them. They will be borderline forever.'" She described being unable to secure inpatient coverage, when faced with psychiatrists who were more reliant on the biomedical understanding of mental health than she was. Conditions that could be stabilized with medications were prioritized over conditions that required ongoing care, even in a crisis situation.

CONSEQUENCES OF THE BIOMEDICAL MISMATCH

Crisis Reinstitutionalization

Due to the poor fit of BPD with the current treatment paradigm, patients with BPD continue to use inpatient services in high numbers. As their suffering goes unchecked and un(der)treated, patients are often voluntarily and involuntarily routed into more intensive, yet brief, crisis-intervention forms of care (see Sulzer, 2015b). As one provider explained, "We realized, and anyone with half a brain has realized that these are the patients that utilize our emergency services and inpatient hospitalizations the most." Due to high rates of suicidality and suicide completion, many providers feel that inpatient care is necessary on a frequent basis. The same clinician explained her claim in detail,

> Uhm, oh my goodness, probably when I was in emergency services because what would happen, we called them *frequent fliers*, back then. I'm sure they call them the same thing now. But these are the people that were in and out of the emergency room with suicidal ideation all the time. I mean, I would see the same people over and over again for two, three years in a row, at least once, maybe sometimes twice a month. And you know, you have to err on the side of caution. We would always hospitalize them. And I think at that point in time, I realize that more needed to be done than just putting them in the hospital.

It was not just providers in our sample who held this impression: the evidence base suggests persons with BPD have a high prevalence of suicidality and self-harming behaviors, and are frequent utilizers of medical facilities; indeed, these are among the criteria for having the disorder (APA, 2013a, 2013b; Skodol, Gunderson, & McGlashan, 2002). Although population estimates for the disorder range from 1% to 3% (Carpenter & Trull, 2012; Grant et al., 2008; Lenzenweger, Lane, Loranger, & Kessler, 2007; Swartz, Blazer, George, & Winfield, 1990; Torgersen, Kringlen, & Cramer, 2001), this condition makes up a third of inpatient resources today (Biskin & Paris, 2012), and 20% of total mental health visits (Carpenter & Trull, 2012; Leichsenring, Leibing, Kruse, New, & Leweke, 2011; Lieb, Zanarini, Schmahl, Linehan, & Bohus, 2004; Widiger & Weissman, 1991). One study found patients with BPD were 4.95 times more likely to be hospitalized than patients with Major Depressive Disorder (Bender et al., 2001), and another found they were equally as likely as patients with Schizophrenia to be hospitalized, but more likely to have shorter stays and higher rates of outpatient contacts (Skodol, Buckley, & Charles, 1983). Another study found a mean of nine psychiatric hospitalizations across a three-year period (Clarke, Hafner, & Holme, 1995). These high rates of psychiatric hospitalizations are also a correlated with higher emergency room usage (see Bender et al., 2001; Clarke et al., 1995). Skodol et al. (1983) found that patients with BPD appear to utilize psychiatric emergency rooms with a greater frequency than patients with Axis I disorders, though they did not report rates.

However, because of their ongoing high usage rates, patients face ongoing pushback from providers. This can manifest as patients with personality disorders being the subject of clinical jokes. As a psychologist described, in the hospital she had been working at, "They're almost like infamous people that were like 'oh, hey how are you doing again?' And so, usually, it was lots of personality stuff." While jokes alone might seem less than ideal, but not alarming, they represented a small indication of a larger phenomenon. Patients were not only subject to crisis reinstitutionalization in an era of deinstitutionalization, they were also subject to a *discourse of untreatability*.

A Discourse of Untreatability

Perhaps the original naming of patients as Borderline because they did not fit into the categories of treatable patients has persisted more significantly than any other aspect of patient care. This may be the implicit rule that most fundamentally drives all of the results previously discussed. Provider after provider either described patients with BPD as untreatable, or acknowledged this was the prevailing view among those not well-versed in the evidence base. A clinician believed that this stigma was perpetuated through generations of professional education,

> Even during my own training, the professor said people don't get better, they just suck your time and energy and you know, you can never get away from them. Obviously now I know that's not accurate, but think about all the other clinicians that … don't have that perception broadened like I have, you know, who still perhaps believe that.

As one clinical social worker explained, "Historically, not empirically, that once a borderline, always a borderline, and they're untreatable." This is a *discourse of untreatability*, a final rule that providers must navigate if they engage with patients who have BPD.

Providers also explained that a history of being labeled as untreatable had modern day consequences, which they directly linked with care provision. The same clinical social worker further stated, "People with borderline, when they are diagnosed with borderline, know that many clinicians do not want to work with them." A patient that seems to be untreatable may seem to have no real place in a biomedical model based mental health treatment system. One psychologist cut straight to the point:

> Most clinicians that I know and have worked with for many years really shy away from personality disorders. And they don't think there's really an awful lot that you can do with them because, you know, medication doesn't work. But skills do. Cognitive behavioral therapy to a point.

In a post DSM 5 era, despite the removal of the axial system, and in spite of a compelling evidence base of treatment options, BPD still suffers from a discourse of untreatability. While this feminized population has perhaps been saved from being placed in mental institutions against their will for extended periods of time, they retain the problem of the original group Stern studied: clinicians in our sample still express concerns that patients are not getting better and treatment isn't working. Since Stern's time, effective interventions have been found, but remain fraught with barriers, which leads to consequences that ripple through the system.

INTRODUCING THE SOCIAL TO THE BIOMEDICAL

There are compelling reasons that biomedicine falls short for BPD, all of which are primarily social in nature. The first is that some experts argue BPD is linked in many cases with a history of trauma. The second is that there is a failure to consider gender as a meaningful aspect of the experience of patients with BPD. Given that women are diagnosed at three times the rate as men, it is astonishing that more attention is not paid to how gender may influence care provision. Lastly, the stigma of BPD is unique within the mental health care field, and the social process of stigmatizing this particular group of patients for their care seeking behaviors may have a pronounced effect. These factors cannot be captured within a biomedical discourse or disease model wherein disorders are understood as having a primarily biological origin with a primarily chemical solution.

HISTORIES OF TRAUMA

Patients with BPD fail to fit within the biomedical model because, as many scholars have argued, this condition has a clear overlap with childhood abuse or trauma. Approximately 91% of BPD individuals report experiencing sexual, physical, and emotional childhood abuse (Kuo, Khoury, Metcalfe, Fitzpatrick, & Goodwill, 2015). Social context and family attachments may be important considerations when working with this patient group, and those considerations fall outside of a healthcare model that focuses primarily on biological causes of mental health. One psychologist explained that in relation to BPD,

> We're gonna be thinking more longer term ... identifying with that personality difficulties that these disorders began very early in life, and have a lot of attachment roots with this sort of like how people interacted in their family and there are a lot of developmental pieces to it, that just simply cannot be really managed in a short-term setting.

Because BPD may be intimately linked to attachment issues in childhood, it could be a long-term process to regain the ability to trust persons of authority, as well as to manage and build relationships in adulthood. Another provider explained "all of their attachments are unstable and chaotic. Very intense, followed by very distant, which is the definition of chaotic. So, you know, basically the core dynamic of borderline is chaotic attachment patterns." In this sense, the biopsychosocial model, which incorporates social context into health care, is a significantly better fit for BPD. A biopsychosocial approach takes into account an individual's biological, psychological, and social risk factors, and how these interact, when evaluating mental health status (Paris, 1994). While this model exists in the theoretical realm and perhaps in some care-based settings (particularly those outside of the United States), providers in this sample still reported the biomedical, pharmaceutical-based model dominated their field. Therefore, providers faced ongoing pressures to make their treatment of BPD fit with a biomedical treatment paradigm. However, this approach is unlikely to ever be fully effective, because trauma cannot (yet) be treated by taking a pill.

GENDER IN HEALTHCARE

The biomedical model also fails to take into account the gendered nature of BPD diagnosis and treatment. Scholars have demonstrated gender bias in how patients are diagnosed. Women are diagnosed more often than men, even using identical case histories in vignette studies (see Becker, 1997; Wirth-Cauchon, 2001). While space limitations prevent us from having a more extensive discussion of how gender bias may be a confounding variable in the consideration of trauma and stigma, it is evident that medications do not treat gender bias in diagnosis.

In addition to diagnostic issues, the relationship between gender and trauma must be considered. No amount of evaluating the brain chemistry of patients addresses a culture in which women experience higher rates of abuse, rape, poverty, and other traumas. If women are generally more likely to have these experiences, and trauma is so intimately linked to the diagnosis of BPD, we must consider how our society reproduces gendered forms of mental unwellness.

And lastly, the stigma of BPD itself cannot be fully untangled from potential bias in how women are perceived more generally. The most common descriptor providers in our sample used to describe a typical patient was "female," even though men possess the disorder in roughly equal numbers (see Coid, Yang, Tyrer, Robers, & Ullrich, 2006). So long as clinicians more readily diagnose women as having BPD at greater rates than they diagnose men with similar symptoms (see Wirth-Cauchon, 2001) the linkage between gender and stigmatization of BPD bears the markings of a persistent discriminatory practice and discourse.

STIGMA AS A CONSEQUENCE OF A BIOMEDICAL MISMATCH

Lastly, for patients who do get routed into psychiatric care, they may face stigma or mistreatment in the face of their poor fit with the structure of a biomedical mental health system. Providers are conscious of the stigma associated with BPD diagnoses.

> I haven't run into them, any psychiatrists that are nice to [patients with BPD] (laughs). I think because they don't have to (laughs). I mean their role is to give medication. So, since they don't really have to give medication to someone with Borderline Personality Disorder because it really won't do much.

A more experienced clinician added: "I would say the stigma? Huge. It keeps people from getting the treatment they need, it ends up with people getting terrible medical treatment, because they're never taken seriously." One provider tried to explain how this affected patients,

> I think there's a number of people who have borderline personality disorders that have been dismissed in our healthcare and mental healthcare system that they feel additionally stigmatized. Well, when people say "I can't really find a reason why you might not be seeing well," or "I can't really find a reason why your headaches – we're treating your headaches ..." and [the patients] start to say "Oh my God, it's my fault!" And that creates stigma.

Goffman (1963) originally conceptualized stigma as he studied inhabitants of asylums (Goffman, 1962). Perhaps he would not be surprised that all of these years later, deinstitutionalization did not remove the mark of a spoiled identity after all – that stigma retained social consequences, regardless of institutional setting.

DISCUSSION

The case of BPD and the biomedical mismatch may speak to other cases as well. This condition points to evidence that insurance companies may drive clinical practice to a greater extent than might be immediately obvious. Using the concept of structuration to better understand the behavior of clinicians helps to illuminate why this might be the case. Insurance companies are one of the co-creators of rules that clinicians must follow (or rebel against). Biomedical pressures may emerge not only from insurance companies but also through professionalization practices that emphasize pharmacological and technological forms of treatment over social work, and person-intensive treatments.

Reproductive health may be another area of a highly gendered set of health concerns that demonstrates the biomedical rules. The medically inexplicable growth of C-sections as an intervention speaks to the biomedicalization of technological strategies in medicine as well (see Barber et al., 2011; Clark, Mamo, Fosket, Fishman, & Shim, 2010). Here too, providers face pressures to respond in particular ways, which uphold the tenants of biomedicine. Ultimately, actors within the medical establishment encounter a set of daily rules they follow (or take action against) when considering treatment options. They may not explicitly refer to their practices as biomedical in nature, but they are experts in the day-to-day business of practicing healthcare. The day-to-day business they engage in privileges the dispensation of medications, technological interventions, and a downplaying of social factors (Clark et al., 2010).

Actors vary in how they engaged with biomedicine in the context of BPD. Activism, workarounds, and championing the implicit rules all took place. But overall, regardless of strategies, there were consequences for patients with BPD: they faced crisis reinstitutionalization, and were forced to navigate a discourse of untreatability. Ultimately, social factors were evident to clinicians, but not meaningfully integrated into their models of care.

CONCLUSION

Much has changed for patients with BPD from the beginning of deinstitutionalization to the publication of the DSM 5. However, the one theme that remains for patients with BPD is that they continue to face barriers to receiving effective treatment. Evidence-based care for patients with BPD does not parallel the kinds of care biomedicine endorses. Treatment of BPD instead challenges the rules of the biomedical model, leaving patients in a lurch as they are consistently mismatched with the industry tasked with serving them. This has led to unanticipated consequences.

While deinstitutionalization might have offered a promising shift to patient-centered, community-based care, in the case of BPD, we are witnessing a form of reinstitutionalization that is as ineffective as earlier asylums were. Repeated ER visits and 72-hour holds fail to serve a patient population in need of ongoing therapy-intensive treatment. Efforts to save money by moving care to the community are not fully realized when community care is also not well-enough funded to pay to keep patients from frequent emergency hospitalizations. Furthermore, placing clinicians in a catch-22 where they cannot be easily or routinely reimbursed to provide necessary and effective care may be partially responsible for ongoing beliefs about untreatability and other stigma surrounding BPD.

The structure of mental health care in American is not designed to provide care for BPD, and as actors move through the system with great intentions and a patient-centered focus, they still may find themselves frequently defaulting into the patterns well-worn by insurance policies, professional training, and a biomedical model. The failure of the healthcare system to provide a clear pathway for treatment of BPD, despite radical changes over the last century is remarkable. Modern clinician statements about the untreatability of BPD could be mistaken for archaic belief systems, were it not for their active reference to the DSM 5 and the Affordable Care Act. The costs of this are marked in employment absences, disability payments, emergency room costs, incarceration, and perhaps most importantly, a high rate of unnecessarily lost lives as a result of suicidality. This is arguably a social justice issue in that preventative and ongoing care is superior to emergency care for chronic conditions.

50 years after deinstitutionalization, we are seeing a crisis reinstitutionalization of individuals with BPD because of a persistent biomedical mismatch and the ongoing influence of the DSM. Deinstitutionalization might have been a radical step toward freedom for a stigmatized patient group, but a process driven by a biomedical model has real consequences in a socially lived human experience. Any given individual diagnosed with BPD is confined within a system that does not accommodate their etiology, or histories of trauma, or their struggles with interpersonal relationships, within the medical language of synaptic connections, chemical imbalances, and empirically verifiable biological phenomenon. Perhaps many mental health conditions struggle with this fit, but BPD is exceptional in how poorly it fits within our biological understandings of the human condition.

We recommend further research which triangulates data from clinicians-as-experts in their day-to-day practices, insurance company policies, DSM scholars, and most importantly, patient experiences. While there are many conditions worthy of study, the potential benefits of translating the clinical effectiveness research on BPD into daily practice are substantial. And the unique structural reasons this has not occurred-to-date are well worthy of further sociological examination.

REFERENCES

Abraham, J. (2010). Pharmaceuticalization of society in context: Theoretical, empirical and health dimensions. *Sociology*, *44*, 603–622. doi:10.1177/0038038510369368

American Psychiatric Association. (1950). *Diagnostic and statistical manual of mental disorders* (1st ed.). Arlington, VA: American Psychiatric Publishing.

American Psychiatric Association. (1968). *Diagnostic and statistical manual of mental disorders* (2nd ed.). Arlington, VA: American Psychiatric Publishing.

American Psychiatric Association. (1980). *Diagnostic and statistical manual of mental disorders* (3rd ed.). Arlington, VA: American Psychiatric Publishing.

American Psychiatric Association. (1994). *Diagnostic and statistical manual of mental disorders* (4th ed.). Arlington, VA: American Psychiatric Publishing.

American Psychiatric Association. (2013a). *Diagnostic and statistical manual of mental disorders* (5th ed.). Arlington, VA: American Psychiatric Publishing.

American Psychiatric Association. (2013b). *Personality disorders fact sheet*. Retrieved from http://www.dsm5.org/Documents/Personality%20Disorders%20Fact%20Sheet.pdf

Annandale, E. (1998). *The sociology of health and medicine: A critical introduction*. Malden, MA: Polity Press.

Avery, J., Francois, D., Martins, O., Park, S., & Roth, S. (2012). An updated model for the first-time hospitalization of patients with borderline personality disorder: Two illustrative case reports. *Psychiatric Quarterly*, *83*(4), 391–396. doi:10.1007/s11126-012-9209-3

Barber, E. L., Lundsberg, L., Belanger, K., Pettker, C. M., Funai, E. F., & Illuzzi, J. L. (2011). Contributing indications to the rising cesarean delivery rate. *Obstetrics and Gynecology*, *118*(1), 29–38. Retrieved from http://doi.org/10.1097/AOG.0b013e31821e5f65

Bateman, A. W., & Fonagy, P. (2008). 8-year follow-up of patients treated for borderline personality disorder: Mentalization-based treatment versus treatment as usual. *The American Journal of Psychiatry*, *165*(5), 631–638. doi:10.1176/appi.ajp.2007.07040636

Bateman, A. W., Gunderson, J., & Mulder, R. (2015). Treatment of personality disorder. *The Lancet*, *385*(9969), 735–743. doi:10.1016/S0140-6736(14)61394-5

Becker, D. (1997). *Through the looking glass: Women and borderline personality disorder*. Boulder, CO: Westview Press.

Bender, D. S., Dolan, R. T., Skodol, A. E., Sanislow, C. A., Dyck, I. R., McGlashan, T. H., ... Gunderson, J. G. (2001). Treatment utilization by patients with personality disorders. *American Journal of Psychiatry*, *158*(295), 295–302. Retrieved from http://dx.doi.org/10.1176/appi.ajp.158.2.295

Biskin, R. S., & Paris, J. (2012). Diagnosing borderline personality disorder. *Canadian Medical Association Journal*, *184*(16), 1789–1794. doi:10.1503/cmaj.090618

Brown, P. (1990). The name game: Toward a sociology of diagnosis. *Journal of Mind and Behavior*, *11*(3–4), 385–406.

Carpenter, R. W., & Trull, T. J. (2012). Components of emotion dysregulation in borderline personality disorder: A review. *Current Psychiatry Reports, 15*(335). doi:10.1007/s11920-012-0335-2

Charmaz, K. (2006). *Constructing grounded theory: A practical guide through qualitative analysis*. Los Angeles, CA: Sage.

Clark, A., Mamo, L., Fosket, J., Fishman, J., & Shim, J. (2010). *Biomedicalization: Technoscience, health and illness in the US*. Durham, NC: Duke University Press.

Clarke, M., Hafner, R. J., & Holme, G. (1995). Borderline personality disorder: A challenge for mental health services. *Australian and New Zealand Journal of Psychiatry, 29*(3), 409–414. doi:10.3109/00048679509064948

Clarkin, J. F., Levy, K. N., Lenzenweger, M. F., & Kernberg, O. F. (2007). Evaluating three treatments for borderline personality disorder: A multiwave study. *The American Journal of Psychiatry, 164*(6), 922–928.

Coid, J., Yang, M., Tyrer, P., Robers, A., & Ullrich, S. (2006). Prevalence and correlates of personality disorder in Great Britain. *British Journal of Psychiatry, 188*, 423–431. doi:10.1192/bjp.188.5.423

Conrad, P. (2007). *The medicalization of society: On the transformation of human conditions into treatable disorders*. Baltimore, MD: Johns Hopkins University Press.

Conrad, P., & Schneider, J. W. (1980). *Deviance & medicalization: From badness to sickness*. St. Louis, MO: Mosby.

Fiore, R. J. (1988). Toward engaging the difficult patient. *Journal of Contemporary Psychotherapy, 18*(2), 87–106.

Gallop, R., Lancee, W. J., & Garfinkel, P. (1989). How nursing staff respond to the label borderline personality disorder. *Hospital Community Psychiatry, 40*(8), 815–819. Retrieved from http://dx.doi.org/10.1176/ps.40.8.815

Giddens, A. (1984). *The constitution of society*. Berkeley, CA: The University of California Press.

Godderis, R. (2011). From talk to action: Mapping the diagnostic process in psychiatry. In P. J. McGann & D. J. Hutson (Eds.), *Sociology of diagnosis* (pp. 133–154). *Advances in Medical Sociology*. Bingley, UK: Emerald Group Publishing Limited.

Goffman, E. (1962). *Asylums: Essays on the social situation of mental patients and other inmates*. Chicago, IL: Aldine Publishing Company.

Goffman, E. (1963). *Stigma: Notes on the management of a spoiled identity*. New York, NY: Simon & Schuster.

Grant, B., Chou, S. P., Goldstein, R., Huang, B., Stinson, F., Saha, T., … Ruan, W. J. (2008). Prevalence, correlates, disability, and comorbidity of DSM-IV borderline personality disorder: Results from the wave 2 national epidemiologic survey on alcohol and related conditions. *The Journal of Clinical Psychiatry, 69*(4), 533–545. Retrieved from http://www.ncbi.nlm.nih.gov/pmc/articles/PMC2676679/pdf/nihms101410.pdf

Gunderson, J. G., Morey, L. C., & Stout, R. L. (2004). Major depressive disorder and borderline personality disorder revisited: Longitudinal interactions. *Journal of Clinical Psychiatry, 65*(8), 1049–1056.

Horwitz, A. V. (2002). *Creating mental illness*. Chicago, IL: The University of Chicago Press.

Horwitz, A. V., & Wakefield, J. (2012). *The loss of sadness: How psychiatry transformed normal sorrow into depressive disorder*. New York, NY: Oxford University Press.

Ingenhover, T., Lafay, P., Rinne, T., Passchier, J., & Duivenvoorden, H. (2010). Effectiveness of pharmacotherapy for severe personality disorders: Meta-analyses of randomized controlled trials. *Journal of Clinical Psychiatry*, *71*, 14–25.

Karp, D. A. (2007). *Is it me or my meds?: Living with antidepressants*. Cambridge, MA: Harvard University Press.

Kelly, M., & May, D. (1982). Good and bad patients: A review of the literature and a theoretical critique. *Journal of Advanced Nursing*, *7*(2), 147–156. doi:10.1111/j.1365-2648.1982.tb00222.x

Kelly, T. (2009). *Healing the broken mind: Transforming America's failed mental health system*. New York, NY: New York University.

Kirk, S., & Kutchins, H. (1992). *The selling of DSM: The rhetoric of science in psychiatry*. Piscataway, NJ: Aldine.

Koekkoek, B. (2015). Comment on 'does 'difficult patient' status contribute to functional demedicalization? The case of borderline personality disorder.' *Social Science and Medicine*, *145*, 138–139. doi:10.1016/j.socscimed.2015.09.038

Koekkoek, B., van Meijel, B., & Hutschemaekers, G. (2006). "Difficult patients" in mental health care: A review. *Psychiatric Services*, *57*(6), 795–802.

Kuo, J., Khoury, J., Metcalfe, R., Fitzpatrick, S., & Goodwill, A. (2015). An examination of the relationship between childhood emotional abuse and borderline personality disorder features: The role of difficulties with emotion regulation. *Child Abuse and Neglect*, *39*, 147–155. doi:10.1016/j.chiabu.2014.08.008

Kutchins, H., & Kirk, S. A. (1987). DSM-III and social work malpractice. *Social Work*, *32*(3), 205–211. Retrieved from http://www.jstor.org/stable/23715180

Leichsenring, F., Leibing, E., Kruse, J., New, A. S., & Leweke, F. (2011). Borderline personality disorder. *The Lancet*, *377*(9759), 74–84. doi:10.1016/S0140-6736(10)61422-5

Lenzenweger, M. F., Lane, M. C., Loranger, A. W., & Kessler, R. C. (2007). DSM-IV personality disorders in the national comorbidity survey replication. *Biological Psychiatry*, *62*(6), 553–564. doi:10.1016/j.biopsych.2006.09.019

Lieb, K., Vollm, B., Rucker, G., Timmer, A., & Stoffers, J. M. (2010). Pharmacotherapy for borderline personality disorder: Cochrane systematic review of randomised trials. *British Journal of Psychiatry*, *196*(1), 4–12. doi:10.1192/bjp.bp.108.062984

Lieb, K., Zanarini, M. C., Schmahl, C., Linehan, M. M., & Bohus, M. (2004). Borderline personality disorder. *The Lancet*, *364*(9432), 453–461. doi:10.1016/S01406736(04)16770-6

Linehan, M. M. (1987). Dialectical behavior therapy for borderline personality disorder: Theory and method. *Bulletin of the Menninger Clinic*, *51*(3), 261–276.

Linehan, M. M. (1993). *Cognitive-behavioral treatment of borderline personality disorder*. New York, NY: Guilford.

Linehan, M. M., Comtois, K. A., Murray, A. M., Brown, M. Z., Gallop, R. J., Heard, H. L., ... Lindenboim, N. (2006). Two-year randomized controlled trial and follow-up of dialectical behavior therapy vs therapy by experts for suicidal behaviors and borderline personality disorder. *Archives of General Psychiatry*, *63*(7), 757–766. doi:10.1001/archpsyc.63.7.757

Luhrmann, T. M. (2001). *Of two minds: An anthropologist looks at American psychiatry*. New York, NY: Vintage Books.

Manning, N. (2000). Psychiatric diagnosis under conditions of uncertainty: Personality disorder, science and professional legitimacy. *Sociology Health & Illness*, *22*(5), 621–639. doi:10.1111/1467-9566.00223

Metzl, J. M. (2009). *The protest psychosis: How schizophrenia became a black disease*. Boston, MA: Beacon Press.

Miller, L. S., Bergstrom, D. A., Cross, H. J., & Grube, J. W. (1981). Opinions and use of the DSM system by practicing psychologists. *Professional Psychology*, *12*(3), 385–390. Retrieved from http://dx.doi.org/10.1037/0735-7028.12.3.385

Millon, T. (1983). The DSM III: An insider's perspective. *American Psychologist*, *38*(7), 804–814. Retrieved from http://dx.doi.org/10.1037/0003-066X.38.7.804

Morgan, D. L. (2008). Snowball sampling. In L. M. Given (Ed.), *The SAGE encyclopedia of qualitative research methods* (pp. 816–817). Thousand Oaks, CA: Sage.

Nehls, N. (1998). Borderline personality disorder: Stigma, gender stereotypes & limited system of care. *Issues in Mental Health Nursing*, *19*(2), 97–112. doi:10.1080/016128498249105

Nehls, N. (1999). Borderline personality disorder: The voice of patients. *Research in Nursing & Health*, *22*(4), 285–293. doi:10.1002/(SICI)1098-240x.

Oldham, J., Skodol, A. E., & Bender, D. S. (2005). *Textbook of personality disorders*. Arlington, VA: American Psychiatric Publishing.

Orr, J. (2010). Biopsychiatry and the informatics of diagnosis: Governing mentalities. In A. Clark, L. Mamo, J. Fosket, J. Fishman, & J. Shim (Eds.), *Biomedicalization: Technoscience, health and illness in the US* (pp. 353–379). Durham, NC: Duke University Press.

Paris, J. (1994). The etiology of borderline personality disorder: A biopsychosocial approach. *Psychiatry: Interpersonal and Biological Processes*, *57*(4), 316–325. doi:10.1521/00332747.1994.11024696

Schwartz, S. R., & Goldfinger, S. M. (1981). The new chronic patient: Clinical characteristics of an emerging subgroup. *Hospital & Community Psychiatry*, *32*(7), 470–474. Retrieved from http://dx.doi.org/10.1176/ps.32.7.470

Skodol, A. E., Buckley, P., & Charles, E. (1983). Is there a characteristic pattern to the treatment history of clinic outpatients with borderline personality? *Journal of Nervous & Mental Disease*, *171*(7), 405–410.

Skodol, A. E., Gunderson, J. G., McGlashan, T. H., Dyck, I. R., Stout, R. L., Bender, D. S., … Oldham, J. M. (2002). Functional impairment in patients with schizotypal, borderline, avoidant, or obsessive-compulsive personality disorder. *The American Journal of Psychiatry*, *159*(2), 276–283.

Small, M. L. (2009). "How many cases do I need?": On science and the logic of case selection in field-based research. *Ethnography*, *10*(1), 5–38. doi:10.1177/1466138108099586.

Spitzer, R., Williams, J., & Skodol, A. (1980). DSM-III: The major achievements and an overview. *American Journal of Psychiatry*, *137*(2), 151–164.

Stern, A. (1938). Psychoanalytic investigation of and therapy in the border line group of neuroses. *Psychoanalytic Quarterly*, *7*, 467–489.

Sulzer, S. H. (2015a). Challenging the discourse of untreatability for borderline personality disorder: A call for comparative research. *Social Science and Medicine*, *146*, 223–224.

Sulzer, S. H. (2015b). Does difficult patient status contribute to de facto demedicalization? The case of borderline personality disorder. *Social Science and Medicine*, *142*, 82–89.

Swartz, M., Blazer, D., George, L., & Winfield, I. (1990). Estimating the prevalence of borderline personality disorder in the community. *Journal of Personal Disorders*, *4*(3), 257–272. doi:10.1521/pedi.1990.4.3.257

Szasz, T. S. (1961). *The myth of mental illness: Foundations of a theory of personal conduct*. New York, NY: Hoeber-Harper.

Torgersen, S., Kringlen, E., & Cramer, V. (2001). The prevalence of personality disorders in a community sample. *Archives of General Psychiatry*, *58*(6), 590–596. doi:10.1001/archpsyc.58.6.590

Treloar, A. (2009). A qualitative investigation of the clinician experience of working with borderline personality disorder. *New Zealand Journal of Psychology*, *38*(2), 30–34.

Whooley, O. (2010). Diagnostic ambivalence: Psychiatric workarounds and the diagnostic and statistical manual of mental disorders. *Sociology of Health & Illness*, *32*(3), 452–469. doi:10.1111/j.1467-9566.2010.01230.x

Whooley, O., & Horwitz, A. V. (2013). The paradox of professional success: Grand ambition, furious resistance, and the derailment of the DSM-5 revision process. In J. Paris & J. Phillips (Eds.), *Making the DSM-5: Concepts and controversies* (pp. 75–94). New York, NY: Springer.

Widiger, T. A., & Weissman, M. M. (1991). Epidemiology of borderline personality disorder. *Hospital & Community Psychiatry*, *42*(10), 1015–1021.

Wirth-Cauchon, J. (2001). *Women and borderline personality disorder: Symptoms & stories*. New Brunswick, NJ: Rutgers University Press.

Zanarini, M. C. (2004). Update on pharmacotherapy of borderline personality disorder. *Current Psychiatry Reports*, *6*(1), 66–70.

SOLDIER, ELDER, PRISONER, WARD: PSYCHOTROPICS IN THE ERA OF TRANSINSTITUTIONALIZATION

Anthony R. Hatch, Marik Xavier-Brier, Brandon Attell and Eryn Viscarra

ABSTRACT

Purpose – *This chapter uses Goffman's concept of total institutions in a comparative case study approach to explore the role of psychotropic drugs in the process of transinstitutionalization.*

Methodology/approach – *This chapter interprets psychotropic drug use across four institutionalized contexts in the United States: the active-duty U.S. military, nursing homes and long-term care facilities, state and federal prisons, and the child welfare system.*

Findings – *This chapter documents a major unintended consequence of transinstitutionalization – the questionable distribution of psychotropics among vulnerable populations. The patterns of psychotropic use we synthesize suggest that total institutions are engaging in ethically and medically questionable practices and that psychotropics are being used to*

50 Years after Deinstitutionalization: Mental Illness in Contemporary Communities
Advances in Medical Sociology, Volume 17, 291–317

ISSN: 1057-6290/doi:10.1108/S1057-629020160000017010

serve the bureaucratic imperatives for social control in the era of transinstitutionalization.

Practical implications – *Psychotropic prescribing practices require close surveillance and increased scrutiny in institutional settings in the United States. The flows of mentally ill people through a vast network of total institutions raises questions about the wisdom and unintended consequences of psychotropic distribution to vulnerable populations, despite health policy makers' efforts regulating their distribution. Medical sociologists must examine trans-institutional power arrangements that converge around the mental health of vulnerable groups.*

Originality/value – *This is the first synthesis and interpretive review of psychotropic use patterns across institutional systems in the United States. This chapter will be of value to medical sociologists, mental health professionals and administrators, pharmacologists, health system pharmacists, and sociological theorists.*

Keywords: Psychotropics; transinstitutionalization; vulnerable populations; U.S. military; drugs

INTRODUCTION: THE ROLE OF PSYCHOTROPIC DRUGS IN TRANSINSTITUTIONALIZATION

Psychotropic drugs are widely distributed within the United States, a therapeutic practice that has become a cause of great concern. Psychotropics is an umbrella term that encompasses several subclasses of prescription drugs (antipsychotics, antidepressants, mood stabilizers, stimulants, and anti-anxiety drugs) that change brain chemistry and affect the functioning of the central nervous system (CNS). Psychotropic drug use has steadily increased among non-institutionalized adolescent and adult populations in the United States (Gu, Dillon, & Burt, 2010; Jonas, Gu, & Albertorio-Diaz, 2013; Paulose-Ram, Safran, Jonas, Gu, & Orwig, 2007; Pratt, Brody, & Gu, 2011; Smith, 2012). General practitioners, who are not typically trained to recognize and diagnose mental illnesses, are more likely to prescribe psychotropics to patients than are psychiatrists (Glied & Frank, 2009; Mark, Levit, & Buck, 2009). As a result, one in five American adults now take at least one psychotropic drug (Smith, 2012). These contemporary treatment practices stand in the long shadow of the deinstitutionalization of state psychiatric hospitals in the United States. In this chapter, we ask what role did psychotropic drugs play in the process of transinstitutionalization of mentally ill populations in the United States? We use Goffman's concept of total institutions within a comparative case study approach to explore the role that psychotropic drugs have played in the process of transinstitutionalization.

When Thorazine was approved by the Food and Drug Administration (FDA) in 1954, the mass migration of hundreds of thousands of mentally ill people out of state psychiatric hospitals and into other custodial institutions was well underway (Ødegard, 1964; Scull, 1977). While drug companies, hospital staff, and mental health policy makers heralded the great therapeutic transformation the drugs represented at the policy level, the introduction and rapid diffusion of antipsychotic drugs into state psychiatric hospitals in the mid-1950s did not lead to significant increases in hospital discharges (Gronfein, 1985). Rather, psychotropic drugs entered the context of national mental health system reform in the United States at the moment that state psychiatric hospitals became the object of great public and policy scrutiny. Gronfein (1985) makes a useful distinction between operational deinstitutionalization, which refers to the hospital discharge rate, and policy deinstitutionalization, which refers to the formal policy shift from state to federal jurisdictional control over the care and lives of mentally ill people. Antipsychotics may not have "started the engine" of deinstitutionalization, but they "provided the fuel that initially made it run" (Torrey, 2014, p. 33). More generally, psychotropic drugs may not have "opened the back door" of state psychiatric hospitals, but they kept that back door open by providing a means by which to humanely treat mentally ill people in community settings (Paulson, 2012; Torrey, 2014). More importantly, psychotropics followed mental illness out of the back door of the asylum and into the front door of other institutional settings, where they currently constitute the principle treatment modality for mentally ill people (Frank, Conti, & Goldman, 2005).

The failure to establish community mental health centers across the country coupled with the nation's decision to close the great majority of state hospitals created a permanent institutional crisis for hundreds of thousands of mentally ill people (Davis, Fulgniti, Krigel, & Brekke, 2012; Fuller, 2014; Paulson, 2012; Ray & Finley, 1994). The closure of state psychiatric hospitals generated a number of unintended consequences for other social institutions that already served populations with mental illness. While outpatient mental health care provided some relief for milder cases of disorder in community settings (Glied & Frank, 2009), institutions that still provided custodial care constituted a patchwork network of total institutions that could receive more severely impaired populations.

Broad transfers of mentally ill people from state hospitals to other institutions has been described as transinstitutionalization (Bachrach, 1976; Brown, 1985; Warren, 1981). Warren (1981) defines transinstitutionalization as "the transfer of mental patients, juveniles, and the elderly from facilities funded by state and county to facilities organized by entrepreneurs who provide beds, food, and clothing from the various types of welfare payment received by clientele and/or from insurance plans" (p. 726). Transinstitutionalization represented a cyclical effort to shift the financial and political responsibility for mentally ill people from state institutions to federal and private institutions and back again (Morrissey & Goldman, 1986). The process of deinstitutionalization not only had the effect of growing the populations of mentally ill people in nursing homes, jails, and prisons directly, it also created a context in which these total institutions would later become linked, this time indirectly, to one another in new ways that converge around the widespread use of psychotropics.

While custodial institutions vary with respect to their specific institutional practices and bureaucratic aims, they form an interlocking network of total institutions that circulate large numbers of people who already have mental illness and who are exposed to social conditions that create mental illness. Consider the following linkages. Parental deployment as part of the labor of military service men and women, parental imprisonment, and serious mental illnesses all contribute to the number of children in the child welfare system and foster care (Radel & Bramlett, 2014; Roberts, 2012; Vandivere, Yrausquin, Allen, Malm, & McKlindon, 2012). An alarming number of recent military veterans and adults who spent time in the child welfare system find themselves involved with the criminal justice system (Doyle, 2008; Johnson & Waldfogel, 2002; Jonson-Reid & Barth, 2000; Noonan & Mumola, 2007; Tsai, Rosenheck, Kasprow, & McGuire, 2013). Nursing homes quickly became a primary receptacle for formerly hospitalized mentally ill people, and rapidly expanded due to the fact that Medicaid financed much of their care (Fullerton, McGuire, Feng, Mor, & Grabowski, 2009; Mechanic & McAlpine, 2000; O'Connor, Little, & McManus, 2009; Talbott, 1983; Toff & Scallet, 1986). Beginning in the 1970s and continuing to the present day, there is a direct relationship between hospital closure, the lack of adequate inpatient treatment options, and subsequent increases in proportions of jail and prison populations with mental illness (Prins, 2011; Torrey, 2014; Torrey, Kennard, Eslinger,

Lamb, & Pavle, 2010). Large numbers of mentally ill people did not flow to other total institutions, they began lives as America's new homeless populations (Folsom et al., 2005; Goldman & Morrissey, 1985; U.S. Department of Housing and Urban Development, 2009).

Critics have questioned the effectiveness, overall safety, and clinical appropriateness of psychotropics for treating mental health problems in non-institutionalized civilian life (Dumit, 2012; Healy, 2012; Light, 2010). In addition to these challenges, politicians, and community groups have pressed for regulatory reforms and oversight mechanisms for social groups that are particularly vulnerable to mental illness and live within this network of custody. Consider the string of Congressional hearings focused on the linkages of psychotropics to vulnerable groups. Congress first held hearings on the role that psychotropics played in the process of deinstitutionalization in 1983 (United States, 1983). Congress passed the Omnibus Budget Reconciliation Act of 1987 that regulated the distribution of antipsychotic drugs to elders living in nursing homes, which had the intended effect of lowering antipsychotic use, but the unintended effect of increasing antidepressant use among seniors (Snowdon, Day, & Baker, 2006). Or, recall the Congressional hearings in the 2009 intended to highlight the excessive use of psychotropics among children in foster care (United States, 2009). Finally, consider the more recent Congressional attention focused on the high rate of solider and veterans' suicide and potential linkages to psychotropics (Untied States, 2010). The scientific and policy debates advocating for tighter regulations over psychotropics distribution within different institutional settings have unfolded in relative isolation from one another, as if these social formations do not share a common history or purpose.

THEORETICAL FRAMEWORK: GOFFMAN'S TOTAL INSTITUTIONS

Erving Goffman famously used Everett Hughes' concept of "total institutions" to describe an all-encompassing bureaucratic custodial institution that establishes states of social closure and the rationalization of daily life for its inhabitants (including staff and inmates) (Burns, 1991; Goffman, 1961). Total institutions have three principal organizational features. First, they establish forms of physical and psychological closure between the people who live and work within them and the outside world. Second, they organize the conduct of life through a rational plan that schedules the activities of everyday living and limits individuals' autonomy to choose how to live. Third, they are bureaucratically organized and highly regulated institutions characterized by two antagonistic social and cultural worlds, one for the inmates and another for the staff. At the level of social action, total institutions generate the diminishment of individuals' identities and self-mortification, role disposition, and unfitness for the outside world through a series of rituals connected to admission, treatment regimes, and staff/inmate interactions (Burns, 1991). Total institutions are "the forcing houses for changing persons" that serves as a "natural experiment on what can be done to the self" (Goffman, 1961, p. 12).

According to Goffman's original typology, there are five types of total institutions: (1) welfare institutions for the blind, the aged, the orphaned, and the indigent; (2) medical institutions for persons in need of inpatient physical or mental health care (e.g., tuberculosis sanitaria, mental hospitals, and leprosaria); (3) penal institutions like prisons, jails, concentration and war camps; (4) institutions organized around specific kinds of work and labor (e.g., army barracks, ships, boarding schools, work campus, colonial compounds, large mansions); and (5) religious training and practice institutions (e.g., abbeys, monasteries, convents, and cloisters) (Goffman, 1961, pp. 4–5).

The purpose of total institutions is to serve as "storage dumps" for people who require management according to rationally defined bureaucratic aims (Goffman, 1961, p. 7). All aspects of life within them are highly regulated under one official authority, inmates are required to do the same activities together in public, and "the various enforced activities are brought together into a single rational plan purportedly designed to fulfill the official aims of the institution" (Goffman, 1961, p. 6). The great contradiction of total institutions is the tension between their professed goals (caring for the mentally ill or sick, protecting the aged or vulnerable, guarding the dangerous, etc.) and their undeclared use as dumping grounds for society's outcasts (Burns, 1991, p. 157). In accordance with cultural ideas about humane treatment, total institutions do work on people in ways that tend to conflict with bureaucratic efficiency and cost associated with custody. For us, the concept of total institutions is useful theoretically because it highlights the centrality of closure, rationalization, and bureaucracy for contemporary institutions that warehouse large numbers of mentally ill persons.

We use Goffman's concept of total institutions to guide our comparative analysis of psychotropic use patterns in the context of transinstitutionalization.

For our comparative analysis, we have selected four types of total institutions that correspond to four of Goffman's types: state and federal prisons (penal), the foster care system (welfare), nursing homes and assisted care living facilities (medical/welfare), and the active-duty military (labor). Furthermore, we have elected to aggregate large numbers of individual institutions into distinctive "cases" as a strategy to define each case through what they seek to accomplish and the practical means by which they achieve their goals. We recognize that this institutional aggregation into theoretically defined cases potentially obscures a great deal of heterogeneity among institutions. However, we believe that they ought to be critically compared using a robust sociological interpretation of the patterns of psychotropic distribution between them. Taken together, the patterns of psychotropic use we synthesize suggest that total institutions are engaging in ethically and medically questionable practices and that psychotropics are being used to serve the bureaucratic imperatives for social control in the era of transinstitutionalization. In each case, we organize our comparisons around four key findings: (1) high and increasing percentages of psychotropic use; (2) polypharmacy; (3) group disparities in the prescribing of psychotropics; and (4) limited use of psychotherapy.

FOUR CASE STUDIES

Case #1: The Active-Duty Military

The U.S. Armed Forces is made up of five branches: the Army, Air Force, Navy, Marine Corps, and Coast Guard. All branches, except for the Coast Guard fall under the jurisdiction of the Department of Defense (DoD); the Department of Homeland Security controls the Coast Guard. The Department of Defense is the United States' oldest and largest government agency. There are over 1.4 million women and men on active duty and 718,000 civilian personnel, who makes the DoD the nation's largest employer. The overall mission of the Department of Defense is to protect national security and provide the military forces needed to deter war.

In the wake of 9/11, active-duty soldiers have been deployed repeatedly to conduct war operations in the so-called "War on Terror" and, in the process, are exposed to multiple traumas and high levels of enduring stress in live combat zones. Psychotropics are used to help alleviate or control symptoms of insomnia, anxiety, nerves, and post-traumatic stress disorder

(PTSD) symptoms, although estimates vary on the numbers of active-duty soldiers taking these drugs. A June 2010 report from the Defense Department's Pharmacoeconomic Center showed that 213,972 (or 20 percent) of the 1.1 million active-duty troops surveyed were taking some type of psychotropic drug in the form of antidepressants, antipsychotics, sedative hypnotics, or other controlled substances (Brewin, 2011).

In 2001, the Department of Defense changed its long-standing Central Command policy (CENTCOM) forbidding the use of psychotropics by active-duty military and military psychiatrists began to distribute these drugs to manage the traumatic stress of war with the goal of keeping them ready for duty (Benedick, 2007; Bray et al., 2010; Brewin, 2011). The CENTCOM policy allows troops a 90- or 180-day supply of psychotropic drugs that are listed in their Central Nervous System (CNS) formulary before they are deployed for combat. Peter Breggin notes "Drugs such as Valium and Xanax, used to treat depression, [and] the antipsychotic Seroquel, originally developed to treat schizophrenia, bipolar disorders, mania and depression" all appear on the military's formulary (Breggin, 2012). The irony of this policy shift is that prior to 9/11, civilians could not enlist into the armed forces if they were on any of these psychotropic drugs, particularly stimulants (Batasch, 2012; Breggin, 2012). One of the reasons for this policy shift was increased criticism for not prescribing enough medications, especially for pain management, citing that military doctors were prescribing at rates much lower than civilian doctors (Dao, Carey, & Frosch, 2011; Murphy, 2012).

According to documents from the Defense Logistics Agency, the military has spent $1.1 billion dollars since 2001 on psychiatric drugs and pain medications (Dao et al., 2011; O'Meara, 2013). Between 2005 and 2011, there was a 76 percent increase in all psychotropics prescribed to active-duty troops: orders for antipsychotics increased by 200 percent, anti-anxiety drugs by 170 percent, anti-epileptics by 70 percent, and antidepressants by 40 percent (Tilghman & McGarry, 2010). In the words of military officials, psychotropics are openly deployed in combat zones to "conserve the fighting strength" (Benedek, Schneider, & Bradley, 2007, p. 685) and to "enhance performance" (West, 2012). Military psychiatrists argue that psychotropics are helpful and to deprive soldiers of these medications, or to foster fear about these drugs, would be damaging to soldiers' health and their ability to fight war (Batasch, 2012). The military defends this practice by stating that it is necessary to take calculated risks in prescribing these drugs because many service members have three or more deployment operations. Knowlan (2001) surveyed 732 Navy physicians regarding their current use of and attitude toward prescribing psychotropics for deployable personnel. Some Navy physicians support the continued use of psychotropics for active-duty troops because selective serotonin reuptake inhibitors (SSRIs), for example, are seen as less dangerous and highly effective in managing combat stress (Knowlan, 2001). These physicians argue that compared to older drugs, the potential benefits of these newer antidepressants far outweigh the possible side effects (Knowlan, 2001).

As the inability to serve has become an increasingly significant issue over the past two decades for active-duty soldiers, military officials may reserve the right to administer psychotropics involuntarily (Grant & Resnick, 1989). Grant and Resnick (1989) examined the development of federal laws and constitutional principles that inform court decisions regarding soldiers' right to refuse treatment of psychotropic medication. These practices, which may include involuntary hospitalization, could be linked to the U.S. military wanting to expedite the return of troops to duty and maximize hospital stays. At the time of their study, Grant and Resnick (1989) found there were no protocols for the treatment of soldiers for involuntary prescribing and hospitalization. This rationality introduces new risks into the military as a total institution that extend back into civilian society (Smith, 2011). These high rates of psychotropic use and their effects on prisoners' bodies have been linked to subsequent increases in suicide and violent behavior, including sexual assault and violence (Batasch, 2012; Breggin, 2012; Dao et al., 2011; Heyes, 2012; Kuehn, 2010; Murphy, 2012; Sheehan, 2009; Willis, 2012). According to the FDA, all antidepressants have a label stating that young adults (up to the age of 24) have an increased rate of suicidality when taking these drugs in short-term, controlled clinical trials. According to official statistics obtained by the Associated Press (AP), solider suicides were averaging almost one per day in 2012, which is the fastest pace in the nation's decade long war (Burns, 2012). Further, the AP reported that there were 154 suicides for active-duty soldiers in the first 155 days of 2012, which is more than the numbers killed in action in Afghanistan (almost 50 percent more) according to Pentagon statistics (Burns, 2012).

Critics also point to issues such as soldiers being deployed with 180 days of medication, much longer than the common six-week clinical trial (Breggin, 2012), and the ability for soldiers to trade medications freely among themselves (Batasch, 2012; Breggin, 2012; Murphy, 2012). This practice of deploying soldiers with large quantities of psychotropics at their disposal has allowed for troops to "stockpile" medications, which is the common reason for overdoses and inappropriate drug switching or trading (Dao et al., 2011). Further, with active-duty soldiers, the extended time on the battlefield makes it difficult to schedule follow-up appointments or monitor the effects of these drugs. Not only are overmedication and little follow-up serious problems, but many of these soldiers are prescribed several drugs at one time (polypharmacy) and the knowledge of how these drugs interact with each other is still largely unknown, especially in long-term situations (Bray et al., 2010; Breggin, 2012; Dao et al., 2011). Recognizing that these are indeed dire issues, some bases have begun "give back" days, where soldiers can return unused medication; while others have been trying different strategies to help treat issues related to combat (Clark, 2012). Some bases have started trying to extend their therapy programs instead of just relying on drugs alone, which has proven to be effective in helping treat PTSD. While strategies like "exposure therapy" may be effective, both access to and desire to seek psychiatric help may be limited (Clark, 2012).

The military also has a shortage of trained psychiatrists that are available to active-duty troops (Dao et al., 2011; Jeffrey, Rankin, & Jeffrey, 1992). Not only is there a stigma against seeking treatment (Magnezi, Zrihen, Ashkenazi, & Lubin, 2007), but if a soldier does indeed seek out a military psychologist, there is no guarantee of patient privacy rights (Jeffrey et al., 1992). The Department of Defense reserves the right to a patient's records in a "need to know" situation, without operationalizing what exactly constitutes "need to know" (Jeffrey et al., 1992). This lack of confidentiality inevitably leads to service members not seeking out psychologists to address these issues, not only because of the gendered expectations associated with masculine behavior, but also being treated for psychological problems may be detrimental to advancement within the military itself (Jeffrey et al., 1992). All of these issues when examined collectively may contribute to active-duty soldiers being solely reliant on psychotropics for their mental health needs.

Case #2: Elder Long-Term Care Facilities

Elders are admitted to nursing home and assisted care facilities when their social needs and health problems have outstretched their families' ability to care for them. According to the Nursing Home Data Compendium of 2012, an annual survey of nursing homes compiled by the U.S. Government's Centers for Medicare and Medicaid Services, there are approximately 15,683 nursing home facilities in the United States in 2011, and the majority of these facilities are operated by for-profit companies (69 percent). More than 1.4 million senior citizens were living in nursing homes in the United States as of December 2011. Fifteen percent of the nursing home population is under the age of 65, while nearly eight percent is over the age of 95. Women make up nearly two-thirds of the nursing home population. Additionally, non-Hispanic whites also constitute approximately 75 percent of nursing home residents (CMS, 2012).

Psychotropics are used among elders to treat neurological disorders and mental illnesses that plague seniors such as dementia and depression. Bagachi, Verdier, and Simon (2009) found that the most reliable estimates for rates of mental illness in elderly nursing home residents come from the National Nursing Home Survey (NNHS), which estimates that approximately 6.8 percent of residents live with a mental illness. However, most studies of nursing home residents place the rates of mental illness at a much higher percentage. Molinari et al. (2011) found 73 percent of elderly nursing home residents had a psychiatric diagnosis at admission, and 85 percent of the residents had a psychiatric diagnosis three months after admission. Similarly, Hoover et al. (2010) found 54.4 percent of nursing home residents received a diagnosis of depression within the first year of being admitted to the facility: 32.8 percent were diagnosed at admission and a further 21.6 percent were diagnosed later during the first year.

Elders living in nursing homes and assisted care living facilities also face a life on psychotropics. Fears of becoming a "zombie in home" have become realized and are terrifyingly commonplace. The abuse of antipsychotic drugs became so rampant in the United States that Congress passed the *Nursing Home Reform Amendment* as part of the *Omnibus Budget Reconciliation Act of 1987* (OBRA-87) to combat the overuse of antipsychotic drugs in nursing homes (Garrard, Chen, & Dowd, 1995). A review of psychotropic prescribing practices for nursing home residents suggests that while there has been a decrease in the prescribing of antipsychotic medications since the implementation of the OBRA-87 amendment, prescriptions for antidepressants and anxiolytic drugs among nursing home residents have increased (Hughes & Lepane, 2005). Overall, rates of psychotropic drugs use have doubled since the 1990s, especially in facilities in which doctor-patient contact is minimal (Hanlon et al., 2011). Currently, somewhere between 25 percent and 50 percent nursing home residents use psychotropic drugs (Dwyer et al., 2009; Gaboda, Lucas, Siegel, Kalay, & Crystal, 2011). One comprehensive study of over 12,500 nursing homes between 1996 and 2006 documented a doubling in the proportion of residents who received a psychotropic prescription: from 21.9 percent in 1996 to 47.5 percent in 2006 (Hanlon, Handler, & Castle, 2010), and one study found that more than half of the new nursing home residents are prescribed psychotropics within two weeks of their admittance (Voyer & Martin, 2003). These prescribing data are much higher than the reported rates of mental illness in nursing home populations, which suggests the possibility of inappropriate prescribing.

Many seniors are receiving medications for mental illness without appropriate diagnoses. Briesacher et al. (2005) found that approximately one in four residents receive psychotropic medications despite no appropriate indications for psychotropic medication. Other studies have identified discrepancies between residents with legitimate mental diagnoses and rates of psychotropic medication use. A study by Molinari et al. (2011) suggests that 11 percent of nursing home residents are receiving psychotropic medications despite no diagnosis of mental illness. Gaboda et al. (2011) also found that approximately 15 percent of residents were given psychotropic medications without a proper diagnosis. Elder veterans may be at an increased risk of misuse of psychotropic medications. Hanlon et al. (2011) found that nearly 43 percent of elderly veterans were prescribed an antidepressant, despite having no diagnosed mental illness. A 2011 audit of 73 individual nursing home patient records revealed that while only 73 percent of the cases had a mental health diagnosis at admission, 85 percent of these residents were on psychotropics and 19 percent were on four or more drugs simultaneously, while only 50 percent of residents' files recommended behavioral strategies for coping with forms of distress (Molinari et al., 2011).

Furthermore, psychotropic drugs are often given to residents for purposes other than those originally indicated for the medication. A study by Briesacher et al. (2005) found less than half (41.8 percent) of residents received antipsychotic therapy in accordance with prescribing guidelines. Increasingly, atypical antipsychotic medications are being prescribed to elderly patients for off-label indications. Kamble, Chen, Sherer, and Aparasu (2008) found an overall prevalence of 23.45 percent of elderly residents using atypical antipsychotic medications despite increased risk of death, stroke, and neurologic problems. The largest corporate fraud settlement in U.S. history was over this very issue. Janssen Pharmaceuticals, a Johnson & Johnson subsidiary, was forced to pay $2.2 billion dollars for criminal and civil liability for promoting the off-label use of Risperdal for the treatment of dementia (Department of Justice, 2013).

Often, psychotropics are differentially distributed to members of the older adult population along axes of gender and race. White female residents who are younger than 85 years of age are more likely to receive medications and care for mental illness than members of other race and gender groups (Dwyer, Han, Woodwell, & Reichsteiner, 2009; Karkare,

Bhattaharjee, Kamble, & Aparsu, 2011), while members of some subgroups are less likely to be diagnosed and treated for mental illness. Men, non-Hispanic blacks, residents aged 85 and older, and residents with severe cognitive and physical impairments are often not appropriately diagnosed and treated for mental illnesses such as depression (Gaboda et al., 2011; Hoover et al., 2010; Siegel et al., 2012). Additionally, long-term care facilities that have higher proportions of residents with low levels of education and socioeconomic status are less likely to give the appropriate medications to their residents for depression (Siegel et al., 2012). Veterans may be at an even increased risk of misuse of psychotropic medications. Hanlon et al. (2011) found that nearly 43 percent of elderly veterans were prescribed an antidepressant despite having no diagnosed mental illness.

When these psychotropic medications are combined with other medications, the results of polypharmacy can be dangerous for elders (Dwyer et al., 2009). Seniors taking nine or more different medications are 2.33 times more likely to experience adverse health outcomes than those who receive fewer medications (Nguyen, Fouts, Kotabe, & Lo, 2006). These nursing home residents are at increased adverse health outcomes such as the use of potentially inappropriate drugs, adverse drug events, potential drug-drug interactions, hospitalizations, and higher cost (Tamura, Bell, Inaba, & Masaki, 2012). Dwyer et al. (2009) estimated the prevalence of polypharmacy to be 40 percent in a sample of nursing home residents.

Case #3: State and Federal Prisons

The United States currently incarcerates a greater percentage of its population than any other nation with 1,571,013 persons held within a patchwork of thousands of federal and state institutions at the end of 2012 (Carson & Golinelli, 2012). Simultaneously, prisons have become "the new asylums" that warehouse hundreds of thousands of men and women who have been diagnosed with psychiatric disorders, some of which preceded their detention and many that emerged as a result of their imprisonment (Shenson, Dubler, & Michaels, 1990; Torrey, 1995). In 2005, *more than half* of all people incarcerated in federal, state, and jail facilities suffered from some form of psychiatric distress (Glaze & James, 2006). Today, there are more people with serious psychiatric illness in prisons than there are in America's remaining mental hospitals (Torrey et al., 2010). Psychotropics are used not only to manage existing psychiatric symptoms, but also to help prisoners cope with exposure to stressful prison environments (Massoglia, 2008).

While abuses of prescribed psychotropic medications by drug-seeking prisoners have been documented in the case of the antipsychotic Seroquel (Del Paggio, 2005; Pierre, Shnayder, Wirshing, & Wirshing, 2004; Pinta & Taylor, 2007), most psychotropic distribution in prisons occurs through seemingly legitimate pathways inside prison mental health systems.

Distributing psychotropic drugs is the most prevalent and often the only form of mental health treatment available in prisons (Human Rights Watch, 2003). In 2000, 73 percent of state prisons distributed psychotropic drugs to their prisoners. This was the most common form of mental health treatment followed by initial mental health screening (70 percent), therapy/counseling (71 percent), referrals to mental health services upon re-entry (66 percent), conducting psychiatric assessments (65 percent), and providing 24-hour mental health care (51 percent) (Beck & Maruschak, 2001). The institutional use of psychotropics is positively related to increasing levels of confinement: ninety-five percent (95.3) of maximum/high security State prisons distribute psychotropics, compared to eighty eight percent of medium security (88.7), and sixty-two percent (62.1) of minimum/low security prisons (Beck & Maruschak, 2001).

Data from the 2004 Survey of Inmates in State and Federal Correctional Facilities (SISFCF) shows that inmates with a previously diagnosed mental condition who had been treated with a psychotropic drug in the past, 69.1 percent of federal and 68.8 percent of state inmates received a psychotropic during their incarceration (Wilper et al., 2009). In 2006, 46 percent of Vermont prisoners were taking a psychotropic drug (Prison Legal News, 2008). In 2009, over 16,000 federal prisoners received psychotropics – seven percent of the total federal prison population (Senate Subcommittee, 2009). In 2009, the Corrections Center of Northeast Ohio spent half of its medical budget on psychotropics (Torrey et al., 2010). In July 2002, Clark County jail in Ohio spent more on psychotropics than it did on food (Gottschlich & Cetnar, 2002). Prison psychiatrists are much more likely to prescribe psychotropics to women prisoners, accounting for higher rates of psychiatric diagnoses and symptomology among women (Feinman, 1994; Kilty, 2008; Sommers & Baskin, 1990; Zaitzow, 2010). Research conducted by Baillargeon et al. within the Texas Prison System in the late 1990s showed that African American and Hispanic prisoners were more likely to receive older, more outdated antipsychotics and antidepressants or no pharmacotherapy at all when compared to White prisoners (Baillargeon, Black, Contreras, Grady, & Pulvino, 2001; Baillargeon & Contreras, 2001).

As institutions designed for social control, prisons can assert state power by forcing prisoners to take psychotropics, which it can do if the prisoner is classified as dangerous and if the forced drugging is in the best medical interest of the prisoner (Floyd, 1990). Legal scholars have also addressed the civic implications of the fact that forced medication can be used to establish a defendant's competency to stand trial (Herbel & Stelmach, 2007; Winick, 1977) and to be executed (Zonana, 2003). At the same time, prisoners can also refuse to take psychotropics under certain legal conditions that affirm prisoner's constitutional rights to free speech (Sindel, 1991), bodily integrity (Gostin, 2003), due process (Zeigelmuller, 1993), and other constitutional grounds (Cichon, 1992; Dute, 2001; Floyd, 1990).

We would expect that the policies that structure practices inside prisons are organized through a rationality of security and confinement, even in the case of medical practices, but these policies are also designed to provide care and healing for those who suffer (at least theoretically). In this way, psychotropic drugs are used to manage unruly, violent, and dangerous inmates who seemingly represent a threat to themselves and/or others, but also, and perhaps most importantly, to the logic of control and submission that permeates inmate-institution relationships (Rhodes, 2004). However, prisons are also legally obligated to provide a minimum standard of mental health care to inmates and therefore to withhold psychotropic drugs from a prisoner who is suffering might violate inmates' constitutional right to health care under the "deliberate indifference" standard affirmed by the U.S. Supreme Court (*Estelle v. Gamble*, 1976). Unfortunately, no information is available about the racial patterning of psychotropic drugs inside the U.S. criminal justice system.

Case #4: The Child Welfare System

Finally, youth in the foster care system, who have become wards of the state, often live in group homes and in temporary fostered arrangements with families. During the 2012 fiscal year, the U.S. Department of Health and Human Services (USDHHS) reported 399,546 individuals placed in foster care, with a mean age of 9.1 years, 52 percent males and 48 percent females (U.S. Department of Health and Human Services [USDHHS], 2013). The majority of those in foster care are white (42 percent), with smaller percentages of black (26 percent) and Hispanic youth (21 percent) (USDHHS, 2013). Forty-seven percent of those in foster care are placed with a non-relative foster family, 28 percent with a relative foster family, and 6 percent in a group home (USDHHS, 2013). The average length for the amount of time in foster care was 22.7 months, with just over half of all individuals exiting the system by means of reunification with parents or legal guardians (USDHHS, 2013).

The vast majority of these children have already suffered horrific forms of physical and sexual abuse, and continue to face the threat of death while under state protection. Psychotropics are prescribed to lessen their suffering and nurture them back to a state of wellness and wholeness. Due to differences in sampling techniques, there is no consensus on the true prevalence of prescribing practices. However, looking across the literature rates of psychotropic drug use for this population vary from 15 to upwards of 70 percent (Breland-Noble et al., 2004; dosReis, Zito, Safer, & Soeken, 2001; Handwerk, Smith, Thompson, Spellman, & Daly, 2008; Leslie et al., 2011; Raghavan, Lama, Kohl, & Hamilton, 2010), with rates of psychotropic prescriptions increasing over time across the United States (Rubin, Matone, Huang, Feudtner, & Localio, 2012). Furthermore, rates of psychotropic drug use in foster care settings are upwards of 10 times higher than that of community based samples (McMillen et al., 2004). Not only are many children and youth in foster care prescribed psychotropics, they take these drugs concomitantly. Indeed, evidence from state-wide samples of youth in foster care show that anywhere from 13 to 41 percent of these individuals are prescribed more than one psychotropic at the same time (dosReis et al., 2011; Martin, Van Hoof, Stubbe, Sherwin, & Scahill, 2014; Zito et al., 2008).

Research has also shown noted gender, racial, and age differences in psychotropic drug use among those in foster care. Several studies show that males are more likely than females to be prescribed medications (Ferguson, Glesener, & Raschick, 2006; Leslie et al., 2011; Leslie, Raghavan, Zhang, & Aarons, 2010; Martin, et al., 2014; Raghavan et al., 2005). A 2013 analysis of Medicaid claims in a Mid-Atlantic state found that black youth are more likely to concomitantly use psychotropics than whites (dosReis et al., 2011). At the national level, those aged 12–16 are seven times more likely to use psychotropics than those aged 2–5 (Raghavan et al., 2005). Differences have also been noted regarding in home versus out of home residence. For example, drawing on a state-wide sample of children and youth in North Carolina, Breland-Noble et al. (2004) found that those in group homes are 1.8 times more likely to take psychotropics when compared to those living in foster care. Finally, there is also evidence that the use of psychotropics continues even as those in the system "age out." Raghavan and McMillen (2008) found that in one state, 13 percent of individuals leaving the foster care system were still taking at least one psychotropic. Despite these noted rates of psychotropic drug use, many scholars do not question the prescribing practices. In fact, some researchers have argued that certain populations who meet criteria for psychotropic medications had not yet received adequate treatment (Zima, Bussing, Crecelius, Kaufman, & Belin, 1999).

Given the widespread prevalence of psychotropic drug use among children in the American foster care system, scholars and mental health practitioners alike have begun to call into question the ethics, morality, and practicality of these prescribing practices (Crismon & Argo, 2009; Cummings, 2012; Hunt, 2008). For example, Connor, Ozbayrak, Harrison, and Melloni (1998) and Moses (2008) argue that the potency of psychotropics prescribed to this population is much higher when compared to the general population. McMillen, Fedoravicius, Rowe, Zima, and Ware (2007) interviewed 130 child welfare workers and found that concerns were raised regarding overmedicated children, overuse of psychotropic medication, short inpatient stays, and discontinuities in psychiatric treatment. Some critics have also noted the rise in prescribing practice, which have been as high as a three-fold increase in a 10-year period (Zito et al., 2003).

Across the nation, children living under the auspices of child welfare and protective custody are anywhere from 2 to 4 times more likely to be taking a psychotropic drug than children who living outside the system. In Texas, for example, (2003–2004), 37.9 percent of Medicaid enrolled youth in the system used at least one psychotropic, 41.3 percent of them were prescribed three or more psychotropics. Foster care youth in one mid-Atlantic state took an antipsychotic drug on average 222 out of 365 days of 2003. Also controversial is the extent to which these prescribing practices impact the broader society. Given that children and youth in American foster care are more often than not treated via Medicaid funding, some scholars have questioned the fact that taxpayers pay for this psychotropic consumption (Raghavan et al., 2012). There is also concern regarding who should be held responsible for these practices (Leslie et al., 2005; Naylor et al., 2007). Several scholars (Burton, 2010; Camp, 2010; Mello, 2011) place responsibility on state and federal agencies, claiming that their lack of oversight in prescribing practices violates international laws that protect the welfare of children. Longhofer, Floersch, and Okpych (2011) argue that the open system nature of foster care further complicates the collaboration of psychotropic oversight between state, local, and federal agencies. Burns et al. (2004) question if children with complicated mental health issues should be in foster care to begin with; perhaps they would be better suited in an environment that is specialized for their needs, such as an in-patient center (Lyons & Rogers, 2004).

CONCLUSION

To conclude, we first return to our guiding question: What role did psychotropic drugs play in the processes of transinstitutionalization? Furthermore, what is the continuing significance of Goffman's concept for how we understand the institutionalization of mental health care fifty years after deinstitutionalization? These four cases suggest that psychotropics have played a pivotal role in the process of transinstitutionalization of mentally ill people out of state psychiatric hospitals and through a network of interlocking total institutions. While it is not epidemiologically feasible to track individual bodies through this network, by identifying patterns of psychotropic drug use within the nodes of the network, we can draw several interpretations about the questionable use of psychotropics in America's "storage dumps." The depopulation of state psychiatric hospitals was just one moment of a long-term broader institutional shift in U.S. mental health policy through which mental health crises have come to define institutional life. With no discernable mental health infrastructure for the most impaired citizens and the impossible costs of psychotherapy, U.S. citizens have not had many options for mental health care outside of psychotropics.

As people flow from one institutional context to another, with few viable alternative therapies in place, psychotropics have followed them into the military, the prison, the nursing home, and the child welfare system. While the availability of new psychotropics in the 1950s did not initiate the process of deinstitutionalization in the 1950s, psychotropics certainly made it possible for mental health care providers and patients to treat a range of mental illnesses conditions in settings outside state psychiatric hospitals. Unfortunately, many of these treatment settings, like the asylum model they replaced, are based on confinement and custody, and are therefore potential institutional sites for questionable and inhumane treatment. Psychotropic drugs are increasingly distributed to active-duty soldiers, elders living in nursing homes and long-term care facilities, jail inmates and prisoners, and children living within foster care systems – all vulnerable populations with high rates of mental illness.

The active-duty solider who awaits death, dismemberment, or disability; the prisoner who sits warehoused in an overcrowded and overlooked system of mass incarceration; the abandoned elder who fears being a zombie in the nursing home; and the forsaken and problem child – what they share is that they live in a state of disposability made possible by a social structure that cannot recognize or cope with or substantively remedy their suffering. The purpose of each figure – the solider, the elder, the prisoner, and the ward – and the meaning of their institutionalization lies at the boundary of their traumatic continued existence and their fully anticipated, if not accelerated and purposeful civic death inside total institutions. Determining whether a particular medical practice is understood as legitimate because it promotes life and good health, or, conversely, is understood as illegitimate or questionable because it accelerates death and suffering is contingent on the form of political rationality that justifies the enactment of the practice itself. We do not think that the mass distribution of psychotropic drugs inside total institutions is somehow wholly distinct from the broader patterns in so-called free society; rates of psychotropic drug use in non-institutionalized settings has also increased dramatically over the past 50 years. Rather, we believe that as state psychiatric hospital residents spilled out into the community as a result of deinstitutionalization, *psychotropics came with them* and thus helped to establish a new institutional practice through which social order might be maintained.

REFERENCES

Bachrach, L. (1976). *Deinstitutionalization: An analytical review and sociological perspective.* Washington, DC: National Institute of Mental Health.

Bagachi, A. D., Verdier, J. M., & Simon, S. E. (2009). How many nursing home residents live with a mental illness? *Psychiatric Services, 60*, 958–964.

Baillargeon, J., Black, S. A., Contreras, S., Grady, J., & Pulvino, J. (2001). Anti-depressant prescribing patterns for prison inmates with depressive disorders. *Journal of Affective Disorders, 63*, 225–231.

Baillargeon, J., & Contreras, S. (2001). Antipsychotic prescribing patterns in the Texas prison system. *Journal of the American Academy of Psychiatry and the Law, 21*(1), 48–53.

Batasch, M. (2012). *Report: Army psychotropic drug use on the rise.* Retrieved from http://dailycaller.com/2012/04/11/report-army-psychotropic-drug-use-on-the-rise/

Beck, A., & Maruschak, L. (2001). *Mental health treatment in state prisons.* Washington, DC: Bureau of Justice Statistics.

Benedek, D., Schneider, B., Bradley, J., & Benedek, D. (2007). Psychiatric medications for deployment: An update. *Military Medicine, 172*, 681–685.

Bray, R., Pemberton, M., Lane, M., Hourani, L., Mattiko, M., & Babeu, L. (2010). Substance use and mental health trends among US military active duty personnel: Key findings from the 2008 DoD health behavior survey. *Military Medicine, 175*, 390–399.

Breggin, P. (2012). *Military to hold conference on escalating suicides: Drugs not allowed.* Retrieved from http://www.huffingtonpost.com/dr-peter-breggin/military-suicide_b_1602927.html

Breland-Noble, A., Elbogen, E., Farmer, E., Dubs, M., Wagner, H., & Burns, B. (2004). Use of psychotropic medications by youths in therapeutic foster care and group homes. *Psychiatric Services, 55*, 706–708.

Brewin, B. (2011). *Military's drug policy threatens troops' health, doctors say*. Retrieved from http://www.nextgov.com/health/2011/01/militarys-drug-policy-threatens-troops-health-doctors-say/48321/

Briesacher, B., Limcangco, M., Simoni-Wastila, L., Doshi, J., Levens, S., Shea, D., & Stuart, B. (2005). The quality of antipsychotic drug prescribing in nursing homes. *Archives of Internal Medicine*, *165*, 1280–1285.

Brown, P. (1985). *The transfer of care: Psychiatric deinstitutionalization and its aftermath*. New York, NY: Routledge.

Burns, B., Phillips, S., Wagner, H., Barth, R., Kolko, D., Campbell, Y., & Landsverk, J. (2004). Mental health need and access to mental health services by youth involved with child welfare: A national survey. *Journal of the American Academy of Child and Adolescent Psychiatry*, *43*, 960–970.

Burns, R. (2012). *As suicides rise, military struggles to respond*. Retrieved from http://www.armytimes.com/article/20120608/NEWS/206080308/As-suicides-rise-military-struggles-to-respond

Burns, T. (1991). *Erving Goffman*. London: Routledge.

Burton, A. (2010). 'They use it like candy': How the prescription of psychotropic drugs to state-involved children violates international law. *Brooklyn Journal of International Law*, *35*, 454–513.

Camp, A. (2010). A mistreated epidemic: State and federal failure to adequately regulate psychotropic medications prescribed to children in foster care. *Temple Law Review*, *83*, 369–404.

Carson, A., & Golinelli, D. (2012). *Prisoners in 2012 – Advance counts (NCJ 242467)*. Washington, DC: Bureau of Justice Statistics.

Center for Medicare and Medicaid Services (CMS). (2012). *Nursing home compendium 2012*. Retrieved from http://www.cms.gov/Medicare/Provider-Enrollment-and%20Certification/CertificationandComplianc/downloads/nursinghomedatacompendium_508.pdf

Cichon, D. (1992). The right to "just say no": A history and analysis of the right to refuse antipsychotic drugs. *Los Angeles Law Review*, *53*, 283–426.

Clark, H. (2012). *Fort Campbell's warrior care clinic offers integrative therapies*. Retrieved from http://www.army.mil/article/72673/Fort_Campbell_s_Warrior_Care_Clinic_offers_integrative_therapies/

Connor, D., Ozbayrak, K., Harrison, R., & Melloni, R. (1998). Prevalence and patterns of psychotropic and anticonvulsant medication use in children and adolescents referred to residential treatment. *Journal of Child and Adolescent Psychopharmacology*, *8*, 27–38.

Crismon, M., & Argo, T. (2009). The use of psychotropic medication for children in foster care. *Child Welfare*, *88*, 71–100.

Cummings, M. (2012). Sedating forgotten children: How unnecessary psychotropic medication endangers foster children's rights and health. *Boston College Journal of Law & Social Justice*, *32*, 357–389.

Dao, J., Carey, B., & Frosch, D. (2011). For some troops, powerful drug cocktails have deadly results. *The New York Times*, February 13.

Davis, L., Fulgniti, A., Krigel, L., & Brekke, J. (2012). Deinstitutionalization? Where have all the people gone? *Current Psychiatry Reports*, *14*, 259–269.

Del Paggio, D. (2005). Psychotropic medical abuse in correctional facilities. *Psychopharmacology newsletter*, *June*, 1–5.

Department of Justice. (2013). *Johnson and Johnson to pay more than $2.2. billion to resolve criminal and civil investigations*. Retrieved from http://www.justice.gov/opa/pr/johnson-johnson-pay-more-22-billion-resolve-criminal-and-civil-investigations

dosReis, S., Yoon, Y., Rubin, D. M., Riddle, M. A., Noll, E., & Rothbard, A. (2011). Antipsychotic treatment among youth in foster care. *Pediatrics*, *128*, e1459–e1466.

dosReis, S., Zito, J. M., Safer, D. J., & Soeken, K. L. (2001). Mental health services for youths in foster care and disabled youths. *American Journal of Public Health*, *91*, 1094–1099.

Doyle, J. (2008). Child protection and adult crime: Investigator assignment to estimate causal effects of foster care. *Journal of Political Economy*, *116*(4), 746–770.

Dumit, J. (2012). *Drugs for life: How pharmaceutical companies define our health*. Durham, NC: Duke University Press.

Dute, J. (2001). Compulsory medication within the prison system. *Medicine & Law*, *20*, 221–226.

Dwyer, L., Han, B., Woodwell, D., & Reichsteiner, E. (2009). Polypharmacy in nursing home residents in the United States: Results of the 2004 national nursing home survey. *The American Journal of Geriatric Pharmacotherapy*, *8*, 63–72.

Estelle v. Gamble, 429 U.S. 97 (1976).

Feinman, C. (1994). *Women in the criminal justice system*. Westport, CN: Preager Publishers.

Ferguson, D., Glesener, D., & Raschick, M. (2006). Psychotropic drug use with European American and American Indian children in foster care. *Journal of Child and Adolescent Psychopharmacology*, *16*, 474–481.

Floyd, T. (1990). The administration of psychotropic drugs to prisoners: state of the law and beyond. *California Law Review*, *78*, 1243–1285.

Folsom, D., Hawthorne, W., Lindamer, L., Gilmer, T., Bailey, A., Golshan, S., … Jeste, D. (2005). Prevalence and risk factors for homelessness and utilization of mental health services among 10, 340 patients with serious mental illness in a large public mental health system. *American Journal of Psychiatry*, *162*, 370–376.

Frank, R., Conti, R., & Goldman, H. (2005). Mental health policy and psychotropic drugs. *The Milbank Quarterly*, *83*(2), 271–298.

Fuller, E. F. (2014). *American psychosis: How the federal government destroyed the mental illness treatment system*. New York, NY: Oxford University Press.

Fullerton, C., McGuire, T., Feng, Z., Mor, V., & Grabowski, D. (2009). Trends in mental health admissions to nursing homes. *Psychiatric Services*, *60*(7), 965–971.

Gaboda, D., Lucas, J., Siegel, M., Kalay, E., & Crystal, S. (2011). No longer undertreated? Depression diagnosis and antidepressant therapy in elderly long-stay nursing home residents, 1999 to 2007. *Journal of the American Geriatrics Society*, *59*, 673–680.

Garrard, J., Chen, V., & Dowd, B. (1995). The impact of the 1987 federal regulations on the use of psychotropic drugs in Minnesota nursing homes. *American Journal of Public Health*, *85*(6), 771–776.

Glaze, L. E., & James, D. J. (2006). *Mental health problems of prison and jail inmates*. Washington, DC: Bureau of Justice Statistics.

Glied, S., & Frank, R. (2009). Better but not best; recent trends in the well-being of the mentally ill. *Health Affairs*, *28*(3), 637–647.

Glied, S. A., & Frank, R. G. (2009). Better but not best: Recent trends in the well being of the mentally ill. *Health Affairs*, *28*(3), 637–648.

Goffman, E. (1961). *Asylums: Essays on the social situation of mental patients and other inmates*. New York, NY: Anchor Books.

Goldman, H., & Morrissey, J. (1985). The alchemy of mental health policy: Homelessness and the fourth cycle of reform. *American Journal of Public Health*, *75*, 727–731.

Gostin, L. (2003). Compulsory medical treatment: The limits of bodily integrity. *The Hastings Center Report*, *33*(5), 11–12.

Gottschlich, J., & Cetnar, G. (2002). Drug bills at jail top food costs. *Springfield News Sun*.

Grant, W., & Resnick, P. (1989). Right of active duty military personnel to refuse psychiatric treatment. *Behavioral Sciences & the Law*, *7*, 339–354.

Gronfein, W. (1985). Psychotropic drugs and the origins of deinstitutionalization. *Social Problems*, *32*(5), 437–454.

Gu, Q., Dillon, C., & Burt, V. (2010). *Prescription drug use continues to increase: U.S. prescription drug data for 2007–2008*. NCHS Data Brief, 42. Hyattsville, MD: National Center for Health Statistics.

Handwerk, M., Smith, G., Thompson, R., Spellman, D., & Daly, D. (2008). Psychotropic medication utilization at a group-home residential facility for children and adolescents. *Journal of Child and Adolescent Psychopharmacology*, *18*, 517–525.

Hanlon, J., Handler, S., & Castle, N. (2010). Antidepressant prescribing in US nursing homes between 1996 and 2006 and its relationship to staffing patterns and use of other psychotropic medications. *Journal of the American Medical Directors Association*, *11*, 320–324.

Hanlon, J., Wang, X., Castle, N., Stone, R., Handler, S., Selma, T., … Dysken, M. (2011). Potential underuse, overuse, and inappropriate use of antidepressants in older veteran nursing home residents. *Journal of the American Geriatrics Society*, *5*, 1412–1420.

Healy, D. (2012). *Pharmageddon*. Berkeley, CA: University of California Press.

Herbel, B., & Stelmach, H. (2007). Involuntary medication treatment for competency restoration of 22 defendants with delusional disorder. *Journal of the American Academy of Psychiatry and the Law*, *35*, 47–59.

Heyes, J. (2012). *More than 110,000 US soldiers remain on antidepresssants and sedatives*. Retrieved from http://www.naturalnews.com/036001_soldiers_psychiatric_drugs_veterans.html#ixzz2AjAq4XJ2

Hoover, D., Siegel, M., Lucas, J., Kalay, E., Gaboda, D., Devananda, D. P., & Crystal, S. (2010). Depression in the first year of stay for elderly long-term nursing home residents in the U.S.A. *International Psychogeriatrics*, *22*, 1161–1171.

Hughes, C. M., & Lepane, K. L. (2005). Administrative initiatives for reducing inappropriate prescribing of psychotropic drugs in nursing homes-how successful have they been? *Drugs & Aging*, *22*(4), 339–351.

Human Rights Watch. (2003). *Ill equipped: U.S. prisons and offenders with mental illness*. New York, NY: Human Rights Watch.

Hunt, J. (2008). Analysis of children in foster care finds high prescribing of psychotropic meds. *The Brown University Child & Adolescent Psychopharmacology Update*, *10*, 1–3.

Jeffrey, T., Rankin, R., & Jeffrey, L. (1992). In service of two masters: The ethical-legal dilemma faced by military psychologists. *Professional Psychology: Research and Practice*, *23*, 91–95.

Johnson, E., & Waldfogel, J. (2002). Parental incarceration: Recent trends and implications for child welfare. *Social Service Review*, *76*, 460–479.

Jonas, B. S., Gu, Q., & Albertorio-Diaz, M. (2013). *Psychotropic drug use among adolescents: United States, 2005–2010*. NCHS Data Brief, 135. Hyattsville, MD: National Center for Health Statistics.

Jonson-Reid, M., & Barth, R. (2000). From placement to prison: The path to adolescent incarceration from child welfare supervised foster or group care. *Children and Youth Services Review*, *22*(7), 493–516.

Kamble, P., Chen, H., Sherer, J., & Aparasu, R. R. (2008). Antipsychotic drug use among elderly nursing home residents in the United States. *American Journal of Geriatric Pharmacotherapy*, *6*, 187–197.

Karkare, S., Bhattaharjee, S., Kamble, P., & Aparsu, R. (2011). Prevalence and predictors of antidepressant prescribing in nursing home residents in the United States. *American* Journal of Geriatric Pharmacology, *9*(2), 109–119.

Kilty, J. (2008). Governance through psychiatrization: Seroquel and the new prison order. *Radical Psychology*, *2*(7), 1–24.

Knowlan, M. (2001). A survey of navy physicians' attitudes toward the use of selective serotonin reuptake inhibitors in active duty military personnel. *Military Medicine*, *166*, 526–559.

Kuehn, B. (2010). Military probes epidemic of suicide. *Journal of the American Medical Association*, *304*, 1427–1430.

Leslie, L., Gordon, J., Lambros, K., Premji, K., Peoples, J., & Gist, K. (2005). Addressing the developmental and mental health needs of young children in foster care. *Journal of Developmental and Behavioral Pediatrics*, *26*, 140–151.

Leslie, L., Raghavan, R., Hurley, M., Zhang, J., Landsverk, J., & Aarons, G. (2011). Investigating geographic variation in use of psychotropic medications among youth in child welfare. *Child Abuse & Neglect*, *35*, 333–342.

Leslie, L., Raghavan, R., Zhang, J., & Aarons, A. (2010). Rates of psychotropic medication use over time among youth in child welfare/child protective services. *Journal of Child and Adolescent Psychopharmacology*, *20*, 135–143.

Light, D. (2010). *The risks of prescription drugs*. New York, NY: Columbia University Press.

Longhofer, J., Floersch, J., & Okpych, N. (2011). Foster youth and psychotropic treatment: Where next? *Children and Youth Services Review*, *33*, 395–404.

Lyons, J., & Rogers, L. (2004). The US child welfare system: A de facto public behavioral health care system. *Journal of the American Academy of Child & Adolescent Psychiatry*, *43*, 971–973.

Magnezi, R., Zrihen, I., Ashkenazi, I., & Lubin, G. (2007). The cost of preventing stigma by hospitalizing soldiers in a general hospital instead of a psychiatric hospital. *Military Medicine*, *172*(7), 686–689.

Mark, T. L., Levit, K., & Buck, J. A. (2009). Data points: Psychotropic drug use prescriptions by medical specialty. *Psychiatric Services*, *60*(9), 1167.

Martin, A., Van Hoof, T., Stubbe, D., Sherwin, T., & Scahill, L. (2014). Multiple psychotropic pharmacotherapy among child and adolescent enrollees in Connecticut Medicaid managed care. *Psychiatric Services*, *54*, 72–77.

Massoglia, M. (2008). Incarceration as exposure: The prison, infectious disease, and other stress-related illnesses. *Journal of Health and Social Behavior*, *49*, 56–71.

McMillen, J., Fedoravicius, N., Rowe, J., Zima, B., & Ware, N. (2007). A crisis of credibility: Professionals' concerns about the psychiatric care provided to clients of the child welfare system. *Administration and Policy in Mental Health and Mental Health Services Research*, *34*, 203–212.

McMillen, J., Scott, L., Zima, B., Ollie, M., Munson, M., & Spitznagel, E. (2004). Use of mental health services among older youths in foster care. *Psychiatric Services*, *55*, 811–817.

Mechanic, D., & McAlpine, D. (2000). Use of nursing homes in the care of persons with severe mental illness: 1985–1995. *Psychiatric Services, 51*, 354–358.

Mello, M. (2011). Psychotropic medication and foster care children: A prescription for state oversight. *Southern California Law Review, 8*, 395–428.

Molinari, V., Chiriboga, D., Branch, L., Schinka, J., Schonfeld, L., Kos, L., & Hyer, K. (2011). Reasons for psychiatric medication prescription for new nursing home residents. *Aging & Mental Health, 15*, 904–912.

Morrissey, J., & Goldman, H. (1986). Care and treatment of the mentally ill in the United States: Historical developments and reforms. *T*he Annals of the American Academy of Political and Social Science, *484*, 12–27.

Moses, T. (2008). Psychotropic medication practices for youth in systems of care. *Journal of Child and Family Studies, 17*, 567–581.

Murphy, K. (2012). *Soldiers at war in fog of psychotropic drugs.* Retrieved from http://seattletimes.com/html/nationworld/2017944964_drugsofwar10.html

Naylor, M., Davidson, C., Ortega-Piron, D., Bass, A., Gutierrez, A., & Hall, A. (2007). Psychotropic medication management for youth in state care: Consent, oversight, and policy considerations. *Child Welfare, 86*, 175–192.

Nguyen, J., Fouts, M., Kotabe, S., & Lo, E. (2006). Polypharmacy as a risk factor for adverse drug reactions in geriatric nursing home residents. *The American Journal of Geriatric Pharmacotherapy, 4*, 36–41.

Noonan, M., & Mumola, C. (2007). *Veterans in state and federal prison, 2004.* Washington, DC: US Department of Justice, Office of Justice Programs.

O'Connor, D., Little, F., & McManus, R. (2009). Elders with serious mental illness: Lost opportunities and new policy options. *Aging & Social Policy, 21*(2), 144–158.

Ødegard, Ø. (1964). Patterns of discharge from Norwegian psychiatric hospitals before and after the introduction of psychotropic drugs. *American Journal of Psychiatry, 120*, 772–778.

O'Meara, K. (2013). *Drugs, wired warriors and "virtual" insanity.* Retrieved from http://www.cchrint.org/2013/01/23/cchr-exposes-psychiatrys-military-spending-to-create-drugged-out-super-soldiers-by-kelly-omeara/

Paulose-Ram, R., Safran, M. A., Jonas, B. S., Gu, Q., & Orwig, D. (2007). Trends in psychotropic medication use among US adults. *Pharmacoepidemiology and Drug Safety, 16*, 560–570.

Paulson, G. (2012). *Closing the asylum: Causes and consequences of the deinstitutionalization movement.* Jefferson, NC: McFarland & Company, Inc. Publishers.

Pierre, J., Shnayder, I., Wirshing, D., & Wirshing, W. C. (2004). Intranasal quetiapine abuse. *The American Journal of Psychiatry, 161*, 1718.

Pinta, E., & Taylor, R. (2007). Quetiapine addiction? *The American Journal of Psychiatry, 16*, 174–175.

Pratt, L., Brody, D., & Gu, Q. (2011). *Antidepressant use in persons aged 12 and over: United States, 2005–2008.* NCHS Data Brief, 78. Hyattsville, MD: National Center for Health Statistics.

Prins, S. (2011). Does transinstitutionalization explain the overrepresentation of people with serious mental illness in the criminal justice system? *Community Mental Health Journal, 47*, 716–722.

Prison Legal News. (2008). *Vermont DOC: Nations biggest prison dispenser of psychotropic medication.* Retrieved from https://www.prisonlegalnews.org/news/2008/jan/15/vermont-doc-nations-biggest-prison-dispenser-of-psychotropic-medication/. Accessed on January 15, 2008.

Radel, L., & Bramlett, M. (2014). *Children in non-parental care: Findings from the 2011-2012 national survey of children's health.* Washington, DC: U.S. Department of Health and Human Services, Office of the Assistant Secretary for Planning and Evaluation.

Raghavan, R., Brown, D. S., Thompson, H., Ettner, S. L., Clements, L. M., & Key, W. (2012). Medicaid expenditures on psychotropic medications for children in the child welfare system. *Journal of Child and Adolescent Psychopharmacology, 22*, 182–189.

Raghavan, R., Lama, G., Kohl, P., & Hamilton, B. (2010). Interstate variations in psychotropic medication use among a national sample of children in the child welfare system. *Child Maltreatment, 15*, 121–131.

Raghavan, R., & McMillen, J. (2008). Use of multiple psychotropic medications among adolescents aging out of foster care. *Psychiatric Services, 59*, 1052–1055.

Raghavan, R., Zima, B. T., Andersen, R. M., Leibowitz, A. A., Schuster, M. A., & Landsverk, J. (2005). Psychotropic medication use in a national probability sample of children in the child welfare system. *Journal of Child & Adolescent Psychopharmacology, 15*, 97–106.

Ray, C., & Finley, J. (1994). Did CMHC's fail or succeed? Analysis of the expectations and outcomes of the community mental health movement. *Journal of Rehabilitation, 67*(2), 16–21.

Rhodes, L. A. (2004). *Total confinement: Madness and reason in the maximum security prison.* Los Angeles, CA: University of California Press.

Roberts, D. (2012). Prison, Foster Care, and the Systematic Punishment of Black Mothers. *UCLA Law Review, 59*, 1474.

Rubin, D., Matone, M., Huang, Y. S., Feudtner, C., & Localio, R. (2012). Interstate variation in trends of psychotropic medication use among Medicaid-enrolled children in foster care. *Children and Youth Services Review, 34*, 1492–1499.

Scull, A. (1977). *Decarceration: Community treatment and the deviant—A racial view.* Englewood Cliffs, NJ: Prentice Hall.

Senate Subcommittee on Human Rights and the Law. (2009). *Human rights at home: Mental illness in U.S. prisons and jails.* Serial No. J-111-45. Washington, DC: U.S. Government Printing Office.

Sheehan, D. (2009). *Suicide gets army's attention.* Retrieved from http://www.army.mil/article/28744/suicide-gets-armys-attention/

Shenson, D., Dubler, N., & Michaels, D. (1990). Jails and prisons: The new asylums? *American Journal of Public Health, 80*(6), 655–656.

Siegel, M. J., Lucas, J. A., Akincigil, A., Gaboda, D., Hoover, D. R., Kalay, E., & Crystal, S. (2012). Race, education, and the treatment of depression in nursing homes. *Journal of Aging and Health, 24*, 752–778.

Sindel, P. E. (1991). Fourteenth amendment – The right to refuse antipsychotic drugs masked by prison bars. *Journal of Criminal Law and Criminology, 81*(4), 952–980.

Smith, B. (2012). Inappropriate prescribing. *Monitor on Psychology, 43*(6), 36.

Smith, S. (2011). Introduction: Health legacies of war on and beyond the battlefield. *The Journal of Law, Medicine & Ethics, 39*, 5–7.

Snowdon, J., Day, S., & Baker, W. (2006). Current use of psychotropic medication in nursing homes. *International Psychogeriatrics, 18*, 241–250.

Sommers, I., & Baskin, D. R. (1990). The prescription of psychiatric medications in prison: Psychiatric versus labeling perspectives. *Justice Quarterly, 7*, 739–755.

Talbott, J. (1983). A special population: The elderly deinstitutionalized chronically mentally ill patient. *Psychiatric Quarterly, 55*, 90–105.

Tamura, B., Bell, C., Inaba, M., & Masaki, K. (2012). Outcomes of polypharmacy in nursing home residents. *Clinics in Geriatric Medicine, 28*, 217–236.

Tilghman, A., & McGarry, B. (2010). Medicating the military: Use of psychiatric drugs has spiked; concerns surface about suicide, other dangers. *ArmyTimes*, March 17.

Toff, G., & Scallet, L. (1986). *The mentally ill in nursing homes*. Washington, DC: National Institute of Mental Health.

Torrey, E. (1995). Jails and prisons—America's new mental hospitals. *American Journal of Public Health, 85*(12), 1611–1613.

Torrey, E. (2014). *American psychosis: How the federal government destroyed the mental illness treatment system*. New York, NY: Oxford University Press.

Torrey, E., Kennard, A., Eslinger, D., Lamb, R., & Pavle, J. (2010). *More mental ill persons are in jails and prisons than hospitals: A survey of the states*. Arlington, VA: Treatment Advocacy Center.

Tsai, J., Rosenheck, R., Kasprow, W., & McGuire, K. (2013). Risk of incarceration and other characteristics of Iraq and Afghanistan era veterans in state and federal prisons. *Psychiatric Services, 64*(1), 36–43.

United States. Congress. House. Committee on the District of Columbia. Subcommittee on Fiscal Affairs and Health. (1983). *Deinstitutionalization of the mentally ill: Hearings before the subcommittee on fiscal affairs and health of the committee on the District of Columbia*, November 2, 17, 18, 1981. Washington, DC: U.S. Government Printing Office.

United States. Congress. House. Committee on Veterans' Affairs. (2010). *Exploring the relationship between medication and veteran suicide: Hearing before the committee on veterans' affairs, U.S. house of representatives, one hundred eleventh congress, second session*, February 24, 2010. Washington, DC: U.S. Government Printing Office.

United States. Congress. House. Committee on Ways and Means. Subcommittee on Income Security and Family Support. (2009). Prescription psychotropic drug use among children in foster care: Hearing before the subcommittee on income security and family support of the committee on ways and means, U.S. house of representatives, one hundred tenth congress, *second session*, May 8, 2008. Washington, DC: U.S. Government Printing Office.

U.S. Department of Health and Human Services. (2013). *The Adoption and Foster Care Analysis and Reporting System (AFCARS)*. Report, 20. U.S. Department of Health and Human Services, Administration for Children and Families, Washington, DC.

U.S. Department of Housing and Urban Development. (2009). *The 2008 annual homeless assessment report to Congress*. US Department of Housing and Urban Development, Washington, DC.

Vandivere, S., Yrausquin, A., Allen, T., Malm, K., & McKlindon, A. (2012). *Children in non-parental care: A review of the literature and analysis of data gaps*. Washington, DC: U.S. Department of Health and Human Services, Office of the Assistant Secretary for Planning and Evaluation.

Voyer, P., & Martin, L. (2003). Improving geriatric mental health nursing care: Making a case for going beyond psychotropic medications. *International Journal of Mental Health Nursing, 12*(1), 11–21.

Warren, C. (1981). New forms of social control: The myth of deinstitutionalization. *American Behavioral Scientist, 6*, 724–740.

West, K. (2012). *Psychotropic medications issues in military and Veterans: Public health implications*. Retrieved from http://weblaw.usc.edu/centers/saks/documents/KWest-PMediacal IssueInMilitaryAndVeterans.pdf. Accessed on March 22–23, 2012.

Willis, A. (2012). *Prescribed drugs 'to blame over spate of violence among US soldiers'*. Retrieved from http://www.telegraph.co.uk/news/worldnews/northamerica/usa/9193850/Prescribed-drugs-to-blame-over-spate-of-violence-among-US-soldiers.html

Wilper, A., Woolhandler, S., Boyd, J., Lasser, K., McCormick, D., Bor, D., & Himmelstein, D. (2009). The health and health care of US prisoners: Results of a nationwide survey. *American Journal of Public Health*, *99*, 666–672.

Winick, B. J. (1977). Psychotropic medication and competence to stand trial. *Law & Social Inquiry*, *2*, 769–816.

Zaitzow, B. H. (2010). Psychotropic control of women prisoners: The perpetuation of abuse of imprisoned women. *Justice Policy Journal*, *7*(2), 1–37.

Zeigelmuller, W. P. (1993). Sixth amendment due process on drugs: The implications of forcibly medicating pre-trial detainees with antipsychotic drugs. *Journal of Criminal Law and Criminology*, *83*, 836–867.

Zima, B., Bussing, R., Crecelius, G., Kaufman, A., & Belin, T. (1999). Psychotropic medication use among children in foster care: Relationship to severe psychiatric disorders. *American Journal of Public Health*, *89*, 1732–1735.

Zito, J., Safer, D., Gardner, J., Magder, L., Soeken, K., Boles, M., … Riddle, M. (2003). Psychotropic practice patterns for youth: A 10-year perspective. *Archives of Pediatrics & Adolescent Medicine*, *157*(1), 17–25.

Zito, J., Safer, D., Sai, D., Gardner, J., Thomas, D., Coombes, P., … Mendez-Lewis, M. (2008). Psychotropic medication patterns among youth in foster care. *Pediatrics*, *121*, e157–e163.

Zonana, H. V. (2003). Competency to be executed and forced medication: Singleton v. Norris. *Journal of the American Academy of Psychiatry and the Law Online*, *31*, 372–376.